ID0205750

Dementia and Social Work Practice

Carole B. Cox, PhD, is professor at the Graduate School of Social Service, Fordham University. She is a fellow of the Gerontological Society of America and the author of more than 50 journal articles and chapters dealing with various aspects of aging and caregiving. She has done extensive research on caregivers for persons with Alzheimer's disease, their needs, and use of services with a particular focus on ethnicity. In the past few years, she has expanded her interest in caregiving to that of grandparents raising their grandchildren. She has developed a program and curriculum for empowerment training for grandparents, *Empowering Grandparents Raising Grandchildren: A Training Manual for Group Leaders* (Springer Publishing, 2000), and is also the editor of *To Grandmother's House We Go and Stay: Perspectives on Custodial Grandparents* (Springer Publishing, 2000). Her other books include *Home Care for the Elderly: An International Perspective* (Greenwood, coauthor Abraham Monk, 1991), *The Frail Elderly: Problems, Needs, and Community Responses* (Auburn House, 1993), *Ethnicity and Social Work Practice* (Oxford University Press, coauthor, Paul Ephross, 1998), and *Community Care for an Aging Society: Policies and Services* (Springer Publishing, 2005).

Dementia and Social Work Practice

Research and Interventions

Carole B. Cox, PhD, Editor

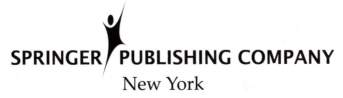

SPRINGER PUBLISHING COMPANY
New York

Springer Publishing Company, LLC.
11 West 42nd Street
New York, NY 10036

Acquisitions Editor: Jennifer Perillo
Production Editor: Carol Cain
Cover design by Joanne E. Honigman
Typeset by Apex Publishing, LLC

07 08 09 10/ 5 4 3 2 1

Library of Congress Cataloging-in-Publication Data

Dementia and social work practice : research and intervention / Carole Cox, editor.

   p. ; cm.
   Includes bibliographical references and index.
   ISBN-13: 978-0-8261-0249-2 (alk. paper)
   ISBN-10: 0-8261-0249-2 (alk. paper)
1. Dementia. 2. Psychiatric social work. 3. Social work with older people. I. Cox, Carole B.
[DNLM: 1. Alzheimer Disease—therapy. 2. Dementia—therapy. 3. Aged. 4. Caregivers—psychology. 5. Social Support. 6. Social Work, Psychiatric—methods.
   WT 155 D3755 2007
   RC521.D45338 2007
   616.8'3—dc22   2006036613

Printed in the United States of America by Bang Printing.

This book is dedicated to all those who care,
all those who receive care,
and all those who will ...

Contents

PART 3: DIVERSITY AND DEMENTIA
Carole B. Cox

PART 4: COMMUNITY CARE
Carole B. Cox

Contributors

María P. Aranda, PhD, LCSW
Associate Professor
School of Social Work
University of Southern California

Edna L. Ballard, MSW, ACSW
Educational Core Faculty
Bryan Alzheimer's Disease Research Center
Duke University Medical Center

Elizabeth Baxter, MPH
Project Director
The Archimedes Movement
Portland, Oregon

Kun Chang, MSW
Associate Executive Director, Greater Boston Chinese Golden Age Center
Regional Director, National Association of Asian and Pacific Islanders

Victoria Cotrell, GSSW
Portland State University

Nancy Emerson Lombardo
Senior Research Scientist
Adjunct Research Assistant of Neurology
Rogers Memorial Hospital
Bedford, Massachusetts

Cynthia Epstein, MSW, ACSW
Family Counselor/Clinical Investigator
William and Sylvia Silberstein Institute for Aging and Dementia
Department of Psychiatry
New York University
School of Medicine

Lynn Friss Feinberg, MSW
Deputy Director, National Center on Caregiving
Family Caregiver Alliance
San Francisco, California

Marilyn Hartle, MSW, LCSW
Partner
Jentle Harts Consulting
Indianapolis, Indiana

Jeanne Heid-Grubman, MSW, LNHA
Healthcare Administrator
The Holmstad, Covenant Retirement Community
Batavia, Illinois

Jennifer K. Hohnstein, BA, JD
Project Coordinator
Wellesley College Center for Research

Jed Johnson, MSW, MBA
Assistant Vice President
Adult and Senior Services
Easter Seals National Office
Washington, DC

Teorrah Kontos, MSW
Program Manager
Cognitive Dementia and Memory Service
Eastern Health Care, The Peter James Centre
Victoria, Australia

Daniel Kuhn, MSW
Director, Professional Training Institute
Greater Illinois Chapter
Alzheimer's Association
Skokie, Illinois

Jill Manthorpe, MA
Professor of Social Work
Social Care Workforce Research Unit
King's College, London
London, England

Katie Maslow, MSW
Associate Director
Public Policy Division
Alzheimer's Association
Washington, DC

Rhonda J. V. Montgomery, PhD
Helen Bader Professor of Applied Gerontology
University of Wisconsin, Milwaukee

Carmen Morano, PhD
Hunter College School of Social Work
Brookdale Center on Aging

Darby Morhardt, MSW, LCSW
Research Assistant Professor
Director of Education
Cognitive Neurology and Alzheimer's Disease Center
Northwestern University
Feinberg School of Medicine
Chicago, Illinois

Jo Moriarty
Kings College
London, England

Lisa Peters-Beumer, MPH
Project Director
Adult and Senior Services
Easter Seals Headquarters
Chicago, Illinois

Jeannine M. Rowe, MSW
University of Wisconsin, Milwaukee

Nina M. Silverstein, PhD
Associate Professor Gerontology
University of Massachusetts, Boston
Boston, Massachusetts

Lisa Snyder, MSW, LCSW
University of California, San Diego
Shiley-Marcos Alzheimers Research Center
La Jolla, California

Sandra Weintraub, PhD, ABPP-CN
Professor of Psychiatry and Behavioral Sciences and
Professor of Neurology
Cognitive Neurology and Alzheimer's Disease Center
Northwestern University Feinberg School of Medicine

Carol J. Whitlatch, PhD
Assistant Director
Margaret Blenkner Research Institute

Bei Wu, PhD
West Virginia University
Health Sciences Center
Center on Aging and Department of Community Medicine

Sheryl Zimmerman, PhD
Professor of Social Work, Epidemiology, and Public Health
Codirector, Program on Aging, Disability, and Long-Term Care
Cecil G. Sheps Center for Health Services Research
University of North Carolina at Chapel Hill

Preface

Dementia is one of the most devastating illnesses, as it involves a progressive decline in mental functioning leading to eventual total incapacity. Thus, it affects all aspects of diagnosed individuals—eventually robbing them of their very identities. There are many types of dementia, but the most common form is Alzheimer's disease, which affects over 4 million Americans, the majority of whom are age 65 or older. However, although associated with aging, the illness is also found in persons in midlife, where the impact can be particularly severe, as it affects employment, income, and the expected life course.

The toll associated with dementia is not restricted to the individual with the diagnosis. Families who provide the majority of care become increasingly burdened throughout the course of the illness. Additionally, many insurance plans do not cover services such as day care, respite, and home care, forcing caregivers to use their own funds for these supports. The toll is also transmitted to society through the financial costs of care as well as the lost productivity, absenteeism, and reduced employment of caregivers.

Social workers, whose focus and skills relate to the individual, the environment, and the interactions between them, are perhaps the most appropriate professionals to serve the growing population of persons with dementia and their caregivers. But, in order to do so, social workers themselves must be knowledgeable about the illness, its course, and its myriad effects on the individual, the family, and society. Unfortunately, education on dementia is noticeably absent in graduate schools of social work, where gerontology courses tend to be very limited and those that do exist spend perhaps one or two sessions focusing on the illness.

This book seeks to fill a major gap in the education and development of gerontological social workers whose skills are sorely needed by persons with dementia and their caregivers. But beyond specific gerontological courses, this book should also be a valuable resource to practitioners working with diverse populations in a variety of settings, ranging from the home to the institution.

As all members of a family are affected by dementia, the problems associated with the illness are intergenerational. Practitioners dealing with adults and children will find that this book offers valuable insights regarding interventions that can help clients cope with the complex issues related to the disease. From the time of initial diagnosis to the final stages of dementia, families must make transitions and decisions that can truly be helped by a social worker's skills, understanding, knowledge, and empathy.

The theme of this book underscores the many factors associated with dementia and its care and the ways in which social work involvement can be most valuable. The chapters, written by leaders in the field of dementia care, examine the development and impact of dementia and the many ways in which social work expertise can be most effectively utilized by clinicians, researchers, and advocates.

Throughout the 21 chapters of this book, the social and psychological ramifications of the illness are stressed. Within each chapter are implications and suggestions for social work involvement. The book begins with a chapter that describes Alzheimer's disease and other dementias, then continues to chapters that focus on the early stages of the illness and particular services, and concludes with models of care in other countries and challenges to the profession.

Dementia is an all-encompassing illness that affects many spheres of the affected individual, his or her family, and society. This book is divided into five sections, each of which deals with one of these spheres.

Part One, "Setting the Stage for Social Work," includes an overview of dementia, assessment instruments, and its association with other chronic illnesses. As discussed earlier, Alzheimer's disease is not the only cause of dementia; Darby Morhardt's chapter describes the many different types of dementias and their manifestations. It underscores the importance of how understanding these differences is crucial for effective practice.

Many instruments are available for the assessments of dementia. The chapter by Victoria Cotrell describes these instruments, the differences between screening and diagnosis, and the roles that social workers must play in multidimensional assessments of persons with dementia to ensure the identification of all of their complex needs.

Persons with dementia are not immune from other chronic conditions that cause them increased debilitation and suffering—while also placing further demands on the health care system. Katie Maslow's chapter discusses the increased burden and complexity associated with chronic illness and dementia and their management.

Part Two, "The Early Stage and Interventions With Families," is devoted to understanding the impact of a dementia diagnosis on both the individual and his or her family. The chapter by Lisa Snyder introduces social workers to the emotional, physical, and social issues that persons face in the early stage of the illness. The chapter by Dan Kuhn explores the challenges faced by caregiving families and the important roles that social workers can play in assisting them.

Carol Whitlatch and Lynn Feinberg discuss the impact of caregiving on the family, the types of decisions families must confront throughout the illness, and the importance of developing interventions targeted to their specific needs. Cynthia Epstein describes the research and clinical interventions with families developed at New York University's Aging and Dementia Research Center. Her findings have vast implications for improving the caregiving relationship and the care that is provided.

Part Three, "Diversity and Dementia," consists of five chapters that examine dementia with regard to culture and ethnicity and model programs from other countries that may offer suggestions for replication in the United States. My chapter is an overview of the ways in which cultural diversity often impacts the illness, from the recognition of symptoms to the use of services. It emphasizes the knowledge and understanding that social workers must have in working with diverse populations while also stressing the importance of guarding against stereotypes.

María Aranda and Carmen Morano offer considerations and suggestions for social workers in adapting psychosocial interventions for Latino caregivers. Nancy Emerson Lombardo describes a service model created for Chinese caregivers that can be replicated for use with other populations. The chapter by Jill Manthorpe and Jo Moriarty discusses the tasks and roles of social workers in the developing world, Europe, and Japan. Teorrah Kontos focuses on dementia care and programs in Australia. These last two chapters offer ideas from other countries that could be incorporated into our own systems of care.

Part Four, "Community Care," includes chapters on the primary community services that can assist both afflicted individuals and their caregivers. As caregivers struggle to understand and cope with dementia, they are often overwhelmed by the demands of the illness, their lack of understanding, and their need for additional resources.

Skilled care management, as discussed in the chapter by Liz Baxter, can help to strengthen caregivers by offering them support and resources. Nina Silverstein and Lisa Peters-Beumer examine the important subject of community mobility and dementia and how social workers can help clients transition from being in the "driver's seat" to accepting the "passenger seat."

The role that social work can play in adult day services for persons with dementia is described in the chapter by Jed Johnson and Marilyn Hartle. Edna Ballard's chapter uses examples from her work at the Duke University Family Support Program to discuss the roles that support groups can play in meeting caregiver needs. Finally, the chapter by Montgomery and Rowe describes the roles of social workers in respite care programs, which can offer immense relief to caregiving families.

Part Five, "Residential Care and Other Models," is composed of two chapters that focus on institutional care for the person with dementia. The chapter by Sheryl Zimmerman examines research on the factors related to the quality of care of persons in residential settings. The following chapter by Jeanne Heid-Grubman discusses how research on quality can be translated into effective social work practice in the institution.

The final chapter of the book concludes with challenges to the profession that must be met if social work is to be truly effective in meeting the myriad needs faced by persons with dementia and their caregivers.

It is hoped that this book will encourage and stimulate social workers to not only increase their involvement with persons with dementia and their families but also educate those currently working with this population. As the number of persons with dementia multiplies in the coming decades, there is an urgent and immediate need for the profession's commitment to strengthen and improve the quality of the systems affecting these persons.

Foreword

Alzheimer's disease and related disorders have been called "equal opportunity destroyers" because they cut a swath not only through persons with progressive losses (and, notably in this book, retained capacities) but also entire families whose lives are forever changed by their effects. Actor David Hyde Pierce aptly labeled as "collateral damage" the often silent but insidious health and relationship losses faced by multigenerational families who must deal with dementia. Carole Cox and her contributors, all leaders in social work and dementia research and practice, provide a cohesive and definitive roadmap that addresses the direct and collateral damage of progressive memory disorders.

These seasoned clinicians and researchers offer practical strategies for enhancing quality of life and relationships as well as quality of services for affected persons and their concerned families. Readers will be convinced of the centrality of the recognition of cognitive decline through long-term care to the future of adult development and aging. This is the first volume of its kind to demonstrate how the profession of social work must be poised to meet the immediate, long-term, and future needs, preferences, and values of persons and families coping with memory disorders from recognition through bereavement.

In this era of "translational medicine" there is an equally great need to translate well-designed and rigorously evaluated social work interventions for broad community application. Cox and her colleagues offer an authoritative, theoretically sound, dementia-friendly, practice-feasible and policy-relevant systems perspective. The effects of Alzheimer's disease and other dementias on individuals and communities demand a collaborative interdisciplinary approach, and nowhere are the social work leadership and communication strengths requisite to this approach more evident than in the carefully woven chapters of this tightly edited compendium.

From early-stage programs through bereavement and from clinical to support groups to community respite and advanced dementia care programs, this single volume offers practical, tested, and meaningful person-centered and family-friendly strategies. Even better, all authors incorporate culturally sensitive suggestions for adaptation to diverse ethnic, cultural, and regional strengths, preferences, and needs.

To adapt a wise quote from Rosalynn Carter about family caregivers: in the future there will be only four kinds of social workers—those who work with Alzheimer's families, those who are part of Alzheimer's families, those who will work Alzheimer's families, or those who will face Alzheimer's in their immediate personal circles. That future is now, and this book should be required reading for all student and practicing social workers in all specialties and settings.

Lisa P. Gwyther, MSW, LCSW
Associate Clinical Professor, Department of
Psychiatry and Behavioral Sciences
Education Director, Bryan Alzheimer's Disease Research Center
Duke University Medical Center
Durham, North Carolina

Dementia and Social Work Practice

PART I

Setting the Stage for Social Work

CHAPTER ONE

Social Work and Dementia

Carole B. Cox

INTRODUCTION

It is common knowledge that the population of the United States is aging. In 2004, 12.4% of the population was 65 years or older, and this proportion is expected to increase to 20% by 2030 (National Institute on Aging, 2006). An aging population has ramifications throughout society, and one of particular concern is the impact it will have on the social work profession. Accordingly, the Council on Social Work Education (2001) estimates that between 60,000 and 70,000 gerontological social workers will be needed by 2030 to meet the needs of the elderly. These professionals will require specific knowledge, competency, and skills, particularly the ability to work with those coping with dementia.

Dementia is not a necessary part of aging, but its prevalence increases with age. *Dementia* refers to a loss of mental functions in two or more areas (such as language, memory, visual and spatial abilities, and judgment) to the extent that the person's daily life is affected. Alzheimer's disease, which affects more than 4.5 million persons in the United States, is the most common source of dementia. The risk of developing Alzheimer's doubles every 5 years after age 65, affecting approximately 2% of the population aged 65 to 74, 19% of those aged 75 to 84, and 47% of those 85 and older (Evans, Funkenstein, & Albert, 1989). By

2050, between 11 million and 16 million persons may be diagnosed with the illness.

There is probably no greater cause of anxiety and stress than receiving the diagnosis of dementia. A recent survey of Americans found that, next to cancer, Alzheimer's is the most feared disease among all age-groups; after age 55, the fear of Alzheimer's supersedes that of cancer. In addition, three out of five persons worry that they will be responsible for the care of someone with the illness (MetLife Foundation, 2006).

The impact of dementia is pervasive as its effects are felt through-out society. A recent reevaluation of Alzheimer's annual cost to business (from $33.1 billion in 1998 to $61.1 billion in 2002) underscores the economic impact of the illness, mostly due to the caregivers' loss of productivity, absenteeism, and eventual job replacement (Koppel, 2002). In addition, persons with the illness place large burdens on the medical care and long-term care systems, where their many demands have been linked to increases in staff burnout and turnover (Weinberg, 2003).

The impact of the illness is particularly great on the informal caregiver, the family member who continues to provide the bulk of care throughout the course of the illness. These caregivers have been termed "the hidden victims" (Zarit, Orr, & Zarit, 1985). In comparison to other caregivers, they spend more time per week providing care and also report greater strain and impact on employment, mental and physical health, and leisure time (Alzheimer's Association and National Alliance for Caregiving, 2004). The needs of persons with the dementia and their families have direct implications for the social work profession because social work knowledge, skills, and roles can be critical throughout the course of the illness.

UNDERSTANDING DEMENTIA

Dementia is not a disease; it is a group of symptoms that are so severe that they interfere with an individual's ability to function normally in everyday life. Dementia affects intellectual abilities so that functions such as thinking, remembering, and reasoning are impaired to the extent that the individual has difficulty carrying out normal activities. The symptoms also frequently cause changes in mood, behavior, and personality.

It is important to recognize that although some slowing in cognitive functions and memory loss often accompanies aging, these conditions do not constitute dementia. They are usually mild and do not interfere with daily functioning (although they can be troubling and cause anxiety about developing dementia). It is most important for social workers to recognize that although dementia is more prevalent in older persons, it is not a normal part of aging.

Many conditions—such as depression, delirium, alcohol or drug use, malnutrition, vitamin use, hormone imbalance, and infections—can cause dementia-like symptoms. In such cases, once the cause is discovered and treated, the symptoms may disappear. Dementia is considered irreversible in that there is no existing cure for the condition. Consequently, it is critical that any diagnosis of dementia exclude conditions whose symptoms could mimic those of dementia.

Medications are a particularly notable cause of reversible dementia, particularly since older people may not be able to process medications effectively or may suffer from multiple drug interactions. Other causes of reversible dementia include metabolic abnormalities that affect the thyroid, hypoglycemia, pernicious anemia, nutritional deficiencies including dehydration, emotional problems, and infections such as meningitis and encephalitis.

ALZHEIMER'S DISEASE

The exact cause of Alzheimer's disease, the most common form of dementia in older persons, is still not known, although the greatest risk factors are increasing age and a family history of the illness. Other possible risk factors are high cholesterol, hypertension, diabetes, and low levels of the vitamin folate. Although there are no clear preventive measures against Alzheimer's disease, research is examining the roles that mental, physical, and social activities may play in protecting against it (National Institute on Aging, 2006).

Memory loss is the most notable symptom, but Alzheimer's disease also affects language, object recognition, and functioning. Common behavioral symptoms include psychosis, depression, agitation, and wandering. Unfortunately, early symptoms of the disease may be frequently ignored by family members who perceive them as a normal part of the aging process. A study of more than 800 families who eventually sought help found that the mean time from the onset of symptoms to seeking assistance was 36 months (Cox & Albisu, 2003). Such delayed responses mean that early-stage interventions and therapies, which could delay the progression of the illness or reduce symptoms, are frequently not used.

According to the Alzheimer's Association (2006), the 10 warning signs that indicate Alzheimer's include the following:

- Memory loss
- Difficulty performing familiar tasks
- Problems with language

- Disorientation of time and place
- Poor or decreased judgment
- Problems with abstract thinking
- Misplacing things
- Changes in mood and behavior
- Personality changes

Although these changes become frequent as people age, they are more extreme and progressive in persons with Alzheimer's disease.

As the disease progresses, symptoms become so severe that they prohibit normal functioning. Eventually, persons with Alzheimer's disease are unable to recognize familiar people or places, forget how to do simple tasks, and have difficulty speaking, reading, and writing. Often they have pronounced personality changes, becoming aggressive or paranoid. Eventually, they will require total care. The progressive nature of the illness makes early diagnosis critical because it is in the early stages that the person will be most able to decide his or her own course of care and participate in important decisions.

In addition, during the early stages, medications are most effective in controlling symptoms. *Cholinesterase inhibitors* prevent the breakdown of *acetylcholine,* a chemical in the brain that affects memory. People taking these drugs may experience improvement in their cognitive symptoms. *Memantine* is a drug that regulates *glutamate,* a brain chemical that affects learning and memory. It may also have benefits on cognitive and psychomotor functioning in tune with mild to moderate Alzheimer's disease.

Given that persons with dementia are often desperate for cures and effective therapies, they are vulnerable to claims of unsubstantiated treatments. Moreover, certain supplements including herbal and natural medicines may have uncertain quality and potency and may also have harmful interactions with prescribed medications. Social workers can help to educate persons about managing the illness, the risks of alternative treatments, and the need for compliance with prescribed medication.

SOCIAL WORKERS AND DEMENTIA

Given the vast dimensions of life that dementia impacts, social workers—with their micro- and macroperspectives of the helping process—can assume a major role in care. As the illness affects entire families and reverberates throughout the community, social workers can directly assist individuals with dementia while also ensuring that the systems with which they interact are supportive and responsive to their needs.

Social work skills in assessment and counseling can help persons with dementia meet the challenges of the illness throughout its devastating course. At the microlevel, social workers can enable persons with dementia to explore their feelings, fears, and concerns associated with the diagnosis. Their ability to understand individuals and to develop trusting relationships can be vital in helping clients cope with the challenges that dementia entails.

Stress is a major component of dementia, as it robs individuals of their identity and ability to function; it also robs their families of the person they loved. Stress further ensues as the illness progresses; relationships alter, and demands increase. Social work interventions can reduce this stress as they help clients understand the problems they face, develop new responses, and formulate goals and care plans that can increase their capacity to adjust.

In addition, social workers' knowledge of service delivery systems is important for identifying gaps and problems in programs that either deter their use or limit their effectiveness. Throughout the course of the illness, social workers must be able to ensure that programs are accessible and acceptable, that resources are available, and that they are compatible with their clients' needs. Social workers can reduce barriers to service utilization and thus make sure that the environment itself is supportive rather than a further source of stress.

Social work research is required to further explore the needs of people with dementia as well as the needs of their caregivers. Research on issues such as service delivery, intervention, and quality care is critical for the development of effective services. As program evaluators, social workers must be involved in assessing the outcomes of programs and identifying the areas in which change may be needed in order to improve services.

Advocacy is an important task for social workers involved with dementia. This involves advocating not only for individual clients but also for critical policies and services that are essential if needs are to be effectively met. Advocacy can help ensure that persons with dementia are not ignored and that their concerns are heard. Advocacy is also important for the development of further supports, funding, and resources for these persons and their families.

BASIS FOR INTERVENTIONS

The ecological perspective, the strengths perspective, family systems theory, and systems theory are among the theories that can provide bases for social work interventions with dementia. The skilled practitioner will use each in various phases of assessment, in problem solving, and in the development of care plans. Consequently, social work interventions can empower and enable caregivers as they strengthen their functioning and well being.

Examples of the applicability of the social work approach include genograms and ecomaps that may be used in the initial contact phase with the individual and the caregivers. Both of these tools can aid in assessments, as they clarify the relationships between the person with dementia and their caregivers as well as with other systems. In addition, the participation of clients in the development of these measures is an immediate way to develop rapport and increase their involvement in the helping process.

A *genogram* depicts the family's history, major life events, marriages, relationships, occupations, mobility, and health status. Through this description of the family context, both the practitioner and the client are able to better understand the functioning of the family and its history. As the genogram will also document any history of dementia in the family, it can also help elicit any anxieties and concerns that the caregiver may have about developing the illness.

The *ecomap* depicts the ties and types of relationships that the individual and the caregiver have with supports and resources. It describes the qualitative nature of relationships and indicates which types of relationships are absent or malfunctioning. Developing an ecomap can also help family members gain insights into their present situation and plan for the future as they are made aware of the resources that are available, those that they lack, and those that may need strengthening.

Dementia, Loss, and Relationships

A diagnosis of dementia can cause severe reactions among both the afflicted individual and the family. Such reactions are similar to those associated with the grieving process: the stages of denial, fear, pain, sadness, and acceptance. In the early stage of the illness, the person with dementia typically experiences a sense of loss and anticipatory grief over the diagnosis and what it signifies. Many will engage in anticipatory grief as they attempt to cope with the losses that they know they will experience. As cognition declines, feelings of loss may weaken, but feelings of stress, depression, and unease often continue.

Feelings of loss and grief are common among the family as they too struggle with a diagnosis that suggests an ongoing cognitive decline and increasing impairment of their loved one. This grief becomes more intense as the illness continues and symptoms intensify (Ponder & Pomeroy, 1996). As the personality changes, families often experience the loss or psychological death of the patient, even though he or she is still alive. Grief also results from the loss of many roles including that of spouse, child, and friend.

Social work interventions can assist both the individual with the illness and the family to adapt to the diagnosis and deal with the resultant feelings of grief and loss. Ensuring that individuals have the appropriate information and are knowledgeable about available resources is a primary task. Helping them understand that anger, fear, pain, and sadness are normal feelings can be critical for their continued functioning. It is equally important to help the diagnosed individual make plans and decisions regarding his or her own future and to make sure that those desires are communicated and recognized.

Doka (2004) suggests several measures that practitioners can use to assist families in coping. This begins with having them explain how their lives have changed and then helping them explore ways that these losses or changes may be restored. They should examine their support systems, coping skills, and willingness to ask for help. As care plans are developed, social workers should be involved in helping families make decisions about employment, services, and eventual placement.

Dementia can also strain many family relationships. The primary caregiver may feel overwhelmed and resentful toward siblings who they feel are not adequately involved in the caregiving process. Marital relationships can be strained as caregivers may become exhausted by meeting the demands of the person with dementia. Children may feel neglected and caregivers increasingly guilty that they are not meeting their needs. Moreover, families may disagree about the type of care that is required particularly with regard to institutionalization. Social work interventions can support families by identifying areas of stress, facilitating the expression of feelings and expectations, developing plans, and increasing mutual support.

Culture and Ethnicity

Ethnicity is a major factor in considering reactions to dementia. Culture strongly affects the ways in which symptoms are perceived and people's willingness to use services. Whether cognitive impairment is viewed as a normal part of aging will affect the willingness of families to seek assistance. In the same way, culture affects the roles that caregivers play and their interest in using services. In addition, as initial symptoms (such as forgetfulness) may be more acceptable to certain cultures, they may not seek out services until a later stage of the illness. Consequently, medications that could benefit persons in the early stage are less likely to be used.

Caregivers may be strongly influenced by the cultural values and traditions that dictate their caregiving roles. Consequently, formal services that could assist them with many of their tasks may not be used if they conflict with the norms that mandate informal care and alternative treatments.

To work effectively with diverse populations, social workers must understand the way in which the illness is viewed, as well as the family's concept of caring and responsibility. It is only through this knowledge that they can develop interventions that are appropriate and acceptable to a specific group. Without such knowledge, it is difficult to sensitively respond to the needs of these individuals.

Ethical and Legal Issues

As dementia progresses and cognition declines, the individual's comprehension, judgment, and ability to make appropriate decisions also become impaired. Consequently, a serious ethical dilemma arises with respect to protecting the autonomy of the individual and the obligation to protect him or her from harm. This concern reflects the core principles of the social work profession, which underscore self-determination, defending the rights of the client, and safeguarding his or her well-being (National Association of Social Workers, 1999). A diagnosis of dementia can easily override these values as the person is judged incompetent to make decisions, thus seriously jeopardizing their autonomy.

At the same time, social workers are mandated to ensure safeguards for clients who lack decision-making ability. Persons with dementia are often unable to make decisions regarding their assets or other financial matters but still are able to make decisions regarding their medical care and treatment. Thus, as a means of recognizing their capacity and protecting their independence, competency assessments need to evaluate many areas of functioning.

Consequently, practitioners must be knowledgeable about assessing the capacity of the individual as well as the process of determining legal competency and its outcomes. They must be sure that the preferences of the client are heard and, as much as possible, adhered to, as a diagnosis of dementia does not invalidate all of a person's capabilities. Moreover, to do so will further erode the client's self-esteem, possibly leading to a downward cycle in his or her ability to function.

The legal and financial issues that develop as a result of dementia are of primary concern to many families. Obtaining assistance early in the course of the illness can enable the individual to be involved in financial planning and decisions regarding future care. As cognitive status declines, so too do comprehension, judgment, and the ability to make decisions.

Practitioners must help ensure that the rights and interests of the individual are safeguarded and that those handling the affairs are indeed serving the client's best interests. Moreover, they must be prepared to challenge those who may be usurping the patient's rights or providing inadequate care.

A further ethical dilemma confronting social workers is deciding who is the client: the person with the illness, or the family? This is particularly problematic when their desires conflict and meeting the needs of one means offending the other. Helping both work through the decision-making process so that each feels supported requires skills in mediation, flexibility, and the ability to assist persons adapt so that their sense of well-being is supported rather than threatened.

Resources

A major social work role is to educate families about the resources that can assist them. In the earliest stage, caregivers require information about the diagnosis and the course that the illness will take. Referrals may be warranted for memory disorder clinics or specialized geriatric services where the patient can receive a thorough evaluation. If a positive diagnosis of dementia is made, caregivers need to know about supports and services that can assist them. Several of the key services that are important in working with dementia, such as case management, respite, day care, and support groups, are discussed in detail in this book.

However, knowing that services exist does not guarantee that they will be used. Many factors can deter families from using programs, including their own individual characteristics as well as those associated with the services themselves. Consequently, another major task for social workers is to help clients overcome any barriers that may impede utilization so that they may receive needed support. The issues associated with the use of services are discussed in many chapters in this book.

At the federal level, the Family Caregivers Support Program, administered through the Administration on Aging and its state and local offices, provides some financial assistance for families caring for a person with dementia. However, the amount of funds is limited and varies greatly among the states. Help is also available under Medicaid, but eligibility is dependent on state financial and residential criteria. Again, there is great variation among the states with regard to eligibility, services, and the extent of assistance that is offered.

The Alzheimer's Association has chapters throughout the country, and each provides five core services for assisting persons with dementia and their families. These include a 24-hour help-line service as well as publications and other resources. Referrals are also made to specific programs and services. The Alzheimer's chapters also offer professional consultation to caregivers, support groups, and educational programs. Safe Return, a program offered through the local chapters, provides assistance when a person with dementia wanders from home. Identification bracelets that can help locate persons if they wander are also available. Finally, the resource section at the end of this book provides a list of resources, organizations, and Web sites that offer valuable information to practitioners and individuals coping with dementia.

CONCLUSION

There is a pressing need for social work knowledge, interventions, and skills in the care of persons with dementia and their families. A significant challenge for the social work profession is to go beyond the role of clinical practitioner to that of researcher and advocate. Research is needed to continue to elucidate the many factors associated with well-being and coping. Advocacy is critical for ensuring that policies and programs that can benefit persons with dementia and their caregivers are adequately funded and implemented.

REFERENCES

Alzheimer's Association. (2006). *Fact sheet: 10 warning signs of Alzheimer's disease.* Chicago: Author.

Alzheimer's Association and National Alliance for Caregiving. (2004). *Families care: Alzheimer's caregiving in the United States, 2004.* Chicago: Alzheimer's Association.

Council on Social Work Education/SAGE/SW. (2001). *A blueprint for the new millennium.* New York: Author.

Cox, C., & Albisu, K. (2003). The impact of caring for a relative with dementia: A comparison of those caring for persons living alone, spousal caregivers, and co-resident adult children. *Journal of Mental Health and Aging, 8*, 216–230.

Doka, K. (2004). *Living with grief: Alzheimer's disease.* Washington, DC: Hospice Foundation of America.

Evans, D., Funkenstein, H., & Albert, M. (1989). Prevalence of Alzheimer's disease in a community population of older persons: Higher than previously reported. *Journal of the American Medical Association, 262*(18), 2552–2556.

Koppel, R. (2002). *Alzheimer's disease: The costs to U.S. business in 2002.* Washington, DC: Alzheimer's Association.

MetLife Foundation. (2006). *MetLife Foundation's Alzheimer's survey: What America thinks.* New York: Author.

National Association of Social Workers. (1999). *Code of ethics.* Washington, DC: Author.

National Institute on Aging. (2006). *What causes AD?* Washington, DC: Author.

Ponder, R., & Pomeroy, E. (1996). The grief of caregivers: How pervasive is it? *Journal of Gerontological Social Work, 27*, 3–21.

Weinberg, A. (2003). Quality care indicators and staffing units in a nursing facility subacute unit. *Journal of the American Medical Directors Association, 3*, 1–4.

Zarit, S., Orr, N., & Zarit, J. (1985). *The hidden victims of Alzheimer's disease.* New York: New York University Press.

CHAPTER TWO

Alzheimer's Disease and Non-Alzheimer's Dementias

Darby Morhardt and Sandra Weintraub

INTRODUCTION

Alzheimer's disease and related dementias that arise in old age present issues that greatly affect the entire family system and society at large. In spite of the long-predicted growth in the older adult population, few courses on aging and gerontology exist in many schools of social work in the United States. The importance of social work assessment and intervention has been given even less attention, even though the problems related to dementia affect at least two and often three generations. The social worker who understands the basics of differential dementia diagnosis will be better equipped to educate and counsel individuals and families on the course of the disease. Combining neuroscientific knowledge about dementia with the social work process, particularly a systems and interpersonal theoretical approach, will prepare the effective practitioner in this growing field.

Alzheimer's disease (AD) is the leading cause of dementia among the elderly (Evans, Funkenstein, Albert, Scherr, Cook, et al., 1989). Increased public awareness of memory loss as a first symptom of AD has brought patients to medical attention much earlier in the course of their disease than was true even 10 years ago. As a result of increased knowledge of AD as a distinct disease, much has been learned about the proper ways to treat and care for affected individuals. This has resulted in a multitude of books and articles (scientific, medical, clinical, and psychosocial) targeted at those who provide care and treatment for the person with Alzheimer's disease, especially caregiving families.

Over the past 10 years, the recognition of non-Alzheimer's dementias has also increased; however, research, treatment, and education for patients and families coping with these less common forms of dementia lags far behind the progress made with AD. Information on management and intervention for diagnosed persons and families is needed as these non-Alzheimer's dementias are different in their early symptomatology and often emerge at an earlier age of onset.

It is the task of this chapter to inform and equip social workers with a solid understanding of Alzheimer's and non-Alzheimer's dementias, how these illnesses affect the brain, how they progress, and how they affect both the diagnosed individuals and the families who care for them. Descriptions of how families cope with different forms of dementia illustrate the importance of comprehensive individual assessment in approaching the work.

UNDERSTANDING THE HUMAN BRAIN

To begin to understand AD and related dementias, it is important to have a basic understanding of the brain and how it is organized. This discussion is not a substitute for a course in neuroanatomy. However, a working knowledge of brain anatomy is the basis for further understanding dementia because the symptoms are a direct reflection of the effects of disease on different parts of the brain. Different brain regions control different aspects of cognition and behavior (Figure 2.1). Thus, the symptoms that an individual with dementia expresses are a direct result of neuropathology in specific brain regions that control those cognitive functions and behavior in the normal state. This knowledge allows the social worker to explain changes in behavior and reasoning in ways that can potentially lessen the burden that families feel by helping them understand that they are not to blame for what the disease is doing to their family member.

The human brain has two hemispheres joined by a bridge of fibers, the *corpus callosum,* that allow them to communicate. Each area of the brain has a different set of functions, so damage to a particular area will determine the type of symptoms expressed. This concept is best understood in the context of a stroke. A stroke occurs when a blood vessel in the brain is blocked or bursts. This destroys the brain tissue that is fed by that vessel. In neurodegenerative disease, the mechanism for brain tissue

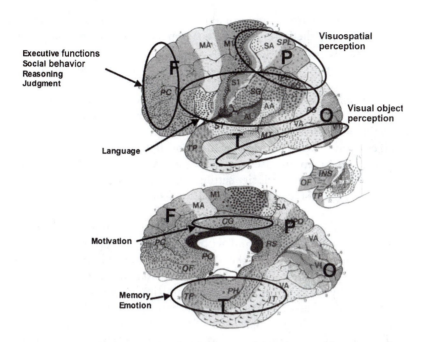

FIGURE 2.1   Behavioral neuroanatomy: Functional networks for cognition and behavior. The upper portion of the figure shows the left side of the brain (front of the brain is on the left side of this figure). The lower portion of the figure shows the medial surface of the right side of the brain. The different shades of gray represent different functions for the different sections of the brain. Thus, sections M1, S1, A1, and V1 are the "primary" areas of the brain that mediate movement, touch, hearing, and vision, respectively. Adjacent regions are known as "association cortex." Thus, MA, SA, VA, and AA are areas where the signals from the primary regions are elaborated. They are responsible for perception, that is, for example, knowing whether a sound is music or speech. The next areas of the brain, PC, AG, and TP, are essential for integrating information from hearing, touch, and vision. Thus, knowing that a specific bird makes a certain sound relies on these regions. Finally, on the medial surface of the brain, PH (known as paralimbic cortex) integrates sensory and motor information with the needs, goals, and motivations of the individual. Memory, emotional regulation, and motivation rely on this area. F = frontal lobe; T = temporal lobe; P = parietal lobe; O = occipital lobe. Adapted from Mesulam (2000).

damage is the formation of abnormal proteins that invade different brain regions and cause the brain cells to die. Depending on the region of the brain where the degeneration begins, symptoms may vary dramatically from one person to another and from one form of neuropathology to another.

The *frontal lobes* (right and left), the largest of the brain regions to be described, are concerned with reasoning, planning, organizing, problem solving, selective attention, personality, and movement, and other higher cognitive functions that include social behavior and emotions. Some of these functions also are known as *executive functions.* In lay terms, multitasking and priority setting are examples of executive functions. Some parts of the left frontal lobe are also important for our ability to speak.

The frontal lobes also play a role in our ability to adapt our behavior to the social situation at hand and act in ways that are appropriate. Damage that causes dysfunction of the frontal lobes can result in disinhibited behavior, poor judgment, impaired ability to plan and organize activities, extreme apathy (also known as *abulia*), and impulsive behaviors. Not all affected individuals will experience all these symptoms. Some may be overly disinhibited, for example, while others may lack any initiative.

The *parietal lobes* contain the *primary sensory cortex,* which is concerned with perception of stimuli related to touch, pressure, temperature, and pain. Damage to some regions in the right parietal lobe can cause visuospatial deficits (e.g., the individual may have difficulty finding his or her way around new or even familiar places). Damage to the left parietal lobe may disrupt the individual's ability to understand spoken and/or written language.

The *temporal lobes* contain regions that process short-term memory. Other parts of the temporal lobes are involved in our ability to recognize objects and faces. Additional areas allow us to comprehend words that others speak or that we read. The right temporal lobe is involved mainly in visual memory (i.e., memory for pictures and faces). The left temporal lobe is involved mainly in verbal memory (i.e., memory for words and names). Damage to the temporal lobes can cause severe short-term memory loss (*amnesia*), difficulty naming even common objects, and difficulty recognizing faces and objects. Again, individuals may experience similar or differing symptoms depending on the exact location of the degenerative damage.

Finally, the *occipital lobe* is the part of the brain that processes primary visual information. Our ability to see and experience both color and movement, therefore, relies on the area within the occipital lobes. Damage to this region can cause visual deficits. Individuals with damage in regions right next to this primary region may often be mistakenly thought to need new glasses when the problem lies in their *perception* of the information rather than the simple reception of light waves.

This brief review of behavioral neuroanatomy is critical to understanding the symptoms of diseases that affect the brain. In the next section, we discuss one class of illness, namely, neurodegenerative disease, that causes dementia by progressively damaging different brain regions, eventually leading to widespread cognitive and behavioral deficits and complete inability to function independently.

WHAT IS DEMENTIA?

According to the *Diagnostic and Statistical Manual of Mental Disorders* (4th ed.), dementia is characterized by progressive memory loss and additional cognitive deficits. However, this definition no longer accommodates all the forms of dementia that have been recently identified. In fact, there are many forms of dementia that do not begin with memory loss, such as frontotemporal dementia, which is discussed later in the chapter. Therefore, the definition of dementia that will be used is the following: "Dementia" is a clinical syndrome that is characterized by the insidious onset and gradual progression of cognitive and/or behavioral symptoms that constitute a departure from the individual's customary way of thinking and/or behaving. The changes can occur in memory, reasoning, judgment, language, visual perception, or features of personality and emotional responsiveness. The change is progressive and the deficits are at a level that ultimately interferes with routine activities of daily living, independence, and social relationships (Mesulam, 2000; Wicklund & Weintraub, 2005).

Identifying the Causes of Dementia

Dementia is not a disease or diagnosis itself. Instead, it is only a symptom, much like fever. Fever indicates that there is an illness but not what the illness is. Thus, you can have fever in response to the flu, or you can have fever in response to an infected sore. Similarly, while dementia indicates that the brain is not functioning normally, it does not indicate the source of the malfunction. Pinpointing the source requires neurological and neuropsychological evaluation to define the domains of cognition and behavior that are affected, tests of neuroimaging to determine if there has been a stroke or tumor that can produce symptoms of dementia, and blood tests to detect medical illnesses (such as thyroid dysfunction) that could cause a disturbance of mental function. Figure 2.2 illustrates the differential diagnosis of dementia based on

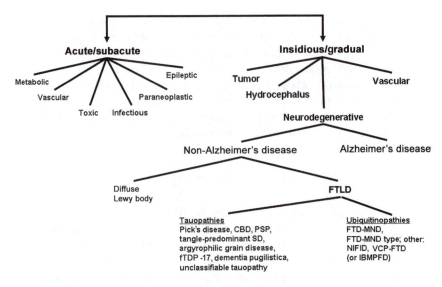

FIGURE 2.2   Differential diagnosis of dementia. "Dementia" is a
clinical diagnosis based on the examination of the patient. There
are many causes of dementia in older individuals. This branching
diagram shows that the causes can be divided according to the
nature of the onset of symptoms. An acute (minutes to hours) or
subacute (weeks to months) onset signals the entities branching
to the left. These sources of dementia are often treatable and
also referred to as "reversible." In contrast, a more gradual onset
(months to years) signals other causes represented on the right
side of the branch. Neurodegenerative brain diseases are the most
common causes of dementia of gradual onset. Alzheimer's disease,
the most common cause of dementia in individuals over age 65,
is one type of neurodegenerative disease. On the left side of the
neurodegenerative branch are a variety of "non-Alzheimer's" forms of
neurodegeneration.

whether the symptoms begin suddenly (acute or subacute) or gradually
and insidiously.

   The major causes of dementia covered in this chapter fall under the
general category of neurodegenerative diseases and vascular disease. We
do not discuss sources of dementia that are due to medical conditions
and are potentially reversible with medical treatment, as mentioned in
chapter 1. Other neurodegenerative disorders that can cause dementia

not covered in this chapter include Parkinson's disease, Huntington's disease, and acquired immunodeficiency syndrome (AIDS).

The diagnosis of any dementia is based on the combination of a detailed clinical history (including a collateral source of information in addition to the patient), physical examination, neuropsychological testing, and neuroimaging. To date, there are no blood tests that specifically detect the different causes of dementia. Thus, all the tests that a patient undergoes are done to rule out causes other than neurodegenerative disease. Even the magnetic resonance imaging (MRI) scan is done to rule out tumors and strokes since the neurodegenerative changes are not visible on the MRI itself. The neuropsychological examination provides the only proof of the dementia symptoms. A detailed discussion of assessment can be found in chapter 3.

As noted previously, some individuals may have symptoms that, while they mimic neurodegenerative dementia, instead are caused by certain medical problems. These other sources of dementia symptoms include stroke, brain tumor, infection, significant head trauma, alcoholism, depression, vitamin B12 deficiency, and hypothyroidism (see Figure 2.2). Infectious causes of dementia include chronic fungal meningitis, encephalitis, syphilis, and AIDS. Additionally, Creutzfeldt-Jakob disease, or spongiform encephalopathy, is caused by *prions,* proteins that have been altered so that they behave like viruses that infect the brain and cause neuronal degeneration.

Clinical Profiles of Dementia

While the name of a particular illness, such as Alzheimer's disease or Huntington's disease, is the most common method for classifying and understanding diseases, another way one can label neurodegenerative dementias is by the classification of the initial symptomatology. As noted previously, the initial symptoms are a clue to the region of the brain that is undergoing early stages of neurodegeneration.

Weintraub and Mesulam (1993) described four *neuropsychological profiles* of dementia, each distinguished by their presenting symptoms, neuroanatomical locus of disease, and neuropathological findings at brain autopsy. Weintraub and Morhardt (2005) used these four profiles to illustrate how different types of clinical symptoms of dementia could provide a framework for health care providers/clinicians to tailor education for patients and families in the clinical setting. Their specific management strategies appear in Table 2.1. Others have also provided information that can be used for tailoring educational programs (Farmer & Grossman, 2005).

TABLE 2.1   Neuropsychological Profiles of Dementia

Primary Mental Domains and Examples of Normal Abilities Included in Each	Symptoms of Impairment in This Domain That Persons With Dementia Experience	Strategies for Addressing These Symptoms
Attention		
Ability to sustain attention and concentrate without being distracted	Loses train of thought	Break information down into small portions—do not give more than one instruction at a time
	Can't concentrate for long periods of time	
Ability to grasp a normal amount of information from a conversation or set of instructions	Can't grasp all of the information (e.g., in a lengthy conversation)	Repeat instructions as the task is being done
Ability to persevere at a task	Easily distracted	Check on progress in a task and remind patient of what comes next
	Can't carry through on a task	Provide written instructions
Explicit (Volitional) Learning and Memory		
Ability to learn new information and retain it over time into the future	Repetitive questions and conversations	Repeat instructions, information; immediately ask patient leading questions about information (i.e., say, "Today is Sunday," then ask patient, "What day is it today?")
Orientation: knowledge of time, date, location, people's identities	Inability to recall events from immediate past (a few hours, days)	
Knowledge of current news events	Inability to retrieve a short list of items	
Knowledge of current personal events	Inability to recognize familiar places or faces (need to make sure that visual perception is intact before concluding that this is a memory deficit)	Write information in a portable format—provide patient with a "locket" or belt device containing a short list of the day's activities and times; teach patient to use it
Ability to remember facts and information from the distant past (usually preserved in early stages)	Gets lost in neighborhood (also need to rule out visual perceptual cause for this symptom)	Use patient's favorite spot as "Orientation Center" and include a calendar and digital clock

TABLE 2.1 *(Continued)*

Primary Mental Domains and Examples of Normal Abilities Included in Each	Symptoms of Impairment in This Domain That Persons With Dementia Experience	Strategies for Addressing These Symptoms
	Not aware of the day or the date	Make sure patient has a digital watch
		Maintain a consistent daily routine
		Provide patients with identifying information (Medic Alert, Alzheimer's Association Safe Return bracelets)
		Give patient a cell phone and call at regular intervals to check on location
Language		
Normal speech and ability to convey messages effectively	Hesitation in conversation; pausing to grope for words (this can also be due to poor concentration)	Speak in simple sentences, one at a time
Able to understand what others are saying		If a patient cannot come up with the right words, try to figure out the context of what he or she might be trying to say—don't allow your own perceptions to sway your interpretation
Able to name familiar objects without groping for words or substituting lengthy descriptions	Asks for sentence to be repeated (this can also be due to poor concentration, so need to differentiate)	
Able to understand what is read	Can't name familiar objects	Construct a communication notebook—if a patient has difficulty saying names of family members, provide a book of photos labeled with names and relevant information
Able to write meaningfully	Speech contains errors in word usage or pronunciation	
	Unable to understand what is read	
	Unable to write properly, makes errors	Devise a strategy for emergency situations bypassing the need to use the telephone—alert devices, automatic dialing to police, etc.

Continued

TABLE 2.1 *(Continued)*

Primary Mental Domains and Examples of Normal Abilities Included in Each	Symptoms of Impairment in This Domain That Persons With Dementia Experience	Strategies for Addressing These Symptoms
		Seek intervention from a speech language pathologist in order to devise alternative communication system—not to focus on restoring lost skill
Visual Perception		
Able to look at objects and recognize them	Difficulty finding objects that are in full view, especially when they are in a visually distracting environment (i.e., a closet or refrigerator)	First make sure that acuity is as good as it can be (i.e., if glasses are needed)
Able to tell two different objects apart		Keep personal items (objects, clothing) in the same location and simplify the visual environment; remove distracting things
Able to find objects in a cluttered array	Goes into the wrong rooms in the house	
Able to judge distance, spatial relations (e.g., the type of skill that is used in parking a car)	Takes wrong turn in familiar neighborhood	
Able to draw simple geometric forms	Can't recognize own face in the mirror	Arrange clothing within different categories by color or group outfits together for easy access
Able to navigate through a familiar space (home, neighborhood)	Thinks images in the mirror are other people (can also be confused with hallucination-type behaviors)	Do not use large letters to label information—use smaller letters
		Use verbal labels for rooms and objects around the house (i.e., "Door," "Susan's Room," etc.)
Comportment/Executive Functions		
Socially appropriate behavior	Behaves in an embarrassing way (too familiar or does things in public that should be done in private)	Provide regular schedule of structured activity to overcome motivational inertia
Awareness of one's own deficits and the changes in mental ability that are taking place		

TABLE 2.1 *(Continued)*

Primary Mental Domains and Examples of Normal Abilities Included in Each	Symptoms of Impairment in This Domain That Persons With Dementia Experience	Strategies for Addressing These Symptoms
Ability to make sound judgments regarding one's own safety and safety of others Ability to make good decisions about living and financial arrangements Ability to initiate activities and to carry them out	Unaware of memory and other cognitive deficits; denies them Not able to assess safety risk of things such as driving or managing finances Not able to appreciate need for supervision and rejects help Cannot get started on a project and carry it out (i.e., loses the "get-up-and-go")	Educate institutional staff about symptoms and alert staff to the need for outside motivation and encouragement to do small steps of a task Provide reassurance and include patient in negotiations about changing living situation or level of support but be firm—offer choices between helpful options ("Do you want a housekeeper one day a week or two?"—"No housekeeper" is not an option if indicated) Consult with physician for medications to manage difficult behavioral symptoms Consult with care professionals to assist in planning

Emotional Regulation (there are large individual differences in normal emotional capacity—the important factor is that emotions remain characteristic for the individual)

Able to control emotions (doesn't laugh, cry, or anger easily) Emotional reactions are in line with the precipitating event Able to read the emotional state of others	Typical emotional reactions no longer occur—replaced by either absence of emotion, exaggerated emotion, or "mellowing" of previously high emotionality	Caregivers need to recognize that the patient lacks the ability to respond as before and that lack of emotion is not a reflection of how the patient feels toward them

Continued

TABLE 2.1 *(Continued)*

Primary Mental Domains and Examples of Normal Abilities Included in Each	Symptoms of Impairment in This Domain That Persons With Dementia Experience	Strategies for Addressing These Symptoms
Absence of symptoms such as hallucinations, delusion, paranoia, agitation, aggression	Not able to perceive emotional distress in others Inappropriate emotional response to one's own deterioration—patient lacks depth of emotion Development of psychotic behaviors including paranoia, hallucinations (seeing or hearing things that are not actually present), delusions (believing something that is not true, e.g., a spouse is being unfaithful)	Do not challenge the patient's responses—accept them and use techniques to "defuse" potentially volatile interactions (e.g., change the topic)

The four clinical profiles refer to the early stage of the illness only, before other domains have been affected. In these early stages, patients are more likely to be living at home or even still working, and their unique needs are important to address. As neurodegenerative disease progresses, it affects more brain regions than the initial locus of disease, and, correspondingly, more symptoms appear.

The first clinical profile, *amnestic dementia,* is the typical presentation of AD. The earliest symptoms are memory problems and forgetfulness, and this is the most common presenting clinical profile in persons over the age of 65. The reason that memory loss is so salient is that, for reasons that are not well understood, the earliest neuropathological changes of AD (neurofibrillary tangles and senile neuritic plaques) form in the *hippocampus* of the medial temporal lobe, a region that is required for normal short-term memory. With time, however, the pathology spreads to other regions, causing more and more symptoms and, consequently, more functional impairment.

The second clinical profile, *aphasic dementia* or *primary progressive aphasia* (PPA), is characterized early on by progressive difficulty in communication through speech and writing. Despite having difficulty thinking of the proper words to express their thoughts, individuals with PPA show the preservation of other cognitive functions, such as remembering events and being able to function relatively independently. Language suffers in this syndrome because the neuropathology first affects the left side of the brain in the areas that control our ability to use language for communication (Figure 2.1). It is sometimes also considered a form of frontotemporal dementia (FTD) because the frontal and temporal lobes may be affected first. Unlike amnestic dementia, which is a sign of Alzheimer's pathology, aphasic dementia is not closely aligned with a single pathology. Instead, there is a family of neurodegenerative diseases that are also found in other forms of frontotemporal dementia. These are discussed in greater depth later in the chapter. In 30% of cases with PPA, however, there can be autopsy findings of AD for complex reasons we do not understand. Although the aphasia may be the only limiting symptom early on in the course of illness, over time (as in all other forms of dementia) the disease spreads, and symptoms increase.

The third profile includes early changes in behavior and personality, comportment, reasoning, and judgment and is called *executive/comportmental dementia*. Another term in the literature for this type is *FTD— behavioral variant (bv)*. The reason for this type of symptom is that the earliest pathology appears in the frontal and anterior temporal regions of the brain, areas that normally support these functions in the healthy individual.

The fourth clinical presentation is *progressive visuospatial dysfunction*. This presentation is characterized by difficulties in visual perception and recognition despite normal visual acuity. This class has also been referred to as *posterior cortical atrophy*. The changes in visual perception and spatial orientation are caused as the disease first settles in the regions of the brain (occipital, occipito-temporal, and occipito-parietal) involved in these processes. Most often, persons who first present with language, comportmental, and visuospatial difficulties are under the age of 65, in contrast to the older age at onset of individuals with amnestic dementia.

Armed with this information, the clinical social worker is better equipped to educate clients and their families about the relationship of a person's behavior and symptoms to facts about his or her disease. The regional selectivity of different forms of neurodegeneration determines the nature of the clinical symptoms. This explanation makes the symptoms less mysterious and less imbued with underlying personal conflicts and motivations. The social worker can also help families cope with the appearance of more and different symptoms as these diseases progress (Weintraub & Morhardt, 2005).

As already noted, although neurodegenerative disease ultimately affects many brain regions and, therefore, many different types of mental abilities and behavior, it is the early-stage symptoms that are very unique and that require different approaches for education and intervention. Thus, a patient with aphasia, who has trouble thinking of words but who can remember events with high accuracy, will need a very different approach from one who can speak normally yet cannot recall what happened 10 minutes ago. Someone with visuospatial difficulties cannot respond to written notes and instructions in the way that a person with the amnestic profile (memory problems) can. Clinical management strategies based on these different symptoms are outlined in Table 2.1.

WHAT IS ALZHEIMER'S DISEASE?

Alois Alzheimer, a German neuropathologist and psychiatrist, first described the clinical and neuropathological features of what is now known as Alzheimer's disease. He observed the disease in Auguste D., a patient he first saw in 1901, and published his findings in 1906. Her symptoms included "disorientation, impaired memory, as well as trouble in reading and writing." This increased gradually to "hallucinations and a gradual loss of higher mental functions."

A brain autopsy showed the cerebral cortex of her brain to be thinner than normal in addition to other abnormalities, one being the presence of two structures that he called *neuritic plaques* and *neurofibrillary tangles*. These features were known to occur in the brains of much older individuals but were very uncommon to see in such proliferation in the brains of younger people (Auguste D. was only 51 when first admitted to the hospital). For many years after this discovery, AD was known as a "presenile dementia" (before the age of 65). Later on, it was discovered that plaques and tangles in high density were also found in the brains of people whose dementia began in later life. The senile–presenile distinction, therefore, was no longer made, and plaques and tangles were considered to be due to AD regardless of the age at onset.

The differences in brain tissue can be seen in Figures 2.3 and 2.4. Figure 2.3 shows brain tissue taken from an 80-year-old individual who was cognitively normal at the time of death; Figure 2.4 shows tissue taken from the brain of an individual who had developed AD prior to death. The normal tissue contains healthy neurons and very sparse neurofibrillary tangles that appear as darkened elongated structures. In contrast, the tissue from the individual with AD contains numerous tangles and a very large dense amyloid plaque surrounded by degenerating neurons.

These features continue to be the hallmarks that define the diagnosis of definite AD today (Joachim, Morris, & Selkoe, 1988). Toxic to brain cells, the plaques and neurofibrillary tangles cause the cells in the brain

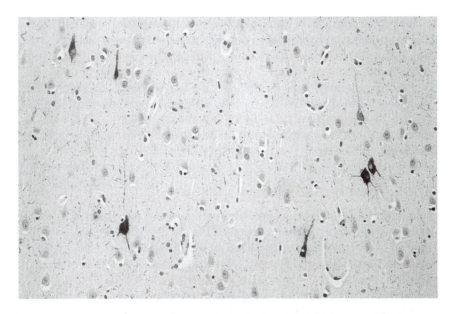

FIGURE 2.3   Brain tissue from a cognitively normal 80 year-old.

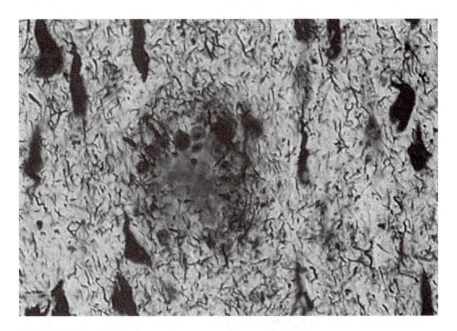

FIGURE 2.4   Brain tissue from a patient with AD.

to lose connections with other nerve cells, stop working, and finally die. The destruction and progressive death of nerve cells causes memory failure, personality changes, problems in carrying out daily activities, and other features of the disease.

Until the 1980s, doctors used the term *organic brain syndrome* as a diagnosis for the confused elderly, and Alzheimer's was not considered a distinct disease entity. Education for families and health care providers on the best methods of caring and communicating with individuals with dementia did not exist.

The Progression of Alzheimer's Disease

In AD, the hippocampus, located in the temporal lobe, is the first affected area. Damage to this memory center of the brain initially affects an individual's recollection of recent events, or what is referred to as short-term memory. As the disease progresses, it travels to other parts of the brain. The route of spread of the disease is governed by the way in which different brain regions are connected with one another. Over time, dysfunction in other brain areas causes problems in visual and verbal memory, changes in personality, atypical emotional reactions, visuospatial deficits, and impairment of language and perception.

In daily life, after the initial short-term memory loss, the affected individual may demonstrate a change in personality; become more irritable or withdrawn; have difficulty organizing and planning, managing money, measuring distance, or finding the right words; become tangential; or blame others inappropriately. Changes in cognitive functions may lead to changes in driving ability, such as less caution, poor judgment, and slowed reaction time. The patient may or may not have insight into the changes and how they are transforming him- or herself and those around him or her. Since the ability to appoint a future decision maker is typically preserved at the very earliest stages of neurodegenerative dementias, planning for the future should begin as soon as possible after diagnosis.

While the anatomical pathway of AD in the brain has been found to be predictable (Braak & Braak, 1998), how the disease manifests itself clinically is experienced as extremely unpredictable by caregiving families who observe and live with the varying levels of functioning from day to day and sometimes hour to hour. Helping families understand this variability and what they can do to appropriately respond and communicate with persons with AD is a major task of the social worker. In so doing, assessing the ability of the caregiving family to organize themselves and intervene accordingly is crucial.

Families need to understand that in the beginning there may be days when the affected individual appears "normal." This apparent normalcy may cause them to question their own observations. However, it is important to explain that neurodegenerative disease is not an "all or none" phenomenon. Instead, it can be likened to a faulty electrical connection that, in the beginning, is "off" sometimes and "on" more frequently. Eventually, there will be more "off" than "on" times—but even in later stages, there may be brief periods of "on" times. It still must be understood that the overall course of the disease is one of increasing disability (Larson et al., 2004).

THE NON-ALZHEIMER'S DEMENTIAS

Although AD is the most common cause of dementia in older individuals, it is now known that there are other forms of dementia that differ from AD. This difference can be seen neuropathologically (at brain autopsy). First, different regions of the brain are affected. Second, the type of cellular pathology seen under the microscope is different from the plaques and tangles associated with AD. Consequently, the types of clinical symptoms manifested by the affected individual at the onset of the disease process are different (Mesulam, 2000). The next section discusses the most common forms of non-Alzheimer's dementias and their implications for treatment and education.

Frontotemporal Degeneration

Frontotemporal degeneration (FTD) is a descriptive name given to a group of conditions that affect primarily the frontal and anterior temporal regions of the brain and, as a result, are characterized by disorders of language and/or social function. As indicated earlier, the frontal lobes are important for our ability to regulate behavior, make decisions, plan, organize, and judge whether our behavior is socially appropriate. They are also important for our ability to inhibit inappropriate thoughts and actions. Thus, people with FTD experience an early decline in social and interpersonal conduct. For example, a person with FTD may demonstrate a decline in manners and social graces, become more disinhibited, use obscene language, be overly familiar with strangers, or make inappropriate sexual remarks.

Individuals with FTD also demonstrate impaired regulation of personal conduct. For example, they may manifest apathy, withdrawal, loss of interest, and lack of motivation and initiative. These symptoms can be misinterpreted as signs of depression. However, they can be distinguished from depression because the affected person does not experience sad feelings. On the other hand, there may be an increase in purposeless activity (e.g., pacing, constant cleaning) or increased talking, laughing, or agitation. The individual may display *emotional blunting*—emotional shallowness and indifference to others coupled with a loss of warmth and empathy. These particular individuals have an early loss of awareness of their symptoms and thus often have a lack of concern regarding the social, occupational, and financial consequences of their behavior. It is common for persons with FTD to lose exorbitant amounts of money because of poor financial decisions at the onset of these symptoms. Some may even end up divorced or jailed because of their inappropriate behavior.

Since the memory area of the brain is not affected in the early stages of FTD, there is no true memory loss as seen in AD. Instead, there are changes in personality, ability to concentrate, social skills, motivation and reasoning, and/or language. Often these symptoms are confused with a psychiatric disorder, and affected individuals are often referred to a psychiatrist before their symptoms are recognized as a dementia caused by brain disease.

FTD Subtypes

FTD is difficult to diagnose, as there are many subtypes, and even within subtypes there can be overlapping clinical features. Signs of parkinsonism due to a mutation on chromosome 17 accompany one form of FTD. This causes abnormal production of a protein known as *tau,* which is found in the brains of patients with this subtype. This form is familial. Taking a family history, therefore, would disclose many affected relatives within and across generations. Nevertheless, not all affected relatives will have exactly the same symptoms. In many cases, however, the disease is *sporadic* (not genetically transmitted).

A very recent report has shown that a mutation in the *progranulin* gene, also on chromosome 17, has been found in patients with FTD who, on brain autopsy, do not have a tauopathy but who instead have another abnormality called *ubiquitin-positive pathology* (Gass et al., 2006). These genetic discoveries are likely to have a major impact on the identification of FTD and its subtypes. Because of the potential implication of these discoveries for hereditary factors, materials are being created to inform patients and families about the meaning of the genetic discoveries and recommending genetic counseling for those at risk for familial forms of FTD, which accounts for approximately 20% of cases.

FTDs also share clinical features with other, more common conditions, such as AD, vascular dementia, and Parkinson's disease. One form of FTD that causes prominent motor symptoms is *corticobasal degeneration* (CBD). Symptoms of CBD can occur very early in the course of illness, making it easier to diagnose. However, motor symptoms can also occur much later, in which case it is harder to diagnose. Individuals with CBD will have increasing difficulty with coordination and walking and may fall easily. They may have problems swallowing and may choke on food or liquids.

Individuals with FTD may often receive faulty diagnoses on the basis of their presenting symptoms. When cognitive and language symptoms dominate, they may receive a diagnosis of AD; when personality change and behavior symptoms rule, they may be told they have a psychiatric disease, such as bipolar disorder. The diagnostic process can be incredibly frustrating and confusing for individuals with FTD and their families. While there is a plethora of material on AD and its management, very little has been written for persons with FTD and their families.

Clinical Diagnoses of FTD

There are several clinical diagnoses that are made during the life of individuals with frontotemporal dementia. These different diagnoses illustrate the complexity of this disorder and reflect the fact that many mechanisms can be affected. In some presentations, language deficits (or aphasia) are the initial symptoms; in others, there are prominent changes in social behaviors and personality; in yet others, there are motor symptoms of the type seen in Parkinson's disease. The names given to the clinical diagnoses include the following:

- Primary progressive aphasia and its subtypes (agrammatic, logopenic, or semantic) (Gorno-Tempini et al., 2004)
- Social FTD (also known as FTD—behavioral variant or FTD—frontal variant)
- Pick's disease
- FTD with motor neuron disease or amyotrophic lateral sclerosis
- Frontotemporal dementia with parkinsonism linked to chromosome 17 (FTDP-17, one of the hereditary forms of FTD)
- CBD
- Progressive supranuclear palsy (an exceedingly rare form of FTD, typified by an inability to execute voluntary eye movements upward and downward)

A consensus conference conducted in 1998 suggested the term *frontotemporal lobar degeneration* (FTLD) as the overall category for these dementias (Neary et al., 1998).

Pathological Diagnosis of FTD

As in AD, the definitive diagnosis of FTD can be made only by postmortem examination of the brain tissue. Sometimes there is a discrepancy between clinical diagnosis and the pathological (tissue) diagnosis. Furthermore, clinical diagnoses do not go by the same names as the pathological diagnoses; this mixture of nomenclature can cause considerable confusion.

For example, the term *Pick's disease* in the clinical arena refers to prominent changes in personality and speech, while the same term is used for a neuropathological diagnosis made when the nerve cells contain globular structures that are stained by a silver chemical. In fact, not all patients who appear to have Pick's disease during their lifetime will be found to have Pick's disease at brain autopsy. The different names given to the type of neuropathology found at the time of brain autopsy are the following, to cite a few (Cairns, Lee, & Trojanowski, in press):

- Frontotemporal lobar degeneration with ubiquitin inclusions, also known as FTD-MND (motor neuron disease)
- Dementia lacking distinctive histology
- Pick's disease
- Frontotemporal dementia with parkinsonism linked to chromosome 17 (FTDP-17)
- CBD
- Argyrophilic grain disease

Prevalence of FTD

FTD typically begins in the fifth or sixth decade of life, although cases have been reported with an onset as young as 21 years and as old as 85 (Grossman, 2002). There is limited prevalence data on FTD. It is seen by some as probably the most common dementia in persons under the age of 60 and as possibly second to AD in the list of neurodegenerative diseases that cause dementia (Ratnavalli, Brayne, Dawson, & Hodges, 2002). Overall, it is recognized that FTD is more common than initially suspected.

Primary Progressive Aphasia

Mesulam (1982) first described *primary progressive aphasia* (PPA) when he published the first report of six cases. Related diagnostic categories are *semantic dementia* and *temporal variant of frontal lobe dementia* (Edwards-Lee et al., 1997; Hodges et al., 1992).

PPA begins with word-finding difficulty, most often observed in conversation, and progresses to involve all aspects of language, including problems with grammar, understanding the speech of others, reading, and writing. Processing of any form of language symbols, including numbers, can also be affected. The limitations in daily activities are the result of language impairments. There are no impairments in memory, visuospatial abilities, visual recognition, executive functions, or comportment for the first 2 or more years after onset (Mesulam, 2004). However, as the disease progresses, these mental skills also become affected. Most individuals with PPA are under the age of 65 at onset.

Subsets of PPA include *semantic dementia,* a form of progressive aphasia that is characterized by difficulty in both the comprehension of single words and the use of single words to name objects, and *progressive nonfluent aphasia,* which is characterized by difficulty initiating speech and agrammatism (inability to produce a grammatical sentence). Fluency of speech is significantly impaired. A third type, *logopenic PPA,* is marked by decreased speech output and difficulty in word finding but no problems with grammar or word comprehension. These fine distinctions among subtypes, however, can be determined only by a careful neuropsychological or speech-language evaluation.

There are two basic approaches to treatment for PPA: one is to focus treatment directly on the impaired language skills, and the other is to provide augmentative/alternative communication strategies or devices. Both are recommended. Beginning in the early stages of the disease, treatment should enhance existing verbal language skills. At the same time, treatment focused on the use of augmentative/alternative communication strategies (such as gestures, drawings, and a communication notebook filled with personal information and relevant information) also should be provided, even though those techniques may not be needed for months or years. These strategies either enhance verbal communication or replace it (Thompson & Johnson, 2005). In recent years, some individuals have found the use of personal digital assistants (known as PDAs) to be helpful in communicating select words or phrases.

A speech and language evaluation will determine which strategy is the best; practice and follow-up treatment with a speech-language pathologist is important in order to further develop the strategy.

The neuropathology of PPA observed at postmortem brain examination is exceedingly complicated. There is much overlap with the neuropathology of the behavioral variant of FTD. In addition, 30% of cases have the neuropathological features of AD. In patients who show AD pathology and symptoms of PPA, investigations are being carried out to determine why they are so different from those with AD pathology and memory loss as the prominent symptom.

Vascular Dementia

Vascular dementia is caused by cerebrovascular disease and in the past has been called *multi-infarct dementia.* Individuals with stroke risk factors—

such as high blood pressure, previous history of strokes, history of heart attack, family history of stroke or heart attack, smoking, high cholesterol (*hyperlipidemia*), diabetes, cardiac arrhythmias, atrial fibrillation, and peripheral vascular disease—are all at risk for vascular dementia.

Cerebrovascular disease causes a blockage of blood flow (*ischemia*) to the deep parts of the brain (the white matter), causing one or more strokes. It is the damage from these strokes that results in cognitive impairment. Unlike large strokes, which affect motor and sensory brain regions and result in visible signs of paralysis or blindness on one side of the visual field, this type of vascular damage affects cognition and behavior. Thus, the only symptoms the patient and family experience are changes in mental abilities and behavior.

The progression of vascular dementia often follows a stepwise course, with periods of stability followed by a decline. Each decline occurs with the cerebrovascular event or stroke, then the patient's condition plateaus, and then, again, it is followed by another decline. Sometimes, however, the course can be gradual and similar to that of AD.

The person with vascular dementia often has particular difficulty sustaining attention and retrieving information. In comparison to AD, which has a predictable anatomical course, the clinical manifestations of vascular disease correspond to the location of the areas damaged by the stroke. Thus, depending on the location of the brain damage, symptoms could also consist of aphasia, visual deficits, or inappropriate social behaviors.

Families caring for someone with vascular dementia may go long periods of time thinking that there may be no further progression. In fact, there may be slight improvement in functioning at times, particularly if the cerebrovascular disease is well controlled and the individual is well supported in his or her environment. Despite plateaus in the course of the illness, it is important for families to plan for future care because vascular dementia continues to get progressively worse over time.

Dementia With Lewy Bodies

Another common cause of dementia in the elderly is *dementia with Lewy bodies* (DLB). Symptoms of DLB include fluctuations in the level of consciousness, visual hallucinations, and parkinsonism (Boeve et al., 2001; McKeith et al., 1996; Turner, 2002). A fourth symptom is *rapid eye movement behavioral disorder*, in which the individual has very vivid nightmares and moves in his or her sleep as if acting out the dreams. Not all of these symptoms need to be present; however, typically two out of four are needed for the diagnosis. Although the visual hallucinations of DLB can take any form, they tend to be nonthreatening and can even be pleasant, such as in one case where a woman saw "fluffy lambs" next to her bed.

DLB progresses more rapidly than AD, and although complex and bizarre delusions are an essential part of the disease, affected individuals do not respond well to neuroleptic medication to manage these symptoms. In fact, neuroleptic medications may actually provoke the parkinsonian symptoms in an individual with DLB who has not yet manifested them spontaneously.

EARLY-ONSET DEMENTIAS

The term *early onset* refers to a dementia in which symptoms begin well below the age of 65. This term has been used interchangeably with the term *early stage,* but the latter really refers to the *stage* or *severity* of *any* type of dementia, whether of early onset (under 65) or late onset (over 65). Thus, people with early-onset dementia may be in any stage of dementia—early (mild), middle, or late.

Maslow (2006) recently presented newly analyzed data from the Health and Retirement Survey. These data indicate that there may be as many as a half a million Americans under age 65 who have dementia. Combining this with data from other studies, the Alzheimer's Association calculates that there are currently between 220,000 and 640,000 people with early-onset Alzheimer's or related dementia in the United States. While additional research is needed to develop a more precise figure, the proposed range provides a plausible first estimate and indicates that the number of Americans with early-onset dementia is much higher than is generally acknowledged.

Since early onset refers to the age of onset and not the specific dementia diagnosis, it is important for the clinician to understand which diagnoses are most likely to be early onset and which are most likely to occur later in life. As stated, it is thought that FTD, PPA, and their subtypes are the most common early-onset diagnoses; the prevalence of these dementias actually decreases with age.

However, the opposite occurs with AD, a disease in which age is the largest risk factor. Persons with early-onset AD have a greater probability of having a familial (i.e., hereditary) form of the disease and/or an atypical presentation of the illness compared to a person over the age of 65.

Since vascular dementia is the result of vascular disease, which is more prevalent with increasing age, this disease has a typically later onset as well, and DLB is typically also a disease of late onset. Thus, although there can be exceptions, a patient with onset of illness before age 50 is far less likely to have AD, vascular dementia, or DLB than to have one of the other neurodegenerative diseases.

Psychosocial Issues in Early-Onset Dementia

Individuals diagnosed with early-onset dementia face far different issues than those who succumb later in life (e.g., in their 70s or 80s). Affected persons in their 40s and 50s are often still working, saving for retirement, and supporting their younger children. The onset of a dementia illness in the prime of their working careers makes these responsibilities daunting (if not impossible) to manage. They may eventually lose employment as a direct result of poor performance that is only in retrospect attributed to their disease symptoms. However, some may be ineligible for employer assistance and have difficulty obtaining disability insurance.

Their spouses and families also face significant financial and emotional stresses. Well spouses may be forced to seek additional work to meet the family's financial needs, or, alternately, they may need to reduce their workload to care for their spouse or assume more responsibility for running the household. Emotionally, the well spouse experiences the loss of intimacy and a coparenting partner. Adolescent children suffer the loss of a parent at a developmentally tumultuous time of life. Young adult children who are normally separating from their family of origin and defining themselves may need to be more involved in their family than their peers. The treating health care team can address these developmental issues by assessing and intervening in the educational and emotional needs of the entire family system.

Most services for people with dementia, such as support groups or adult day services, were designed for and targeted to older people. People with early-onset dementia often feel uncomfortable with these services. Additionally, caregiving families do not feel that they belong in support groups focused on the care of much older people since postretirement issues and the involvement of adult children are not relevant to them.

Conversely, most adult day programs and residential care facilities are not equipped to address the special needs of the younger person, especially if the behavioral symptoms caused by early-onset dementia are difficult to manage. In fact, lack of education about the unmotivated nature of these behaviors hinders care facilities from providing appropriate management. As more is known about these forms of dementia, more policy changes may come into effect. Some residential care and adult day programs recognize the needs of the younger person with dementia and are beginning to offer services to meet their needs.

Difficulties With Diagnosis of Early-Onset Dementia

While the health care community and society at large now have an understanding of AD and its symptoms, non-Alzheimer's dementias remain unknown to many practitioners and are seen as rare or atypical. Affected individuals and their families are often frustrated by physicians who diagnose behavior and personality changes as psychiatric in origin. An accurate diagnosis is further delayed while the patient is treated for a psychiatric disorder. Sometimes, individuals and families must visit many health care providers before they find one who understands what is happening. Specialty clinics that evaluate more unusual forms of dementia often see patients who have had one or more prior evaluations with misdiagnosis. The lack of relevant information not only is frustrating but also puts the patient and family in jeopardy while the patient continues to function without appropriate supervision.

The nature of the symptoms in FTD (i.e., lack of judgment, poor social skills, disinhibition) and in PPA (i.e., inability to verbally express oneself, poor language comprehension, compromised communication skills) leads to embarrassment for family members; they may lose friends and other sources of social support. To further this isolation, families are often reluctant to seek services that are designed primarily for older adults, as mentioned earlier.

The following vignettes illustrate the unique characteristics and needs of people with non-Alzheimer's dementias.

BRUCE AND PATRICIA: FRONTOTEMPORAL DEMENTIA—SOCIAL/BEHAVIORAL VARIANT

Bruce was a 40-year-old businessman, married, with a 10-year-old daughter. He had been suffering from changes in his behavior, personality, and social functioning for at least 4 years prior to being evaluated, most noticeably, however, over the past year. His business partners began noticing changes in Bruce's judgment and decision-making ability. He made an error in his personal finances that cost the family thousands of dollars and when told of the error did not seem perturbed. His workspace became increasingly disorganized. His boss became increasingly frustrated at Bruce's nonchalant attitude and eventually told him that he could no longer continue to work. Again, Bruce expressed no reaction to this news.

Bruce, typically devoted to his daughter, started to demonstrate an inability to properly supervise and care for her. On one occasion he forgot to pick her up after ballet practice; on another, he invited a stranger he met on the street corner in for coffee while only he and his daughter were at home. Always meticulous with finances, Bruce began to lose track of bills and other paperwork. His wife, Patty, assumed that his changes were purposeful and reacted with anger, which resulted in their seeking marital therapy. The couple considered divorce. Bruce's father was confused by the changes in his son's behavior and thought that perhaps it resulted from marital discord.

Initially diagnosed by his physician with depression, Bruce was seen by three other physicians before a diagnosis of FTD was accurately made. Meanwhile, the family conflict became so heated that Bruce's parents and his wife became estranged. Because of poor financial decisions and losses, Bruce and Patty also faced bankruptcy.

This common scenario illustrates a person with early-onset dementia who is at a very different developmental life stage than a person with AD. In this situation, the diagnosed individual has parents in their 60s who are invested in ensuring that he has the care that he needs. Their social worker needs to maintain neutrality by engaging all the parties in a common goal: caring for Bruce. At the same time, the social worker must recognize the personal, emotional, and financial limitations that complicate this situation. The social worker's role as an educator, family counselor, and resource link in partnership with the interdisciplinary team should continue over the course of the illness. The progressive nature of neurodegenerative disease means that Bruce's symptoms will worsen over time, other symptoms will emerge, and his functioning will be increasingly limited. The social worker can help the family adapt to the changes that need to be made throughout the course of the illness.

SARAH AND PAUL: FRONTOTEMPORAL DEMENTIA—PRIMARY PROGRESSIVE APHASIA

Sarah was a 55-year-old writer and high school English teacher. She lived with her recently retired husband, Paul, in their own home. They had three adult children, one who lived in the area and two who lived out of state.

Sarah began having difficulty speaking and delivering her class lectures; in addition, she found that her writing was becoming simplified and lacked the complexity of her previous work. Initially, it was felt that these changes were due to a slowing of mental processes related to "normal aging"; however, as her symptoms progressively worsened over a period of 2 years, her colleagues, students, and family also became concerned regarding the changes.

Sarah sought an evaluation from her primary care physician who recommended psychiatric and neurological evaluations. An in-depth evaluation revealed a diagnosis of primary progressive aphasia, a condition she had never heard of before. She was forced to abandon her teaching position and apply for disability. However, because of the lack of understanding of her condition by the Social Security office, Sarah was denied disability benefits on three different occasions with the recommendation that she would be able to handle a job where she was not required to be verbal.

Social work advocacy on her behalf assisted in assuring that disability (and ultimately Medicare) benefits were obtained. Meanwhile, Paul found himself overwhelmed and frustrated with his increasing sense of isolation. None of his colleagues or friends were experiencing these changes; they were instead anticipating retirement and travel in the next few years.

Paul found little benefit from attending support groups for caregivers of persons with AD, as Sarah's symptoms were different and the other caregivers were at a different stage in their lives. As a result, Paul was motivated to organize and seek out those who would understand. Paul started an online support group for caregivers of persons with PPA. Additionally, speech-language therapy helped Sarah and Paul develop a communication notebook, which was a useful means of communication as Sarah increasingly struggled to give voice to her thoughts and needs. As Sarah's disease progressed, she became involved in adult day services, and Paul attempted to maintain the highest quality of life for both of them in their home for as long as possible. Eventually, as Sarah's disease worsened, Paul made the decision to move her into a long-term care facility.

CLINICAL RECOMMENDATIONS FOR AD AND NON-ALZHEIMER'S DEMENTIAS

The following general recommendations should help social workers who are working with those suffering from AD or non-Alzheimer's dementias as well as their caregivers.

Providing Education

Just as the clinical social worker is unable to assist families without a thorough understanding of dementia and its effects on the brain, families can neither completely understand what is happening nor plan for the future without a similar education. The first question to ask any family caring for a member with dementia is their understanding of the diagnosis. What is the name that has been given to the symptoms? Also recognize that different family members may have different levels of understanding and acceptance of the changes. They may also hear different things from treating health care professionals.

A beginning role is to establish a common understanding and provide as much education regarding the disease as possible and as often as needed. It is helpful to give information in written form as well as verbally. There are many resources for this educational material listed in the back of this book.

Improving the Affected Individual's Mood

Depression is a common symptom in those with dementia, particularly in AD, where short-term memory problems can be especially frustrating in the early stages. Similar frustration levels are found in PPA because the individual is usually aware of how difficult it is to communicate. An initial study in patients with PPA indicates that they may experience depression as a result (Medina & Weintraub, in press). The social worker should be alerted for signs of depression, which include tearfulness, changes in sleeping or eating patterns, irritability, and withdrawal.

While a first intervention may be to increase social supports and activity, if the depression is not lifted, the individual may benefit from an antidepressant medication. Consultation with a neuropsychiatrist or geriatric psychiatrist who is expert in these disorders is important because medications can have unusual effects on individuals with brain disease.

Improving Communication

All dementias challenge the communication abilities of the affected individual. In the early stages of AD, it may help some individuals to keep an appointment book or calendar where they can write things down. It is also helpful to have a central place for keys, eyeglasses, and other items that are frequently used. As the disease progresses, the need for structure and routine is essential. Helping families establish structure in the life of the person with any dementia is an important intervention. The individual may benefit from participating in adult day services or utilizing the help of a companion who can organize and supervise the day.

Communication issues are most profoundly affected in persons with PPA from the beginning. As mentioned earlier, alternate modes of communication should be taught as early as possible to help minimize frustration and get the patient habituated to using them before they may actually be needed. When the disease progresses, it will become more difficult to get the individual to rely on alternate communication methods.

Many families choose to work with a speech-language pathologist knowledgeable about PPA to tailor alternative communication strategies. These strategies may include a communication notebook (filled with photographs of family and friends, emergency information and medications, and pictures of hobbies and commonly visited places) that help bolster independence and allow the person to communicate nonverbally with others. It is recommended that all language-impaired individuals carry a wallet card with a brief explanation of their condition and pertinent emergency information so that they can communicate their situation quickly to anyone with whom they interact (e.g., in a store, at the airport, in an emergency situation).

Avoiding Confrontation

Confrontational situations may emerge in the course of caring for someone with dementia. Persons with AD may be repetitive and have no memory of having asked the same question or repeated the same story. In FTD, individuals may not appreciate that they have experienced changes in personality or behavior. Additionally, poor judgment is common, as are inappropriate behaviors such as telling offensive jokes, approaching strangers, showing sexual disinhibition, and spending indiscriminately. Persons with other forms of dementia in which the frontal lobe becomes affected as the disease progresses may also experience these changes over time.

These behaviors often cause tension with other family members. If a confrontation emerges, it is important that families not respond by arguing or reasoning. It is helpful for them to be told that the patient is not operating under the same rules that most of us have to guide our behavior. Rather, they should try to identify exactly what is causing the situation and understand the triggers or warning signs. Help families pick their battles and intervene in disruptive situations only where the safety of the patient is at stake. Help them figure out how to maintain a sense of humor. Keep the decision-making responsibility of the person with dementia to a minimum to decrease confusion and frustration. Validate feelings and make the patient feel safe. Finally, if needed, certain medications may be introduced to minimize some aberrant behaviors. Except for patients with DLB, those with other forms of neurodegenerative disease may be able to tolerate antipsychotic medications.

Maximizing Activity

Keeping a person with dementia active can be a challenge. However, it is important to maximize cognitive health and improve mood. As earlier described, adult day services and leisure programs provide socialization and structured daily activity. A hired companion who comes to the home may be able to provide some stimulation, help with language practice, or help get the diagnosed individual out of the house for some exercise. It is important to educate companions about the illness and to provide them with activities that they can use to engage the patient. Too often, companions act as "sitters" and do not provide the type of social interaction needed. Nonverbal activities, such as listening to music, art activities, spending time with a pet, or completing puzzles, may be soothing and provide meaningful activity. Persons who have more physical ability and energy may benefit from activities that integrate helpful and stimulating exercise into their day, such as hiking or swimming.

Encouraging Caregiver Health

Caregiving families, regardless of the type of dementia that affects their loved ones, are at risk for increased mental and physical health problems. As a result, they need to maintain their health and fitness. Encourage families to make time for themselves and create breaks by locating friends or family to help or enlisting available community services. Make sure that they remain active and social. Individual, family, and group counseling/support groups can help them cope with the changes and losses they are experiencing in their lives.

CONCLUSION

The descriptions of Alzheimer's disease and non-Alzheimer's dementias presented in this chapter demonstrate the range of symptom variability in persons with these disorders. Working effectively with diagnosed individuals and families requires an understanding of how these disorders manifest themselves in daily life. In addition to the specific diagnosis and symptomatology, the clinician needs to be aware of the myriad number of psychosocial issues inherent in living with and caring for someone with a dementing illness. Social workers with a detailed understanding of the source of the clinical symptoms and their manifestations in daily activities, in addition to a foundation in systems theory and interpersonal dynamics, will be the most suitably prepared for this work.

REFERENCES

Boeve, B. F., Silber, M. H., Ferman, T. J., Lucas, J. A., & Parisi, J. E. (2001). Association of REM sleep behavior disorder and neurodegenerative disease may reflect an underlying synucleinopathy. *Movement Disorders, 16,* 622–630.

Braak, H., & Braak, E. (1998). Evolution of neuronal changes in the course of Alzheimer's disease. *Journal of Neural Transmission, 53*(Suppl.), 127–140.

Cairns, N. J., Lee, V. M., & Trojanowski, J. Q. (in press). Frontemporal dementias: Genetics and neuropathology. In B. Miller & J. L. Cummings (Eds.), *The human frontal lobes* (2nd ed.). New York: Guilford.

Edwards-Lee, T., Miller, B. L., Benson, D. F., Cummings, J. L., Russell, G. L., Boone, K., et al. (1997). The temporal variant of frontotemporal dementia. *Brain, 120*(Pt. 6), 1027–1040.

Evans, D. A., Funkenstein, H. H., Albert, M. S., Scherr, P. A., Cook, N. R., Chown, M. J., et al. (1989). Prevalence of Alzheimer's disease in a community population of older persons: Higher than previously reported. *Journal of the American Medical Association, 262,* 2551–2556.

Farmer, J., & Grossman, M. (2005). Frontotemporal dementia: An overview. *Alzheimer's Care Quarterly, 6,* 225–232.

Gass, J., Cannon, A., Mackenzie, I. R., Boeve, B., Baker, M., Adamson, J., et al. (2006). Mutations in *progranulin* are a major cause of ubiquitin-positive frontotemporal lobar degeneration. *Human Molecular Genetics, 15,* 2988–3001.

Gorno-Tempini, M. L., Dronkers, N. F., Rankin, K. P., Ogar, J. M., Phengrasamy, L., Rosen, H. J., et al. (2004). Cognition and anatomy in three variants of primary progressive aphasia. *Annals of Neurology, 55,* 335–346.

Grossman, M. (2002). Frontotemporal dementia: A review. *Journal of the International Neuropsychological Society, 8,* 566–583.

Hodges, J. R., Patterson, K., Oxbury, S., & Funnell, E. (1992). Semantic dementia: Progressive fluent aphasia with temporal lobe atrophy. *Brain, 115*(Pt. 6), 1783–1806.

Joachim, C., Morris, J. H., & Selkoe, D. J. (1988). Clinically diagnosed Alzheimer's disease: Autopsy results in 150 cases. *Annals of Neurology, 24,* 50–56.

Larson, E. B., Shadlen, M. F., Wang, L., McCormick, W. C., Bowen, J. D., Teri, L., et al. (2004). Survival after initial diagnosis of Alzheimer's disease. *Annals of Internal Medicine, 140,* 501–509.

Maslow, K. (2006). *Early onset dementia: A national challenge, a future crisis.* Washington, DC: Alzheimer's Association.

McKeith, I. G., Galasko, D., Kosaka, K., Perry, E. K., Dickson, D. W., Hansen, L. A., et al. (1996). Consensus guidelines for the clinical and pathologic diagnosis of dementia with Lewy bodies (DLB): Report of the consortium on DLB international workshop. *Neurology, 47,* 1113–1124.

Medina, J., & Weintraub, S. (in press). Depression in primary progressive aphasia. *Journal of Geriatric Psychiatry and Neurology.*

Mesulam, M-M. (1982). Slowly progressive aphasia without generalized dementia. *Annals of Neurology, 11,* 592–598.

Mesulam, M-M. (2000). Aging, Alzheimer's disease, and dementia: Clinical and neurobiological perspectives. In M-M. Mesulam (Ed.), *Principles of Cognitive and behavioral neurology* (pp. 439–522). New York: Oxford University Press.

Mesulam, M-M. (Ed.). (2000). *Principles of cognitive and behavioral neurology.* New York: Oxford University Press.

Mesulam, M-M. (2004). Primary progressive aphasia—A language-based dementia. *New England Journal of Medicine, 349,* 1535–1542.

Neary, D., Snowden, J. S., Gustafson, L., Passant, U., Stuss, D., Black, S., et al. (1998). Frontotemporal lobar degeneration: A consensus on clinical diagnostic criteria. *Neurology, 51,* 1546–1554.

Ratnavalli, E., Brayne, C., Dawson, K., & Hodges, J. R. (2002). The prevalence of frontotemporal dementia. *Neurology, 58,* 1615–1621.

Thompson, C., & Johnson, N. (2005). Rehabilitation of language deficits. In D. Koltai & K. Welsh-Bohmer (Eds.), *Geriatric neuropsychology: Assessment and intervention* (pp. 315–332). New York: Guilford.

Turner, R. S. (2002). Idiopathic rapid eye movement sleep behavior disorder is a harbinger of dementia with Lewy bodies. *Journal of Geriatric Psychiatry and Neurology, 15,* 195–199.

Weintraub, S., & Mesulam, M-M. (1993). Four neuropsychological profiles of dementia. In F. Boller & J. Grafman (Eds.), *Handbook of neuropsychology* (Vol. 8, pp. 253–282). Amsterdam: Elsevier.

Weintraub, S., & Morhardt, D. (2005). Treatment, education and resources for non-Alzheimer dementia: One size does not fit all. *Alzheimer Care Quarterly, 6,* 201–215.

Wicklund, A. K., & Weintraub, S. (2005). Neuropsychological features of common dementia syndromes. *Turkish Journal of Neurology, 11,* 566–588.

CHAPTER THREE

Assessment of Individuals With Dementia

Victoria Cotrell

INTRODUCTION

Dementing illnesses are characterized by cognitive deficits and symptoms caused by disturbances in brain functioning. Each illness is characterized by a pattern, temporal order, and progression of symptoms, but variability within the illness often impacts functioning in unpredictable ways. Symptoms and consequences of these illnesses are often similar to each other and can resemble a number of unrelated physical and psychological conditions. Illnesses also frequently co-occur. This complexity increases the risk of inaccurately attributing cause-and-effect relationships in the process of assessment, especially in older adults who tend to have multiple chronic illnesses to begin with.

Assessment of dementia is a complex task that captures client functioning in multiple spheres and requires a systematic approach to the documentation, interpretation, and transmission of this information. The purpose of an assessment, of course, determines the content and methods to be used. The usual areas of interest include cognitive abilities, functional abilities (i.e., activities of daily living, instrumental activities of daily living, and management of risk and unsafe situations), mood and behavior, and environmental demands and resources, including the status of the caregiver.

Social workers tend to be concerned with *screening* for cognitive impairment rather than diagnosing dementing illness, identifying the *psychosocial needs* of clients and families, and monitoring the individual's *ongoing ability to adapt* to his or her specific environment. Screening for cognitive impairment establishes the presence of a cognitive deficit but does not determine the underlying cause of the loss. Diagnosis usually requires a multidisciplinary effort to address the potential neurological and physiological causes of the deficit(s). This complex process is the basis of the differential diagnosis. Social work knowledge of the individual's functional losses can be particularly useful in this process since functional impairment is an important component of diagnosis and is often best observed in the client's natural environment. Social workers also play an important role in efforts to achieve successful adaptation after the diagnosis.

Both direct observation and the use of objective measurement are important aspects of assessment. In order to document the possible presence of a dementing illness, we must first recognize that the symptoms, behavioral signs, or other events that are observed are suggestive of dementia. These indicators are frequently missed by health professionals in the primary care setting (Boise, Neal, & Kaye, 2004). Additional findings conclude that there is need for improved knowledge of assessment of dementia among all health care professionals, including social workers (Barrett, Haley, Harrell, & Powers, 1997).

The aim of this chapter is to increase sensitivity to the needs and strengths of clients with dementing illness and to present options for documenting and measuring these needs. The primary focus will be on Alzheimer's disease (AD) since it is the most frequently encountered cause of dementia. However, distinctions among other common causes of dementia, especially as they relate to assessment, will be made whenever possible.

In documenting cognitive, functional, and behavioral status, it is important to understand how to administer and interpret objective assessment tools and apply their contextual caveats (including the effects of sociodemographic differences and psychological states on individual measures). Social workers should use commonly accepted and tested screening instruments whenever possible to quantify their observations and to maximize their participation in interdisciplinary collaboration with other professionals. The use by professionals of commonly understood concepts and scores improves the precision of communications about the degree and nature of observed impairments. The reader is referred to the resource section at the back of this book to locate the assessment tools that are discussed in each section. Copyright restrictions should be checked before use. Despite the importance of standardized measures, they should not replace the use of observation and client and collateral interview to guide the assessment.

DIAGNOSIS

The single most important reason to make a referral for a diagnosis of a dementing illness is to ensure that presenting symptoms that are potentially treatable are identified and remedied. A formal diagnosis will also provide the individual and family an opportunity to plan for the future and allow the diagnosed individual time to exercise more control over present and future decision making. This benefit is not without potential social, economic, and psychological consequences, areas in which social work expertise is particularly relevant.

Dementing illnesses can be thought of as stigmatizing, and diagnosed individuals and families should be provided with information and support throughout and following the diagnostic process. For instance, the options for long-term care insurance may be drastically limited after a formal diagnosis of AD. The perceptions that others might have about the diagnosed person's competence should be considered, and an understanding of how information will be shared with others should be reached between the client and individuals who will know of the diagnosis. Care should be taken that clients' personal perceptions of the illness are accurate and do not constrict their ability to maximize their enjoyment of life.

The use of a federally funded Alzheimer's Disease Center for diagnosis assures the client of a comprehensive evaluation and excellent patient and family educational resources. These centers provide expertise in distinguishing the many causes of dementia that afflict older adults. Over 30 such centers, supported by the National Institute on Aging (NIA) and located in major medical institutions across the United States, have been designated to provide clinical services and participate in research on the detection and prevention of dementing illnesses such as AD. The NIA-sponsored Alzheimer's Disease Education and Referral Center sponsors a Web site that lists current AD centers and contact information and also provides a list of available clinical trials and research updates. In addition to providing referral information, this is an excellent resource for social workers interested in remaining current in their knowledge of scientific advances in AD (this Web site is included in the resource section at the back of this book).

If an NIA-funded AD center is not available, a formal evaluation may be done by a local physician, preferably one with geriatric expertise. The physician will determine if the patient has met the criteria for a diagnosis of AD or other dementing illness by performing a comprehensive physical exam (including lab tests), an imaging test, and a thorough medical history. The physician may use a cognitive screening tool such as the Mini-Mental State Exam during the evaluation, but this screening tool should never be used to make a formal diagnosis. A referral to a neuropsychologist for more extensive cognitive testing can be used to confirm the results of initial cognitive screening and to provide more detailed information about the deficits.

Although a *computerized tomography* or *magnetic resonance imaging* scan is typically conducted for an initial evaluation, because of cost and limited benefit to the patient, these scans are not routinely used to monitor the progression of the illness after diagnosis. *Single-photon emission computed tomography* and *positron emission tomography* imaging are generally not recommended for routine diagnosis (Doody et al., 2001).

The specific diagnostic procedures will vary with the suspected cause of the dementia. For instance, imaging is particularly important in the diagnosis of vascular dementias (VaD) to detect and examine the characteristics of cerebrovascular lesions. More detailed evaluation of cardiovascular and pulmonary functioning may also be required. A neurological exam may be particularly important in evaluating the disturbances of movement sometimes present in dementia with Lewy bodies (DLB).

The most commonly accepted guidelines for diagnosing dementia are found in the report of the NINCDS-ADRDA workgroup (McKhann et al., 1984), the *Diagnostic and Statistical Manual of Mental Disorders* (4th ed.; *DSM-IV*) (American Psychiatric Association, 1994), and guidelines prepared by the Presidential Task Force on the Assessment of Age-Consistent Memory Decline and Dementia (American Psychological Association, 1998). In addition, the Quality Standards Subcommittee of the Academy of Neurology recently evaluated the best evidence for the assessment and management of dementing illness (Doody et al., 2001). Together, these documents represent a basic consensus about criteria used to establish a diagnosis of AD and an expanding number of neurological disorders that are likely to be confused with AD (e.g., DLB and frontotemporal dementia [FTD]). These documents are available through the Internet (specific Web sites are listed in the resource section at the back of this book).

As stated earlier in this chapter, the diagnostic process uses a cross-disciplinary approach to rule out competing explanations for presenting symptoms. Identifying individuals appropriate for such a diagnostic work-up is an important first step. Social workers, as part of the health care team, must be knowledgeable about this process.

COGNITIVE STATUS

Cognitive changes are central to the identification of dementia. Certainly a core symptom of dementia—and usually the earliest symptom of AD—is impaired memory. Problems in both acquisition and retrieval of learned information are experienced throughout the courses of AD and LBD. Mild memory loss may not be detected easily unless a family member reports a change. Recent memory loss usually occurs before deficits in memory of important personal history or remote memory. Loss of recent memory is often revealed through repetition of questions and comments, inconsistent knowledge of recently occurring events, chronic loss of objects, missed appointments, and new learning that may require excessive repetition. In VaD, memory may not be severe in comparison to other cognitive deficits, and sometimes a syndrome of dementia does not develop from cerebrovascular disease at all (Read, 2004). The memory is less impaired in dementias of the frontal lobe (i.e., FTD) (Conn, 2004), and memory loss associated with delirium may be similar to AD but is distinguished by the presence of altered consciousness.

Attention and concentration skills, like memory, are critical to all other cognitive domains and are sensitive to changes in neural functioning (Smith & van Gorp, 2004). Attention includes the ability to screen out unnecessary input and focus on relevant incoming stimuli, avoid distraction when necessary, and shift one's attention or focus as demanded by the situation. Severe deficits in memory and attention can severely limit the functioning of the individual.

Early in the course of AD—and, in many cases, of VaD and DLB—deficits of attention can appear as difficulties staying on task and following a conversation. Minor redirection of focus may be needed. More complex behaviors, such as driving, may be affected early in the illness. In delirium, attention is severely impaired, resulting in high levels of distractibility and restlessness.

Language, which becomes increasing impaired with progression of AD, is a complex process that requires many levels of specialized brain functions. In AD, early deficits may include word-finding problems and selection of words with the wrong meaning, an instance of naming disorders called *anomia*. This inaccessibility to a full vocabulary may lead to inefficiency in communication called *circumlocution* (reliance on the use of many, less precise words to describe a thought). Language problems also present as the loss of meaningful content in conversation, worsening with the progression of the illness and ultimately leading to mutism in very advanced AD. However, well-learned social exchanges may be preserved earlier in the illness, reducing the appearance of any type of language deficit.

Aphasia, or language disturbance, is also common in VaD. Depending on the location and degree of cerebral damage, the language impairments may include articulation, fluency, comprehension, naming, repetition, reading, and/or writing. Aphasia is usually a core symptom of FTD. This aphasia is characterized by fluent but empty speech, difficulties in comprehension and object identity, and anomia. Mutism can also develop (Conn, 2004).

Both AD and VaD share the *DSM-IV* diagnostic criteria of memory impairment and the presence of one or more of the following disturbances: aphasia, agnosia, apraxia, and/or disturbed executive functioning (American Psychiatric Association, 1994). *Agnosia,* an inability to correctly identify objects and their correct use (i.e., mind blindness), may be noted in the client's misuse of common objects. Clothing found in the refrigerator and perishable food in the closet may be a sign that the client is having difficulty identifying objects, storing them in an appropriate place, or using them correctly. Sensory input may also be misinterpreted, and some individuals may even complain that something is wrong with their vision, despite an intact visual system. Deficits in awareness of the illness and its consequences, *anosognosia,* may also occur.

Visuoperceptive deficits are related to the agnosias and include visual disruptions that can result in difficulties with directional and distance orientation (Bigler & Clement, 1997). At first, the individual's way-finding problems may be confined to unfamiliar travel, but later the ability to find one's way in familiar settings may also be impaired. Another ability related to perceptual loss is *prosopagnosia,* an inability to recognize familiar faces, including one's own. This rather distressing symptom is seen in both AD and FTD.

Apraxia, the ability to follow through with learned and skilled behaviors, may create problems with following instructions and correctly sequencing the steps of everyday tasks, such as making coffee, handling tools, and cooking. Problems in these more complex behaviors requiring the linking of movements, called *ideational apraxias,* are more commonly seen in earlier stages of AD. The inability to follow through with simple motor behaviors, such as walking or combing one's hair (*ideomotor apraxias*), results from a loss in motor planning and execution and tends to be seen in more advanced AD but much earlier in cases of VaD with neuromuscular involvement (Bigler & Clement, 1997). The inability to perform simple behaviors can become quite profound in advanced dementia, as in the inability to close and open one's eyes intentionally or on command.

Finally, *executive functioning* refers to a set of higher-order skills that are associated with the frontal lobes. The term refers to functions such as abstraction, decision making, problem solving, regulation, organization, monitoring, and planning. Like a conductor in an orchestra, these functions influence and coordinate more basic abilities, such as memory; an individual may demonstrate competence in a basic skill and still be unable to use the skill to accomplish more complex tasks. Executive functioning determines the practical consequences of adaptation to real life, goal achievement, and appropriate behavior.

Disturbance in executive functions is more apparent in frontal lobe disorders with primary symptoms of personality change and motivation, reasoning, and social skill deficits. Individuals with VaD due to cerebrovascular accidents (i.e., strokes) often present with earlier, more abrupt impairment of organization, initiation, and judgment than individuals with AD, where executive functions tend to remain more intact until later in the illness. Still, impaired executive functioning is apparent in the abilities of most individuals with dementia to perform more complex activities of daily living.

Brief Cognitive Measures

When information can be collected directly from the client or a close informant, several brief instruments for screening cognitive deficits are available and have been tested on individuals with dementia. The most frequently used instrument for screening cognitive impairment is the Mini-Mental State Exam (MMSE) (Folstein, Folstein, & McHugh, 1975), which provides professionals with a common language to transmit descriptive information about the status of cognitive functions.

There is a great deal of psychometric information about this instrument, and it has been translated into many languages. Thirty items are used to assess six areas of cognitive functioning: orientation, registration, attention and calculation, recall, language, and figure construction. Scores range from 0 to 30, with a cutoff score of 23 or less indicative of dementia. However, the instrument tends to produce false-negative results among cases of mild impairment and is sensitive to higher levels of education, creating a ceiling effect (Crum, Anthony, Bassett, & Folstein, 1993; Froehlich, Bogardus, & Inouye, 2001). There is also a tendency to produce higher false-positive rates for African Americans than Whites, which is not entirely accounted for by differences in education and socioeconomic status (for a review, see Froehlich et al., 2001).

An adjustment of cutoff scores has been suggested for various populations (Crum et al., 1993), and van Gorp et al. (1999) found that the best overall cutoff score for the dementia group in their study was 26 or less. This adjustment produced no instances of misclassification of undiagnosed cases (false positives) and only 2% undetected dementia cases (false negatives). Higher rates of misclassification were obtained by adjusting cut points according to age and education, as recommended by Crum et al., although both methods yield better accuracy than the traditional cutoff of 23. Use of a higher cutoff score will still produce less accurate results in some individuals with lower levels of education (e.g., less than 8 years of schooling), so consequences of the score, as well as client characteristics, should be considered when interpreting the results (van Gorp et al.). Crum et al. provide a convenient table of cutoff scores on the MMSE by age and educational level; a Web site for this article is provided in the resource section at the back of this book.

Certainly other factors contribute to measurement bias in the use of all brief cognitive measures, such as comorbid illness, psychiatric disorders, and social factors. In a thorough review of the literature, Froehlich et al. (2001) documented a cultural difference for both older African Americans and their caregivers in reporting higher levels of impairment in the physical and mental functioning of the care receiver than White individuals and their caregivers. Consequently, cultural variations need to be considered when using self-report measures with various groups. There is a continued need for the development of instruments that are both appropriate for use with varying levels of cognitive impairment and effective for use with diverse cultural and racial groups. It is important for clinicians to use their judgment in adjusting for the effects of education, culture, and socioeconomic status when using most of the existing instruments.

Reassessment

It has been recommended that cognitive status be reassessed every 6 months since declines of 3 to 4 points per year on the MMSE can occur in progressive dementias such as AD (Cummings et al., 2002). However, use of the MMSE in short intervals of reassessment is controversial since there is much variability in rates of decline on the instrument because of both measurement error and variation in the illness (Clark et al., 1999). Clark et al. suggest not using the MMSE for measuring progression for periods of less than 3 years. Use of longer intervals will increase the accuracy of the score and produce yearly averages that approximate expected declines. Additionally, the need for frequent reevaluation should be considered on an individual basis since cognitive testing can be quite stressful for the individual with progressive cognitive decline.

Informant Measures

Family members often detect changes in the client's cognition or behavior and can be used to supplement information collected from direct evaluation of the client. Family members and other individuals living with the client are in the best position to identify changes in the client's functioning and are generally accurate in their assessment of cognitive status (Cacchione, Powlishta, Grant, Buckles, & Morris, 2003). Cacchione et al. found that collaterals with high levels of interaction with the impaired individual were particularly good at identifying very mild memory problems, even in cases where testing was not sufficiently sensitive to detect changes. A caveat is that closer contact with the individual tends to produce an overreporting of cognitive deficits, while those who spend less time with the individual are more likely to underreport problems. Despite the potential for accurate reporting, collaterals may not recognize some behaviors as indicative of cognitive loss. Thus, it is best to use a semistructured interview that includes questions about memory, orientation, judgment, and problem solving.

Several caregiver rated cognitive assessment instruments with adequate validity and reliability are available. The short form of the *Informant Questionnaire on Cognitive Decline in the Elderly* (Jorm, 1994) is the most widely used informant scale. The short version has 17 items focused on everyday cognitive functions. The caregiver reports the care receiver's improvement or decline on each item using a 5-point scale, with 1 = much improved, 3 = no change, and 5 = much worse in the past 10 years. The results are unaffected by the client's education or language skills but may be biased by the caregiver's characteristics and/or relationship with the individual (Jorm, 2004).

FUNCTIONAL STATUS

Functional status is not only important as an indicator of the presence and progress of dementing illness but is critical in planning for client care as well. The ability to function independently in the home, community, and social sphere is affected by dementia but also by comorbid illness, disability, sensory loss, psychiatric problems, and the social-physical environment. Losses in functional performance due to AD and related disorders are based mostly on deficits in cognitive abilities, such as memory, attention, and specialized functions.

Most activities found in daily living rely on varying degrees and combinations of these cognitive skills. Processing skills are also needed to bring these skills together in an integrated behavior. Knowledge of the status of these underlying cognitive skills alone is not usually very predictive of performance deficits in everyday living. However, identification of specific cognitive components that result in failed performance may lead to successful interventions aimed at compensation. Thus, the use of both cognitive and functional assessments can be useful in finding ways to maximize independence.

A home visit is a particularly good way to observe the functional status of a client. For instance, difficulties in managing meals, cooking, or the intake of adequate nutrition can most efficiently be determined by the status of the kitchen and contents of the refrigerator. Unpaid bills, grooming problems, hoarding, and household disarray are among the items that may signal a need to assess the functional status of the older adult in greater detail.

Two domains of daily activities are usually assessed to determine functional status: basic *activities of daily living* (ADL) and more complex *instrumental activities of daily living* (IADL). ADLs are those behaviors that are basic to personal care and maintenance and include bathing, dressing, toileting, transfer, continence, grooming, and feeding. IADLs include complex skills needed for independent functioning in the home and community. Examples of these tasks are meal preparation, managing currency, shopping, and use of the telephone. Complex tasks that rely on recent memory tend to be affected first, followed by well-learned and practiced activities (Galasko et al., 1995). Thus, IADLs are lost before ADLs, and those IADLs most dependent on memory, such as "recalling recent events," "handling money," and "remembering a list," precede other, less memory-intensive tasks. Similarly, basic ADLs are lost in the order of dressing, toileting and feeding (Galasko et al.).

Functional Measures

MMSE scores tend to decline simultaneously with functional deficits; both can track the short-term progress of dementing illness. However, the floor and ceiling effects that often occur with cognitive testing limit the use of measures such as the MMSE in more severely impaired individuals (Galasko et al., 1995).

The Katz Index is a commonly used instrument for measuring assistance required in each of the six basic ADLs (Katz, Ford, Moskowitz, Jackson, & Jaffe, 1963). Scores range from 0 (complete independence) to 6 (complete dependence in all areas). The two instruments most frequently used to assess IADLs are the Pfeffer Functional Activities Questionnaire (FAQ) (Pfeffer, Kurosaki, Harrah, Chance, & Filos, 1982) and the Lawton IADL Scale (Lawton & Brody, 1969). The FAQ consists of 10 items that measure complex household, occupational, and social competencies. It is scored dichotomously as "no difficulty" and "any difficulty" with a range of scores from 0 to 30. Because the FAQ contains items requiring higher levels of functioning than the Lawton scale, it tends to be more sensitive to changes experienced by very mildly impaired individuals (Tabert et al., 2002). For more severely impaired individuals, the Katz Index may provide a more appropriate measure of functioning.

NONCOGNITIVE SYMPTOMS: BPSD

Individuals with dementia frequently display *behavioral and psychological symptoms* (BPSD). Approximately 66% of individuals with dementia experience BPSD at some time during their illness, although these symptoms are less common to AD than they are to other dementing illnesses (for a review, see Sadavoy, 2004). These symptoms create stress in the caregiver and are a major cause of institutionalization of the afflicted individual (Coen, Swanwick, O'Boyle, & Coakley, 1997).

Reisberg has identified the following seven categories of BPSD and has specified the ways in which the symptoms of AD are likely to be manifested in each category: paranoia and delusions, hallucinations, activity disturbance, aggression, sleep disturbance, affective disturbance, and anxiety and phobias (Reisberg et al., 1986). Affective disturbances are seen earlier in the illness than other symptoms, while the highest frequency of most other BPSD is seen in the moderate to moderately severe stages of the illness. The incidence of BPSD in the severe stage of AD declines significantly (Reisberg & Saeed, 2004).

The presence and order of appearance of BPSD relative to cognitive symptoms is a distinguishing characteristic of frontal lobe dementia, VaD, and delirium. Early changes related to personality are common in FTD and may include socially inappropriate behavior, increased food intake, apathy, lack of inhibition, and ritualistic behavior (Conn, 2004). Frontal lobe injury due to falls and other accidents may result in a frontal lobe personality syndrome of apathy, paranoia, disinhibition, aggression, and *labile affect* (uncontrollable or mood-incongruent laughing, crying, or smiling). Frontal lobe impairment is also associated with depression and anxiety (Conn). Vascular dementias are often associated with depressed or blunted mood, withdrawal, anxiety, and decreased motivation, although noncognitive symptoms of VaD have not been well specified in the literature (Read, 2004). The behavioral symptoms of delirium tend to include instability of mood, belligerence, agitation, suspiciousness, and inability to sleep (Liptzin, 2004). In contrast, cognitive symptoms tend to dominate the clinical picture of AD in the early course of the disorder, with less severe behavioral symptoms occurring later in the illness.

Underlying Causes of BPSD

The symptom manifestations of BPSD suggest a mix of possible causative elements, including premorbid client characteristics (such as suspiciousness or anxiety), neurochemical deficits and structural damage produced by the dementing illness, fears generated by cognitive and functional losses, difficulties perceiving the environment accurately, reduced opportunities for physical and verbal expression, and changes in intimate relationships. The environment, both physical and interpersonal, can create confusion, frustration, boredom, loneliness, and overstimulation and understimulation in the cognitively impaired individual. Medication side effects and toxicity, substance abuse, and comorbid medical conditions, including pain, are also potential sources of BPSD.

Assessment of BPSD

Measurement tools can be used to document the presence and intensity of symptoms and the resulting distress to both client and caregiver. However, thoughtful problem solving is often needed to determine the source or trigger of these symptoms, and an assessment should include a history of the symptom and behavioral and environmental observation whenever possible. The changes that occur with dementing illness challenge the individual in many ways and may ultimately result in problematic responses. If possible, underlying causes should be addressed before pharmacological treatment is attempted.

Health care professionals with little time and no access to the home environment may respond to requests to remedy BPSD with medication and/or referral to a more restrictive environment. Inadequate training about dementia among health care professionals, including physicians, social workers, and nurses, can also contribute to ineffective responses to the illness (Barrett et al., 1997).

The use of psychotropic medications to treat BPSD presents complex problems and risks. Additionally, BPSD often have a different pathophysiological basis than do similar-appearing psychiatric conditions and require a different treatment approach (Sadavoy, 2004). The reader is referred to Sadavoy's useful handbook for considerations about the treatment of BPSD and information on the use of psychotropic medications in older adults.

In assessing the factors that may produce BPSD, the social worker should specify the behavior(s) and determine possible precipitants. The documenting of *antecedent-behavior-consequences* (ABC) is a particularly useful approach for determining the possible contributions to many of these symptoms.

Cohen-Mansfield and Martin (2004) have developed an effective assessment and treatment strategy based on the use of ABC, and the interested reader is referred to their work for more detailed description. The advantage of working with both formal and informal caregivers using this assessment is that it offers the caregiver a systematic way of working through problems (instills a sense of control) and teaches objectivity in interacting with the care receiver with BPSD (prevents emotional reactivity in the caregiver).

BPSD Measures

Measurement tools that document the frequency, severity, and impact of symptoms require the use of collateral reports regarding BPSD, which may produce a biased perspective of the problem. However, validity, reliability and usefulness of tools such as the *Neuropsychiatric Inventory Questionnaire* (NPI) (Cummings, 1997) and the *Behavioral Pathology in AD Rating Scale* (BEHAVE-AD) (Reisberg et al., 1987) have been well established.

The NPI is an easily administered tool that assesses 12 domains of psychiatric disturbance: delusions, hallucinations, agitation, dysphoria, anxiety, apathy, irritability, euphoria, disinhibition, aberrant motor behavior, nighttime behavior disturbances, and appetite and eating. A checklist of the possible behaviors and their severity and frequency is used with the caregiver to rate the severity and frequency of symptoms in each area. An advantage of this tool is that it also assesses the distress to the caregiver produced by each of the domains.

The BEHAVE-AD, basically a structured psychiatric interview of the caregiver, is designed to measure the presence and severity of symptoms as they have appeared in the 2 weeks preceding the interview. It consists of 25 well-defined behaviors grouped into seven areas: paranoid and delusional ideation, hallucinations, activity disturbances, aggression, sleep disturbance, affective disturbance, and anxieties and phobias. If present, the behavior is rated as mild, moderate, or severe. Severity of the symptom is measured on a 4-point scale. Like the NPI, the impact of the symptoms on the caregiver is measured.

Reisberg and Saeed (2004) also provide additional description of the seven categories of BPSD common to AD, distinguishing the clinical presentation of these symptoms from those presented in the cognitively intact psychiatric population and mapping these symptoms onto the Global Deterioration Scale for staging purposes. Psychiatric symptoms exhibited by individuals with dementia, such as paranoia, hallucinations, aggression, sleep disturbance, anxiety and phobias, are superficially similar to those characteristic of the psychiatric population, although they differ somewhat in their presentation (Reisberg & Saeed, 2004). For instance, the nature of paranoia and delusions in AD are more likely to focus on a belief that others are hiding or stealing objects that the individual is, in reality, misplacing. Inability to recognize familiar faces, including one's own, may lead to a host of paranoid beliefs and behaviors in individuals with AD or FTD.

Depression

Depression is a noncognitive symptom that warrants individual assessment because of its complex relationship with cognitive impairment. Relations between the two can be one of three possibilities: (a) *pseudodementia* (where symptoms of depression are mistaken for a nonexistent dementia), (b) symptoms of dementia are mistaken for depression, or (c) the two conditions may coexist. Pseudodementia should be ruled out during the differential diagnosis of dementia to make certain that the depression is treated and to avoid an inappropriate diagnosis of dementia as the cause of cognitive loss.

However, there is disagreement on the extent to which cognitive symptoms associated with depression are of sufficient severity to account for the cognitive losses of dementia (Burt, Zembar, & Niederehe, 1995). Even in the cases where both cognitive disturbance and depressive symptoms remit after treatment of depression, many individuals go on to develop AD (for a review, see Reisberg & Saeed, 2004). Moreover, depression is widely thought to be a risk factor for later development of dementia (Speck et al., 1995; Steffens et al., 1997).

The second relationship is that dementia symptoms are confused with depression and lead to a missed diagnosis of dementia. Common shared symptoms that are likely to be attributed incorrectly to depression include flattened affect, decreased verbalizations, psychomotor slowing, irritability, decreased concentration, and apathy (Alexopoulos, 2004; Purandare, Burns, Craig, Faragher, & Scott, 2001; Reisberg & Saeed, 2004). Many of these symptoms are responses to declining cognitive capabilities and are a result of withdrawal from activities and social interaction, although a slowing of movement has been reported as symptomatic of AD beginning at a relatively early stage of the illness (Reisberg & Saeed).

Finally, dementia and depression may exist together. Depression in the general population of older adults occurs often in the context of illness and is related to increased morbidity and mortality (Alexopoulos et al., 2002). Although the reported rates are highly discrepant, major depression is estimated to occur in approximately 17% of individuals with AD, while the incidence of minor depressive symptoms is considerably higher (Wragg & Jeste, 1989). The incidence of depression in VaD is even higher than in AD (Read, 2004). In AD, depression may further contribute to the progressive neuropathological changes of AD (Alexopoulos et al., 2004), can create excess disability, and certainly decreases the individual's quality of life.

Symptoms that tend to distinguish true depression from symptoms secondary to dementia include sad, downcast mood; self-denigrating thoughts; and nonvegetative symptoms of depression (Alexopoulos et al., 2004; Purandare et al., 2001). Because response to treatment is potentially quite successful, it is advisable to treat depressive symptoms when there is any question as to the etiology.

Depression Measures

Numerous tools designed to identify the presence of depressive symptoms in this population are available. Two commonly used instruments are the *Geriatric Depression Scale* (GDS) (Sheikh & Yesavage, 1986) and the *Cornell Scale for Depression in Dementia* (Alexopoulos, Abrams, Young, & Shamoian, 1988). The GDS is a 30-item scale that can be either self-administered or observer rated, although self-rating should not be considered valid in individuals with an MMSE score of 15 or less (Katz, 1998). When possible, it is best to use both client and collateral responses. Scores of 0 to 10 fall in the normal range and 11 or higher indicate the presence of depression.

The Cornell Scale for Depression is a 19-item measure that is scored primarily on the observation of client behaviors, with less emphasis on the client interview. Scores range from 0 to 38, with higher scores indicating greater severity of depressive symptoms. A score of 13 or more suggests the presence of major depression. A problem with the Cornell Scale, as with the GDS and most depression scales used with older adults, is that they tend to contain items with high somatic and vegetative content (including sleep disturbance), which can be misinterpreted as depression in individuals who have high levels of medical illness, functional disability, and sleep disturbance due to neurological or other physical conditions (Kurlowicz, Evans, Strumpf, & Maislin, 2002). Results of these measures should be treated with greater caution when used with more advanced cases of AD and in individuals with high levels of medical frailty.

PROGRESSION OF AD AND OTHER DEMENTIAS

There is much clinical utility in determining where an individual is in the disease process, and families are particularly interested in identifying their relative's disease status and planning for the future. Since AD progresses in a more predictable fashion and with less variability in symptoms than most other dementing illnesses, staging systems have been developed.

The progression of VaD is distinct from AD and is usually characterized by abrupt changes in mental status that coincide with new damage caused by vascular events. These events may be followed by improvement, stabilization, or decline in functioning. However, AD and VaD often occur together so that abrupt changes may occur in an illness progression characteristic of AD. Moreover, vascular damage that occurs in small vessels located deeper in the subcortical region of the brain may present as a subtle progression of the illness that more closely resembles AD.

Delirium and frontal lobe dementia due to head trauma can also present with abrupt onset and acute changes. Symptoms of delirium may fluctuate considerably in a short period of time, and improvement in mental status can occur, especially when the underlying problem is treated (Liptzin, 2004).

It is important to understand the limitations of a linear perception of AD and to convey these caveats to clients and families whenever appropriate. Staging assumes that progression of the illness is predictable and uniform and that deviation from the pattern of symptom development suggests the presence of a source of disability other than AD. One need not reject these basic assumptions to acknowledge that a great deal of heterogeneity is represented among those with AD, not only with regard to the illness itself but also in the host of comorbid illnesses and psychosocial factors that characterize the geriatric population. Families and clinicians should expect that the progression of the illness, including specific cognitive, functional, and behavioral symptoms, may deviate substantially in individual cases, and staging should not be allowed to demoralize the individual or family.

Global Assessment Measures

The functional, cognitive, and behavioral characteristics of AD can be used to describe a continuum of stages across the levels of dementia severity. The *Clinical Dementia Rating* (CDR) scale (Morris, 1993) and the *Global Deterioration Scale* (GDS) (Reisberg, Ferris, de Leon, & Crook, 1982) are considered the most comprehensive means of staging the progression of the illness. Other clinical staging tools have been developed but are not as well known as these instruments. Both require training to produce formal scores, but even without training, the stages are useful descriptions of the illness progression, and the social worker should be knowledgeable about each instrument. The descriptions are particularly useful in determining progression during later stages of the illness when language impairment is likely to affect the validity of cognitive testing.

Information for the CDR is collected through semistructured interviews with the AD client and an informant. Decline is based on the difference between the client's present and past level of functioning that can be attributed to cognitive loss alone (i.e., disregarding noncognitive factors such as depression or comorbidity). Based on responses, the clinician assesses impairment in six domains: memory, orientation, judgment/problem solving, personal care, community affairs, and hobbies. Each domain is assigned one of four levels of severity: 0 = no dementia, .5 = very mild or questionable, 2 = moderate dementia, or 3 = severe dementia. Memory is weighted heavily in the scoring. A total score corresponds to one of the four levels of impairment or stages.

The GDS rates cognitive status using seven levels of impairment. It is more clinically descriptive than the CDR and assumes that all domains of cognition decline uniformly throughout the illness. An accompanying scale, the *Brief Cognitive Rating Scale* (BCRS), can be used to assist in rating the client on the GDS (Reisberg & Ferris, 1988).

The *Functional Assessment Staging Scale* (FAST) describes functional losses accompanying AD and also corresponds to the stages of the GDS (Reisberg, 1988). When used in conjunction with the GDS, the BCRS, the FAST, and the BEHAVE (described previously) provide a comprehensive cognitive, functional, and behavioral description of the stages of AD. All three of these instruments can be easily accessed through Internet sites that are listed in the resource section at the back of this book.

ENVIRONMENTAL FACTORS

Environmental factors are particularly important in determining the potential for independence and well-being of the individual with dementing illness. Because cognition is compromised, the demands of the environment may quickly exceed the individual's ability to adapt and function without assistance. These environmental demands can result in varying problems with person–environment fit. When the fit is not good and the environment is not adjusted to demand less or support more, the results can include failed adaptation, unacceptable risks, and/or placement in a more restrictive environment. Social workers, with their specific knowledge and understanding of the importance of the environment to the individual, can be critical in evaluating and intervening at this level.

In considering the fit between the person with dementia and the environment, it is useful to consider how much adaptation the environment requires versus how well the individual is equipped to meet those challenges. Environments that tend to be difficult for the cognitively impaired to manage are characterized by situations or tasks that include high-stimulus situations (i.e., multiple sources of high-level stimuli), novel stimuli (unfamiliar situations that require new learning or behavior), tasks that require high levels of attention, and situations that draw heavily on recent and prospective memory (uncued behavior where one must remember to remember, such as remembering to lock the door).

Familiar, organized, and calm environments are less cognitively demanding, although it is important to remember that sufficient stimulation must be provided to maximize remaining functioning. An unsafe neighborhood may require a higher level of judgment and vigilance than the individual possesses, while a safe neighborhood and supportive neighbors extend the safety net beyond the immediate home and family and allow the individual greater freedom to move independently and socialize for a longer duration of the illness.

Cognitive functioning can also be enhanced by supports that reduce demands on the memory, the most effective of which are techniques that the individual used before the illness. These include the use of memory aides or props, such as lists or automatic reminders, contextual cues, and automatic or ritualized behavior. For instance, many individuals have some sort of "memory center" located in their home, a place where the individual keeps appointments, dates of importance, and notes to remember. This memory hub can be used or enhanced to organize appointments, provide instructions, and keep track of client activities and commitments that occur between visits. It is useful to document the client's prior habits regarding memory techniques since efforts to enhance these existing processes will be more effective than attempting to teach the client new methods.

Caregiver Factors

The caregiver is a particularly important aspect of the care receiver's environment. Indeed, the absence of an in-home caregiver is an important predictor of nursing home placement in cases of dementia (Smith, Kokmen, & O'Brien, 2000). The importance of the caregiver is demonstrated by the extensive research and clinical attention given to the emotional and physical status of this individual.

It is important to determine the stability of the caregiving situation, which may be affected by the physical and mental health of the caregiver, the dyadal relationship, and a myriad of other internal and external stressors. Indeed, unusually high levels of burden, depression, physical morbidity, and disrupted family and work relations among caregivers of the cognitively impaired have been widely reported (Schulz, O'Brien, Bookwala, & Fleissner, 1995; Wu et al., 1999). However, much less is known about the role of caregiver characteristics on outcomes for those with dementia.

Assessment measures are available to monitor the caregiver's perceived burden. These instruments are of some value in screening and monitoring the level of distress, but a clinical interview is more likely to reveal the stresses and resources that are unique to the caregiver (Dougherty & Chamblin, 2004). Interviews provide greater elaboration of the caregiver's *perception* of their situation, which is far more predictive than objective measures of stress and support. Additionally, cultural differences in attitudes toward caregiving, family responsibility, and help seeking are not often reflected in formal assessment methods yet have a great deal of influence on the caregiving situation (Dougherty & Chamblin, 2004; Mintzer, Lebowitz, Olin, Miller, & Payne, 2004).

ADAPTIVE STRENGTHS OF PERSON WITH DEMENTIA

An assessment of the person with dementia should include not only a description of what the individual is unable to do but also strengths that indicate restorative or adaptive potential. The strengths perspective, a focus of much social work intervention, should underlie much of the assessment.

Cognitive status is not the only factor that determines the ability to function successfully, and a good psychosocial history should focus on identifying these potential strengths. Here it is important to note existing strengths in the individual's degree of insight and medical/psychiatric status. High levels of insight into everyday living skills increases the likelihood of adaptive responses and safe behavior, enhances cooperation with care providers, and decreases the burden of caregivers (for reviews, see Clare, Markova, Verhey, & Kenny, 2005; Cotrell, 1997).

Absence of comorbid medical conditions, sensory impairments, physical disability, and complex medication regimens means fewer sources of excess disability to compound the losses that occur with dementia, less dependency on others for management, more flexibility in treatment and environmental opportunities, less stress on an impaired communication system, and fewer drug interactions to potentially worsen functioning and present safety issues.

Persons with dementia respond to their illness with a lifetime of unique experiences, personal skills, and perceptions. Responses, therefore, can be expected to vary. For some individuals, these responses are strengths, or successful adaptations, and for others, the challenges are overwhelming. Although we do not usually think in terms of positive adaptations to progressive dementia, early research indicates that many individuals with AD report good quality of life (Albert et al., 1996), that many individuals think a great deal about their illness and consciously pursue behaviors to stabilize their emotional well-being and life satisfaction, and that these responses vary substantially among individuals (Cotrell & Hooker, 2005).

Although much remains unknown about the psychological processes of persons with dementia, it is still useful for the social worker to interview individuals about their experience of the illness and consider the adaptive possibilities inherent in their behaviors and perspectives.

CONCLUSION

The social work assessment is particularly valuable in identifying the complex needs of the individual with dementia. In addition to an understanding of the need for a multidimensional assessment that includes strengths as well as deficits, the social worker also considers the patient's preferences and the social-cultural context of the illness situation. Most important, the social worker is willing to serve as an advocate when the individual with dementia is not receiving proper medical or supportive care because of ageism, devaluation, lack of appropriate knowledge on the part of the provider, or just lack of time.

It is important to develop a broad knowledge base when working with cognitively frail older adults who often present such complex problem situations. When assessing client needs, social workers should have a systematic approach to collecting relevant data and be knowledgeable about appropriate assessment measures and tools and resources. Without a systematic approach, it is possible to become overwhelmed by the sheer number of competing issues and problems. The information collected should be reduced in ways that will accurately represent the ongoing status of the client and that will be understandable and useful to other professionals in an interdisciplinary setting.

Cognitive, functional, and behavioral assessment instruments are helpful in doing much of this work, but they should be used in conjunction with other methods, such as client and collateral interviews and direct observation. In this way, the strengths and weaknesses of all methods are more balanced, and perspectives that tend to be overly represented, such as medicalization of the individual with dementia or Western views concerning caregiving, are moderated.

REFERENCES

Albert, S., Castillo-Castaneda, C., Sano, M., Jacobs, D., Marder, K., Bell, K., et al. (1996). Quality of life in patients with Alzheimer's disease as reported by patient proxies. *Journal of American Geriatrics Society, 44,* 1342–1347.

Alexopoulos, G. (2004). Late-life mood disorders. In J. Sadavoy, L. Jarvik, G. Grossbergt, & B. Meyers (Eds.), *Comprehensive textbook of geriatric psychiatry* (pp. 609–653). New York: Norton.

Alexopoulos, G., Abrams, R., Young, R., & Shamoian, C. (1988). Use of the Cornell Scale in nondemented patients. *Journal of the American Geriatrics Society, 36,* 230–236.

Alexopoulos, G., Buckwalter, K., Olin, J., Martinez, R., Wainscott, C., & Krishnan, K. (2002). Comorbidity of late-life depression: An opportunity for research in mechanisms and treatment. *Biological Psychiatry, 52,* 543–558.

American Psychiatric Association. (1994). *Diagnostic and statistical manual of mental disorders* (4th ed.). Washington, DC: Author.

American Psychological Association, Presidential Task Force on the Assessment of Age-Consistent Memory Decline and Dementia. (1998). *Guidelines for the evaluation of dementia and age-related cognitive decline.* Washington, DC: American Psychological Association.

Barrett, J., Haley, W., Harrell, L., & Powers, R. (1997). Knowledge about Alzheimer's disease among primary care physicians, psychologists, nurses, and social workers. *Alzheimer Disease and Associated Disorders, 11,* 99–106.

Bigler, E., & Clement, P. (1997). *Diagnostic clinical neuropsychology.* Austin: University of Texas Press.

Boise, L., Neal, M., & Kaye, J. (2004). Dementia assessment in primary care: Results from a study in three managed care systems. *Journal of Gerontology: Medical Sciences, 59A,* 621–626.

Burt, D., Zembar, M., & Niederehe, G. (1995). Depression and memory impairment: A meta analysis of the association, its pattern and specificity. *Psychological Bulletin, 117,* 285–305.

Cacchione, P., Powlishta, K., Grant, E., Buckles, V., & Morris, J. (2003). Accuracy of collateral source reports in very mild to mild dementia of the Alzheimer's type. *Journal of the American Geriatrics Society, 51,* 819–823.

Clare, L., Markova, I., Verhey, F., & Kenny, G. (2005). Awareness in dementia: A review of assessment methods and measures. *Aging and Mental Health, 9,* 394–413.

Clark, C., Sheppard, L., Fillenbaum, G., Galasko, D., Morris, J., Koss, E., et al. (1999). Variability in annual Mini-Mental State Examination score in patients with probable Alzheimer's disease: A clinical perspective of data from the CEARAD. *Archives of Neurology, 56,* 857–862.

Coen, R., Swanwick, G., O'Boyle, C., & Coakley, D. (1997). Behavior disturbance and other predictors of carer burden in Alzheimer's disease. *International Journal of Geriatric Psychiatry, 12,* 331–336.

Cohen-Mansfield, J., & Martin, L. (2004). Assessment of agitation in older adults. In P. Lichtenberg (Ed.), *Handbook of assessment in clinical gerontology* (pp. 297–330). New York: Wiley.

Conn, D. (2004). Other dementias and mental disorders due to general medical conditions. In J. Sadavoy, L. Jarvik, G. Grossbergt, & B. Meyers (Eds.), *Comprehensive textbook of geriatric psychiatry* (pp. 545–578). New York: Norton.

Cotrell, V. (1997) Awareness deficits in Alzheimer's disease: Issues in assessment and intervention. *Journal of Applied Gerontology, 16,* 71–90.

Cotrell, V., & Hooker, K. (2005). Possible selves of individuals with Alzheimer's disease. *Psychology and Aging, 20,* 285–294.

Crum, R., Anthony, J., Bassett, S., & Folstein, M. (1993). Population-based norms for the Mini-Mental State Examination by age and educational level. *Journal of the American Medical Association, 269,* 2386–2391.

Cummings, J. (1997). The neuropsychiatric inventory: Assessing psychopathology in dementia patients. *Neurology, 48,* S10–S16.

Cummings, J., Cherry, D., Kohatsu, N., Kemp, B., Hewett, L., & Mittman, B. (2002). Guidelines for managing Alzheimer's disease: Part I. Assessment. *American Family Physician, 65,* 2263–2272.

Doody, R., Stevens, J., Beck, C., Dubinsky, R., Kaye, J., Gwyther, L., et al. (2001). Practice parameter: Management of dementia (an evidence-based review). Report of the Quality Standards Subcommittee of the American Academy of Neurology. *Neurology, 56,* 1154–1166.

Dougherty, L., & Chamblin, B. (2004). Assessment as an adjunct to psychotherapy. In P. Lichtenberg (Ed.), *Handbook of assessment in clinical gerontology* (pp. 91–110). New York: Wiley.

Folstein, M., Folstein, S., & McHugh, P. (1975). Mini-Mental State: A practical method for grading the cognitive state of patients for the clinician. *Journal of Psychiatric Research, 12,* 189–198.

Froehlich, T., Bogardus, S., & Inouye, S. (2001). Dementia and race: Are there differences between African Americans and Caucasians? *Journal of the American Geriatrics Society, 49,* 477–484.

Galasko, D., Edland, S., Morris, J., Clark, C., Mohs, R., & Koss, E. (1995). The consortium to establish a registry for Alzheimer's disease (CERAD). *Neurology, 45,* 1451–1455.

Jorm, A. (1994). A short form of the IQCODE in the elderly: Development and cross validation. *Psychological Medicine, 24,* 135–153.

Jorm, A. (2004). The IQCODE: A review. *International Psychogeriatrics, 16,* 1–19.

Katz, I. (1998). Diagnosis and treatment of depression in patients with Alzheimer's disease and other dementias. *Journal of Clinical Psychiatry, 59,* 38–44.

Katz, S., Ford, A., Moskowitz, R., Jackson, B., & Jaffe, M. (1963). Studies of illness in the aged. The index of ADL: A standardized measure of biological and psychosocial function. *Journal of the American Medical Association, 185,* 914–919.

Kurlowicz, L., Evans, L., Strumpf, N., & Maislin, G. (2002). A psychometric evaluation of the Cornell Scale for depression in dementia in a frail nursing home population. *American Journal of Geriatric Psychiatry, 10,* 600–608.

Lawton, M., & Brody, E. (1969). Assessment of older people: Self-maintaining and instrumental activities of daily living. *The Gerontologist, 9,* 179–186.

Liptzin, B. (2004). Delirium. In J. Sadavoy, L. Jarvik, G. Grossbergt, & B. Meyers (Eds.), *Comprehensive textbook of geriatric psychiatry* (pp. 525–544). New York: Norton.

McKhann, G., Drachman, D., Folstein, M., Katzman, R., Price, D., & Stadlan, E. (1984). Clinical diagnosis of Alzheimer's disease: Report of the NINCDS-ADRDA Work Group under the auspices of Department of Health and Human Services Task Force on Alzheimer's Disease. *Neurology, 34,* 939–944.

Mintzer, J., Lebowitz, B., Olin, J., Miller, K., & Payne, R. (2004). Family issues in mental disorders of late life. In J. Sadavoy, L. Jarvik, G. Grossbergt, & B. Meyers (Eds.), *Comprehensive textbook of geriatric psychiatry* (pp. 1055–1069). New York: Norton.

Morris, J. C. (1993). The Clinical Dementia Rating (CDR): Current version and scoring rules. *Neurology, 43,* 2412–2414.

Pfeffer, R., Kurosaki, T., Harrah, C., Chance, J., & Filos, S. (1982). Measurement of functional activities in older adults in the community. *Journal of Gerontology, 37,* 323–329.

Purandare, N., Burns, A., Craig, S., Faragher, B., & Scott, K. (2001). Depressive symptoms in patients with Alzheimer's disease. *International Journal of Geriatric Psychiatry, 16,* 960–964.

Read, S. (2004). Vascular dementias. In J. Sadavoy, L. Jarvik, G. Grossbergt, & B. Meyers (Eds.), *Comprehensive textbook of geriatric psychiatry* (pp. 511–524). New York: Norton.

Reisberg, B. (1988). Functional assessment staging (FAST). *Psychopharmacology Bulletin, 24,* 653–659.

Reisberg, B., Borenstein, J., Franssen, E., Salob, S., Steinberg, G., Shulman, E., et al. (1987). BEHAVE-AD: A clinical rating scale for the assessment of pharmacologically remediable behavioral symptomatology in Alzheimer's disease. In H. Altman (Ed.), *Alzheimer's disease: Problems, prospects and perspectives* (pp. 1–16). New York: Plenum.

Reisberg, B., Borenstein, J., Franssen, E., Shulman, E., Steinberg, G., & Ferris, S. (1986). Potentially remediable behavioral symptomatology in Alzheimer's disease. *Hospital Community Psychiatry, 37,* 1199–1201.

Reisberg, B., & Ferris, S. (1988). Brief Cognitive Rating Scale. *Psychopharmacology Bulletin, 24,* 629–636.

Reisberg, B., Ferris, S., de Leon, M., & Crook, T. (1982). The global deterioration scale for assessment of primary degenerative dementia. *American Journal of Psychiatry, 139,* 1136–1139.

Reisberg, B., & Saeed, M. (2004). Alzheimer's disease. In J. Sadavoy, L. Jarvik, G. Grossbergt, & B. Meyers (Eds.), *Comprehensive textbook of geriatric psychiatry* (pp. 449–509). New York: Norton.

Sadavoy, J. (2004). *Psychotropic drugs and the elderly: Fast facts.* New York: Norton.

Schulz, R., O'Brien, A., Bookwala, J., & Fleissner, K. (1995). Psychiatric and physical morbidity effects of dementia caregiving: Prevalence, correlates, and causes. *The Gerontologist, 35,* 771–791.

Shiekh, J., & Yesavage, J. (1986). Geriatric Depression Scale: Recent findings in the development of a shorter version. In J. Brink (Ed.), *Clinical gerontology: A guide to assessment and intervention.* New York: Haworth.

Smith, C., & van Gorp, W. (2004). Neuropsychological testing of the older adult. In J. Sadavoy, L. Jarvik, G. Grossbergt, & B. Meyers (Eds.), *Comprehensive textbook of geriatric psychiatry* (pp. 371–390). New York: Norton.

Smith, G., Kokmen, E., & O'Brien, P. (2000). Risk factors for nursing home placement in a population-based dementia cohort. *Journal of the American Geriatrics Society, 48,* 519–525.

Speck, C., Kukull, W., Brenner, D., Bowen, J., McCormick, W., Teri, L., et al. (1995). History of depression as a risk factor for Alzheimer's disease. *Epidemiology, 6,* 366–369.

Steffens, D., Plassman, B., Helms, M., Welsh-Bohmer, K., Saunders, A., & Breitner, J. (1997). A twin study of late-onset depression and apolipoprotein E epsilon 4 as risk factors for Alzheimer's disease. *Biological Psychiatry, 41,* 851–856.

Tabert, M., Albert, S., Borukhova-Milov, L., Camacho, Y., Pelton, G., Liu, X., et al. (2002). Functional deficits in patients with mild cognitive impairment. *Neurology, 58,* 758–764.

Van Gorp, W., Marcotte, T., Sultzer, D., Hinkin, C., Mahler, M., & Cummings, J. (1999). Screening for dementia: Comparison of three commonly used instruments. *Journal of Clinical and Experimental Neuropsychology, 21,* 29–38.

Wragg, R., & Jeste, D. (1989). Overview of depression and psychosis in Alzheimer's disease. *American Journal of Psychiatry, 146,* 577–587.

Wu, H., Wang, J., Cacioppo, J., Glaser, R., Kiecolt-Glaser, J., & Malarkey, W. (1999). Chronic stress associated with spousal caregiving of patients with Alzheimer's dementia is associated with down regulation of B-lymphocyte GH mRNA. *Journal of Gerontology: Medical Science, 54,* 212–215.

CHAPTER FOUR

Social Work and Dementia: Implications of Coexisting Medical Conditions

Katie Maslow

INTRODUCTION

Most people with Alzheimer's disease and other dementias also have other serious medical conditions, such as congestive heart failure, diabetes, chronic obstructive pulmonary disease, and osteoarthritis. This is not surprising since dementia usually occurs in old age when these other medical conditions are common. Yet information for health care and social service professionals about dementia care usually does not address coexisting medical conditions or the implications of these other conditions for the care of people with dementia.

Coexisting medical conditions in people with dementia have important implications for where social workers are likely to encounter these people. Because people with dementia receive medical care for their coexisting conditions, social workers are just as likely to encounter them in health care settings, such as hospitals, emergency rooms, medical clinics, and rehabilitation facilities, as in the residential and community care settings where dementia is more generally expected.

Coexisting medical conditions also have important implications for many aspects of social work practice with people with dementia and their families. The combination of dementia and other medical conditions complicates social work assessment, problem identification, care planning, and care coordination. Assessment is more difficult when the person's cognitive, emotional, and physical functioning are affected simultaneously by dementia and coexisting medical conditions. Identifying the person's and family's most pressing problems, selecting the most appropriate services, and coordinating needed health care and social services are also more difficult in this situation. Even so, the person and family are confronting problems caused by the combination of dementia and other medical conditions. If social workers focus only on the person's dementia or only on his or her other medical conditions, they are likely to miss major issues and provide help that does not meet the needs of the person and family.

This chapter provides information about the prevalence of coexisting medical conditions in people with dementia and the impact of those conditions on their use of health care services. It describes the effect of coexisting medical conditions on the burden of caregiving for families and other informal caregivers, and it discusses the implications of coexisting medical conditions for social work practice in health care, residential care, and community settings.

HOW PREVALENT ARE COEXISTING MEDICAL CONDITIONS IN PEOPLE WITH DEMENTIA?

Until recently, credible information about the proportion of people with dementia who have serious coexisting medical conditions was not available. Most people with dementia do not have a formal dementia diagnosis, and researchers have had difficulty identifying people with dementia in samples large enough to be considered representative of the population. Some researchers and clinicians have assumed that people with dementia are healthier than other people of the same age, and one study conducted in a geriatric community health center supported that assumption for the center's patients with Alzheimer's disease (Wolf-Klein et al., 1988).

Now, information about the prevalence of coexisting medical conditions in people with dementia is available from many studies conducted in samples that represent at least large segments of the population. One study used data from 1999 Medicare claims for a national random sample of 1.2 million fee-for-service Medicare beneficiaries age 65 and over (Bynum et al., 2004). The study found that 8% of the beneficiaries had dementia, and substantial proportions of these beneficiaries also had various coexisting medical conditions (see Table 4.1). Since the proportions in Table 4.1 add up to 266%, it is clear that many people with dementia in this sample had more than one of the listed conditions.

TABLE 4.1   Proportion of Medicare Beneficiaries Age 65 and Older With Alzheimer's Disease and Other Dementias and Specified Coexisting Medical Conditions, 1999 (N = 103,512)

Coexisting Medical Condition	Percentage With Condition
Hypertension	60
Coronary artery disease	30
Congestive heart failure	28
Osteoarthritis	26
Diabetes	21
Peripheral vascular disease	19
Depression	18
Chronic obstructive pulmonary disease	17
Thyroid disease	16
Cancer	11
Osteoporosis	10
Late effects of stroke	10
Parkinson's disease	7

Source: Bynum et al. (2004).

Comparable information from Medicare claims for fee-for-service beneficiaries age 65 and over in 2000 shows that 9% of beneficiaries age 65 and over had dementia (Alzheimer's Association, 2003). Substantial proportions of these beneficiaries also had serious coexisting medical conditions, including coronary artery disease (29%), congestive heart failure (28%), diabetes (23%), and chronic obstructive pulmonary disease (17%). Only 5% of the beneficiaries with dementia had no coexisting medical conditions, and many beneficiaries had more than one of the conditions.

Findings from research in Medicare managed care are similar. A study of almost 4,000 Medicare managed care enrollees age 65 and over with dementia found that serious coexisting medical conditions were common: 39% of the enrollees with dementia also had cerebrovascular disease, 29% had congestive heart failure, 25% had chronic obstructive pulmonary disease, 22% had diabetes, 16% had peripheral vascular disease, 13% had myocardial infarction (heart attack), and 12% had cancer (Hill et al., 2002).

Three other studies had similar findings:

- A study of 5,300 fee-for-service Medicare beneficiaries with dementia, average age 78, found that 30% also had hypertension, 20% had coronary artery disease, and 11% to 15% had diabetes, congestive heart failure, chronic obstructive pulmonary disease, stroke, osteoarthritis, peripheral vascular disease, and/ or cancer (Newcomer, Clay, Luxenberg, & Miller, 1999).

- A study of 680 people with dementia from one large Medicare managed care organization, age 60 and over, found that 37% also had cardiovascular disease, 18% had congestive heart failure, and 13% to 15% had chronic obstructive pulmonary disease, diabetes, and/or cancer (Gutterman, Markowitz, Lewis, & Fillit, 1999).
- A study of 107 people with dementia from a clinic sample in Indianapolis, average age 76, found that 82% also had hypertension, 41% had osteoarthritis, 39% had diabetes, 21% had coronary artery disease, and 8% to 14% had congestive heart failure, chronic obstructive pulmonary disease, renal failure, stroke, and/or cancer (Schubert et al., 2006).

The findings from these studies differ somewhat, depending on the particular medical conditions that were asked about and characteristics of each sample, such as the average age of sample members, their stage of dementia, and whether nursing home residents were included. One study found, for example, that the prevalence of coexisting medical conditions was generally higher in the later stages of dementia (Doraiswamy, Leon, Cummings, Marin, & Neumann, 2002).

Two studies compared the prevalence of coexisting medical conditions in elderly people with Alzheimer's disease versus vascular dementia (Eaker, Mickel, Chyou, Mueller-Rizner, & Slusser, 2002; Hill, Fillit, Shah, del Valle, & Futterman, 2005). As would be expected, these studies found that people with vascular dementia were more likely than people with Alzheimer's disease to have cardiovascular conditions, such as hypertension, congestive heart failure, stroke, and peripheral vascular disease, but there was no difference between the two groups in the prevalence of other medical conditions, such as osteoarthritis, chronic obstructive pulmonary disease, and cancer. In addition, even though people with vascular dementia were more likely than people with Alzheimer's disease to have coexisting cardiovascular conditions, substantial proportions of the people with Alzheimer's disease had these conditions. Eaker et al. (2002) found, for example, that 52% of people with Alzheimer's disease had hypertension, 14% had congestive heart failure, and 14% had stroke.

Despite differences among all these studies, their main findings support two important conclusions:

1. Coexisting medical conditions are common in elderly people with dementia.
2. Many elderly people with dementia have more than one serious coexisting medical condition.

TABLE 4.2   Proportion of People Age 55 to 64 With Disabling Cognitive Impairment and Specified Coexisting Medical Conditions, 2000 (N = 157)

Coexisting Medical Condition	Percentage With Condition
Hypertension	64
Arthritis	55
Heart disease	34
Diabetes	28
Stroke	24
Lung disease	11
Cancer	8

Source: Alzheimer's Association (2006).

Some of the studies described here include people under age 65 with dementia, but their findings are not reported separately for younger versus older people with dementia. A recent analysis of data from the Health and Retirement Study, which includes a nationally representative sample of Americans age 55 to 64, shows that surprisingly large proportions of people with cognitive impairment in that age-group also had serious coexisting medical conditions (Alzheimer's Association, 2006) (see Table 4.2). It is not possible to determine from the survey how many of these people had dementia, but it is likely that many did. Thus, the prevalence of coexisting medical conditions is substantial even in nonelderly people with dementia.

HOW DO COEXISTING MEDICAL CONDITIONS AFFECT THE USE OF HEALTH CARE SERVICES FOR PEOPLE WITH DEMENTIA?

People who have dementia but do not have a particular coexisting medical condition generally use fewer health care services than people who have dementia plus the coexisting medical condition. Figures 4.1a to 4.1c illustrate this relationship for dementia and diabetes in a sample of 1.2 million fee-for-service Medicare beneficiaries age 65 and over.

As shown in Figure 4.1a, beneficiaries with dementia averaged 1,091 hospital stays per 1,000 persons, whereas beneficiaries with dementia plus diabetes averaged 1,589 hospital stays per 1,000 persons. Thus, coexisting diabetes increased the use of hospital care for beneficiaries with dementia. Importantly, this relationship goes both ways. Figure 4.1a also shows that beneficiaries with diabetes but no dementia averaged 587 hospital stays

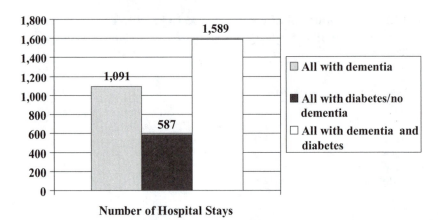

Number of Hospital Stays

FIGURE 4.1a   Average hospital stays per 1,000 Medicare beneficiaries age 65 and older, by dementia, diabetes, and both, 2000.

per 1,000 persons, and beneficiaries with diabetes plus dementia averaged 1,589 hospital stays per 1,000 persons. Thus, dementia also increased the use of hospital care for beneficiaries with diabetes.

Figures 4.1b and 4.1c show the relationship between dementia and diabetes as it affects average number of physician visits and the cost of Medicare home health care. Beneficiaries with dementia had an average of 14.5 physician visits in 2000, beneficiaries with diabetes but no dementia had an average of 15.7 physician visits, and beneficiaries with dementia and diabetes had an average of 17.3 physician visits. Likewise, beneficiaries with

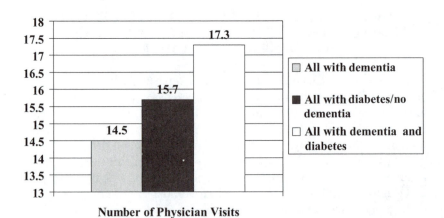

Number of Physician Visits

FIGURE 4.1b   Average physician visits for Medicare beneficiaries age 65 and older, by dementia, diabetes, and both, 2000.

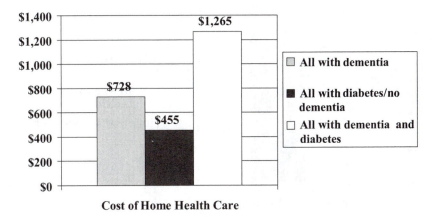

Cost of Home Health Care

FIGURE 4.1c   Average home health care costs per person for Medicare beneficiaries age 65 and older, by dementia, diabetes, and both, 2000.

dementia had average costs for Medicare home health care of $728 in 2000, beneficiaries with diabetes but no dementia had average costs for Medicare home health care of $455, and beneficiaries with dementia and diabetes had average costs for Medicare home health care of more than $1,265.

Figures 4.2a to 4.2c show the relationship of dementia and congestive heart failure in the same sample of 1.2 million fee-for-service Medicare beneficiaries age 65 and over. The combination of dementia and congestive heart failure resulted in more hospital stays and physician visits and higher Medicare home health care costs than either dementia or congestive

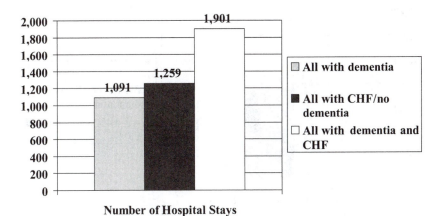

Number of Hospital Stays

FIGURE 4.2a   Average hospital stays per 1,000 Medicare beneficiaries age 65 and older, by dementia, congestive heart failure (CHF), and both, 2000.

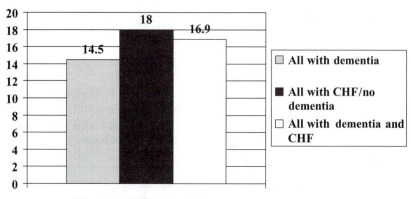

Number of Physician Visits

FIGURE 4.2b   Average physician visits for Medicare beneficiaries age 65 and older, by dementia, congestive heart failure (CHF), and both, 2000.

heart failure without the other. As is true for dementia and diabetes, the difference with respect to number of physician visits is much smaller than the differences with respect to hospital stays and Medicare home health care costs, but it is in the same direction. Many other studies also show that the combination of dementia and particular coexisting medical conditions greatly increases the use of health care services (Eaker et al., 2002; Gutterman et al., 1999; Hill et al., 2002, 2005; Newcomer et al., 1999).

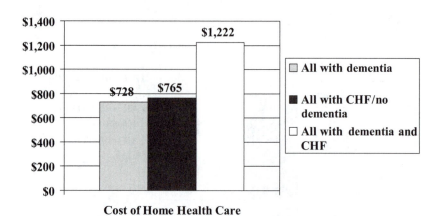

Cost of Home Health Care

FIGURE 4.2c   Average home health care costs for Medicare beneficiaries age 65 and older, by dementia, congestive heart failure (CHF), and both, 2000.

The study noted earlier of 1999 Medicare claims for a national random sample of 1.2 million fee-for-service Medicare beneficiaries age 65 and over found that beneficiaries with dementia and coexisting medical conditions were 2.4 times more likely than beneficiaries with the coexisting medical conditions but no dementia to have a "preventable hospitalization" (Bynum et al., 2004). A "preventable hospitalization" is defined as a hospital stay that could be prevented altogether or the course of which could be mitigated by optimum outpatient medical management. The amount of increase in preventable hospitalizations varied, depending on the particular coexisting medical condition. Beneficiaries with congestive heart failure and dementia were 1.7 times more likely than beneficiaries with congestive heart failure and no dementia to have a "preventable hospitalization." Beneficiaries with diabetes and dementia were 3.5 times more likely than beneficiaries with diabetes and no dementia to have a "preventable hospitalization."

No research is available to explain why the combination of dementia and coexisting medical conditions increases the use of health care services, but it is easy to imagine at least three possible reasons:

1. Dementia complicates the treatment of coexisting medical conditions.
2. Some medical conditions, especially cardiovascular conditions, cause dementia.
3. Many medical conditions and treatments for the conditions increase cognitive impairment, at least temporarily, even if they do not worsen the person's underlying dementia.

One example of the way dementia complicates the treatment of coexisting medical conditions is a case reported in the *Journal of the American Medical Association* (Brauner, Muir, & Sachs, 2000). A woman in her 80s had mild dementia and osteoporosis. Her doctor prescribed a new medication for the osteoporosis and told her and the family members she lived with that she should always take the medication with water and stay upright after taking it. Four weeks later, the woman was brought into the emergency room with symptoms of esophageal rupture secondary to ulceration, which was probably caused by her failure to take the medication as instructed. Despite treatment, she died when the ulcer eroded into a major blood vessel.

A growing body of research supports the second reason; that is, some medical conditions can cause dementia. Hypertension, heart disease, stroke, and diabetes are now known to be risk factors for vascular dementia, and the same conditions are increasingly recognized as risk factors for Alzheimer's disease (Arvanitakis, Wilson, Bienas, Evans, & Bennett, 2004; Breteler, 2000; Honig et al., 2003; Luchsinger, Tang,

Stern, Shea, & Mayeux, 2001; Luchsinger et al., 2005; Nyenhuis & Gorelick, 1998).

With respect the third reason, it is widely recognized that many acute and chronic medical conditions, including infections, fever, dehydration, and thyroid, kidney, and liver disease, can cause at least temporary cognitive impairment. Similarly, medications that are widely used to treat acute and chronic medical conditions can cause cognitive impairment: examples include antiarythmics, antihistamines, antibiotics, antidepressants, antihypertensives, and sedatives. Major surgery and general anesthesia can also cause at least temporary cognitive impairment (American Medical Association, 1999; Lyketsos et al., 2006).

Although the cognitive impairment caused by factors, such as acute and chronic medical conditions, medications, surgery, and anesthesia, does not necessarily worsen a person's underlying dementia, it certainly adds to the difficulty of managing the person's care. Moreover, acute cognitive impairment caused by these factors (usually referred to as delirium) is much more likely to occur in elderly people with underlying dementia than in other elderly people (Fick, Agostini, & Inouye, 2002; Inouye, 2006).

IMPACT OF COEXISTING MEDICAL CONDITIONS ON FAMILIES AND OTHER INFORMAL CAREGIVERS OF PEOPLE WITH DEMENTIA

Families and other informal caregivers of people with dementia and coexisting medical conditions have to manage both the dementia and the coexisting medical conditions. One study found that families of people with Alzheimer's disease and coexisting medical conditions were much more likely than families of people with Alzheimer's disease and no coexisting medical conditions to be providing informal care (Zhu et al., 2006). Each additional coexisting medical condition increased the likelihood that the family would be providing informal care by 62%.

The challenges faced by families and other informal caregivers of people with dementia and coexisting medical conditions are described poignantly in an article by Mary Naylor and her colleagues (Naylor, Stephens, Bowles, & Bixby, 2005). The article reports on interviews with five people with dementia, age 78 to 84, and their informal caregivers. The interviews were conducted in the 6 weeks after the people with dementia were hospitalized for cardiovascular and other serious medical conditions. The article describes the caregivers' intense concern and anxiety about the person's medical condition and many aspects of his or her care, including how to arrange for needed medical equipment, transportation, and home health care; how to obtain needed information from the person's physician(s) and other health care providers; and how to get the person with dementia to take medications and adhere to dietary restrictions and other prescribed treatments for his or her coexisting medical conditions.

The posthospital period is often difficult for families and other informal caregivers of people who do not have dementia (DesRoches, Blendon, Young, Scoles, & Kim, 2002). Dementia adds to that difficulty because the person often does not understand or cannot remember the reasons why he or she must use oxygen or other medical equipment, adhere to dietary and exercise requirements, or limit movement following hip or other surgery. The person is unlikely to be able to help with arranging medical appointments and other needed care and may not be able to recognize or report important symptoms. As a result, families and other informal caregivers of people with dementia probably experience more burden and stress in the posthospital period than families and informal caregivers of people who do not have dementia.

Even without hospitalization, the ongoing, day-to-day burden and stress associated with caregiving for a person with dementia is probably greater if the person also has coexisting medical conditions. Helping with and monitoring medications is a good example. People who take multiple medications often have difficulty remembering to take them as instructed, that is, at the right time, in the right dose, and with whatever other precautions are required. Family caregivers of older people who do not have dementia report many kinds of "hassles" associated with helping the person with medications (Travis, Bernard, McAuley, Thorton, & Kole, 2003). Dementia compounds medication-related hassles because a person with dementia is much more likely to have difficulty remembering the medication schedule, doses, and other precautions. The person with dementia is also more likely to take too little or too much of prescribed medications and then to be unable to tell the family caregiver what he or she has taken. Even mild dementia can affect a person's ability to take medications correctly (Insel, Morrow, Brewer, & Figueredo, 2006).

Families report that part of the difficulty of providing care for a person with dementia is the need for constant vigilance (Mahoney, 2003). Many families say they are always "on duty," especially in health care situations. They feel they must be present during all medical visits to provide information the person with dementia cannot remember or report, hear and remember treatment instructions, and make sure the person receives appropriate care. Families are anxious about whether they will recognize important medical symptoms, including adverse reactions to medications that may or may not have been taken as prescribed. All these feelings add to the difficulty of providing care for a person with dementia and increase families' feelings of being overwhelmed.

A demonstration project conducted in Veterans Administration medical centers in upstate New York found that families of veterans with dementia and coexisting medical conditions benefited less than families of veterans with dementia but no coexisting medical conditions from the extra information and support provided through the project (Maslow et al., 2005). This difference is understandable given the difficulty and high levels of stress and burden associated with managing care for a person with dementia and coexisting medical conditions. These families need more and perhaps different kinds of help.

IMPLICATIONS FOR SOCIAL WORKERS

As noted at the beginning of this chapter, coexisting medical conditions in people with dementia have important implications for many aspects of social work practice with these people. Five general implications are relevant in all settings where social workers see older people, their families, and other caregivers:

1. Social workers should be aware that many people with dementia also have serious coexisting medical conditions and, conversely, that older people with serious medical conditions may also have dementia.
2. Social work assessments should include both dementia and coexisting medical conditions, and social workers should consider both when prioritizing the problems facing the person and family.
3. Social work care plans for people with dementia and coexisting medical conditions should include interventions and services that take into account the relationship between the dementia and coexisting conditions, that is, interventions and services for the person's dementia that are appropriate given the person's coexisting medical conditions and, conversely, interventions and services for the coexisting medical conditions that are appropriate given the person's dementia.
4. Social workers should help people with dementia and coexisting medical conditions and their families and other caregivers navigate the often complex health care and social service systems that provide needed services for the person.
5. Social workers should help coordinate the medical and nonmedical care needed by people with dementia and coexisting medical conditions. In particular, they should make sure that important information about both the dementia and the coexisting medical

conditions goes with the person as he or she transitions between health care, residential care, and community care settings.

In addition to these implications for social work practice, all health care and social service professionals, including social workers, should be aware of the growing body of research showing that cardiovascular conditions and diabetes are risk factors for dementia. They should encourage concerted medical management of these conditions to avoid or delay worsening of the person's underlying dementia (Boksay, Reisberg, Torossian, Boksay, & Krishnamurthy, 2005; Lyketsos et al., 2006).

The following sections note some specific implications of dementia and coexisting medical conditions for social work practice in health care, residential care, and community settings. Social workers in each setting will undoubtedly think of additional and more detailed implications for their practice.

Implications for Social Workers in Health Care Settings

As described earlier, coexisting medical conditions in people with dementia mean that social workers are likely to encounter these people in virtually all health care settings. On average, 25% of elderly hospital patients have dementia (Maslow, 2006). Data are not available on the proportion of elderly patients with dementia in other health care settings (e.g., emergency rooms and medical clinics), but these proportions are undoubtedly substantial.

Dementia is frequently not recognized in elderly patients who come into hospitals, emergency rooms, medical clinics, and rehabilitation settings for treatment of their coexisting medical conditions. Thus, an important first step for social workers in these settings is recognition of possible dementia.

Findings from Medicare claims data may be useful in this context as a reminder to social workers and others of the prevalence of dementia in older people with particular medical conditions. Relevant data show, for example, that in 2000, 17% of the Medicare beneficiaries age 65 and older had diabetes; of these beneficiaries, 12% also had dementia, with the proportion increasing from 5% of beneficiaries age 65 to 74 to almost one-third of beneficiaries age 85 and older (Alzheimer's Association, 2003). Likewise, 12% of Medicare beneficiaries age 65 and older had congestive heart failure, and 21% of these beneficiaries also had dementia, with the proportion increasing from 10% of those age 65 to 74 to more than one-third of those age 85 and older. Social workers should expect to see dementia in similar proportions of elderly patients with other serious medical conditions.

Social workers in health care settings should be aware of the signs and symptoms of possible dementia. They should ask families and other caregivers of older patients who may have dementia but do not have a dementia diagnosis in their medical record whether the person has ever received such a diagnosis and, if not, whether the caregiver has noticed a significant decline in the person's cognitive functioning that might indicate dementia. Social workers should communicate relevant findings to others who are providing medical care for the person, and they should document the findings in the person's medical record. They should also encourage the establishment of routine procedures for recognition of possible dementia in all health care settings (see, e.g., Mezey & Maslow, 2004).

Social workers should be aware and remind others of the many ways that dementia can complicate treatment of a person's medical conditions. In all health care settings, dementia interferes with the person's ability to report symptoms, provide an accurate medical history, and make treatment decisions. In hospitals and emergency rooms, dementia increases the risk of patient wandering, delirium, inadequate food and fluid intake, falls, and physical restraints (Inouye, 2006; McKay, Farrell, Ennis, & Binstadt, 2006; Michelson, 2006). As noted earlier, many medications and other treatments that are commonly used to treat acute and chronic medical conditions can cause at least temporary cognitive impairment and worsen cognitive functioning in people with dementia, thus further reducing the person's ability to understand and remember treatment recommendations and adding to the difficulties caregivers face in getting the person to comply with the recommendations. Awareness of these issues can help all staff members in health care settings plan for and avoid problems that can result in negative health outcomes.

Most people with dementia have family members or friends who can provide needed information and help with treatment decisions and ongoing care. Social workers in health care settings should contact and involve these people. Clearly, involvement of family members is an important component of social work practice with many kinds of clients and in many settings. It is critical for people with dementia. Yet families and friends are not always contacted and encouraged to be involved, and they may not be routinely identified in some health care settings.

Some people with dementia do not have family members or friends. Social workers in health care settings should be aware and make other staff members aware of this situation and the increased risks it creates for the person's health and safety. Drebing and Harden (2006) describe two client situations that illustrate these risks. One man with dementia who lived alone showed a visitor a drawer full of empty medication containers for prescriptions that had been filled only 2 days earlier; he could not remember what happened to the medication. Another man with dementia who lived alone was told in the hospital that he should use a moisturizer for the psoriasis on his legs; he did not remember the recommendation accurately and put kerosene on his legs because he believed his doctors told him to do so.

In part because of concerns about health-related risks like these, people with dementia who live alone are more likely than those who live with a family caregiver to be placed in a nursing home after hospitalization (Mahoney, Eisner, Havighurst, Gray, & Palta, 2000). Drebing and Harding (2006) describe an exciting project that attempted to avoid such placements by creating a support system in the community for individuals with dementia who live alone. The project required a substantial commitment of time and resources that, unfortunately, may be beyond current capacities in many communities. Even so, by being aware of and informing other staff members about the person's situation, social workers in health care settings may be able to help devise ways to maintain the person's health at home and avoid unnecessary nursing home placements.

Implications for Social Workers in Residential Care Settings

At least half of all elderly residents of nursing homes and assisted living facilities have dementia (American Health Care Association, 2006; Centers for Medicare and Medicaid Services, 2005; Rosenblatt et al., 2004; Sloane, Zimmerman, & Ory, 2001). Dementia and coexisting medical conditions are probably more likely to be recognized and documented in nursing homes than in assisted living or other residential care facilities. Social workers in all residential care settings should be sure that both dementia and coexisting medical conditions are identified and documented in resident records.

Even if the conditions are documented in resident records, however, staff members who work directly with residents in these facilities may not have access to the information or understand its importance. Social workers can help to communicate relevant information about dementia and coexisting medical conditions to direct care staff. Social workers can also help to train direct care staff, for example, to notice and report changes in a resident's physical condition even if the resident is not aware of the changes because of his or her cognitive impairment. Likewise, social workers can help train direct care staff to notice and report changes in residents' cognitive functioning that may indicate either worsening dementia or an acute physical health problem that is causing temporary confusion.

Residential care facilities differ in their capacity to provide care for people with various conditions, and some facilities are not able to manage a resident with dementia and serious coexisting medical conditions. Social workers who participate in admission decisions can help administrators, on the one hand, and families, on the other hand, to decide whether a given individual with dementia and other medical conditions is appropriate for a particular residential care facility.

Transfers of residents with dementia and coexisting medical conditions to a hospital or emergency room are risky if the resident is sent alone, without a staff or family member (Hyde, 2006; Michelson, 2006). Yet many residential care facilities cannot spare a staff member to accompany the resident. If the resident has a family member or friend in the community, the social worker can help by talking with that person ahead of time about the probability that the resident will sometime have to be transferred to the hospital or emergency room for treatment of his or her medical conditions and the importance of having a plan about who will accompany the resident if such a transfer is needed. Social workers can also facilitate transfers back to the residential care facility, in particular by helping to ensure that necessary information about the person's hospital stay or emergency room visit is received promptly by the facility and conveyed to staff members who work directly with the resident.

Finally, federal legislation enacted in early 2006 creates financial incentives through the "Money Follows the Person" program for states to discharge Medicaid-funded nursing home residents to less restrictive settings, including other residential care facilities and home. Social workers in nursing homes can help determine which residents can be safely discharged and what services they will need in the other residential care facility or at home. Although a resident's coexisting medical conditions may be manageable in the other setting, his or her dementia may not and vice versa. The resident's needs related to both his or her dementia and coexisting medical conditions must be addressed if the discharge is to be safe and beneficial for the person.

Implications for Social Workers in Community Settings

At any one time, about 70% of people with dementia are living at home, with or without an informal caregiver. Many of these people receive home and community-based care from agencies that employ social workers. One-quarter of people of all ages who receive Medicare or Medicaid-funded home health care have moderate to severe cognitive impairment consistent with dementia (U.S. Department of Health and Human Services, 2004). At least half of elderly adult day care participants have dementia (Partners in Caregiving, 2002). National data are not available on the proportion of people with dementia among those who receive services through state home and community-based waiver programs, but data from Michigan and Florida show that 37% of people who received home care services through those states' waiver programs had cognitive impairment consistent with dementia (Hirdes et al., 2004; Mitchell, Salmon, Polivka, & Soberon-Ferrer, 2006). Social workers in all these community settings will encounter people with dementia and coexisting medical conditions. Geriatric case managers and social workers in senior centers and other community organizations that serve older people will also encounter people with dementia and coexisting medical conditions.

Dementia may not be recognized in community-dwelling people. Even if dementia is recognized, the relationship between a person's dementia, the person's other serious medical conditions, and the consequent difficulty of managing his or her care may not be understood. Social workers in community settings should be aware of the likelihood of dementia and coexisting medical conditions, include both in their client assessments, and create care plans that account for both.

If the person with dementia and coexisting medical conditions has a family or other informal caregiver, social workers should be aware of the likely impact of the coexisting conditions on the caregiver's feelings of stress and burden. Interventions and services should be provided to support the caregiver and reduce stress and burden. If the person with dementia and coexisting medical conditions is alone, social workers should attempt to devise a community support system that can help reduce risks to the person's health and safety, on the one hand, and avoid premature nursing home placement on the other hand.

As described earlier, people with dementia and coexisting medical conditions are much more likely than people with the coexisting medical conditions but no dementia to have "preventable hospitalizations," that is, hospitalizations that could be prevented altogether or whose course could be mitigated by optimum outpatient medical management. The reasons for these preventable hospitalizations are not known, but one factor is undoubtedly the difficulty of managing coexisting medical conditions in a person with dementia. Social workers in community settings can help by making sure the person's physician(s) and other health care providers are aware of the person's dementia and its impact on the person's ability to provide accurate information about his or her medical history, report symptoms, and understand and comply with treatment recommendations.

Finally, social workers in community settings should make sure that relevant information about the person's dementia and coexisting medical conditions goes with the person when he or she is sent to the hospital or emergency room. Availability of this information can help hospital and emergency room staff understand the person's situation more rapidly, diagnose his or her medical problems more accurately, and avoid unnecessary medical tests. Up-to-date information about how to contact family and other informal caregivers should also be sent with the person so that hospital and emergency room staff can reach these caregivers quickly to involve them in treatment decisions and discharge planning.

CONCLUSION

Social workers will encounter people with dementia and coexisting medical conditions in many practice settings. By being aware of the impact of dementia on treatment of other medical conditions and, conversely, the impact of other medical conditions on dementia, social workers can help ensure the best possible care and outcomes for these people and reduce the often overwhelming stress and burden experienced by their families and other informal caregivers. To achieve these objectives, social workers in all settings should include both dementia and coexisting medical conditions in their assessments, consider both when prioritizing the problems facing the person and his or her caregivers, and select interventions and services that address those problems. Coexisting medical conditions complicate social work practice with people with dementia, but focusing only on the dementia or only on the other medical conditions ignores the reality of the person's situation and results in less appropriate care and less-than-optimal outcomes.

REFERENCES

Alzheimer's Association. (2003). *Alzheimer's Disease and Chronic Health Conditions: The Real Challenge for 21st Century Medicare.* Available at http://www.alz.org

Alzheimer's Association. (2006, June). *Early Onset Dementia: A National Challenge, a Future Crisis.* Available at http://www.alz.org

American Health Care Association. (2006). USDHHS Nursing Home data for June 2006. Available at http://www.ahca.org/research/oscar/rpt_MC_mental_status_200606.pdf

American Medical Association. (1999). *Diagnosis, management, and treatment of dementia.* Chicago: Author.

Arvanitakis, Z., Wilson, R. S., Bienas, J. L., Evans, D. A., & Bennett, D. A. (2004). Diabetes mellitus and risk of Alzheimer's disease and decline in cognitive function. *Archives of Neurology, 61,* 661–666.

Boksay, I., Reisberg, B., Torossian, C., Boksay, E., & Krishnamurthy, M. (2005). Alzheimer's disease and medical disease condition: A prospective cohort study [Letter to the editor]. *Journal of the American Geriatrics Society, 53,* 2235–2236.

Brauner, D. J., Muir, J. C., & Sachs, G. A. (2000). Treating nondementia illness in patients with dementia. *Journal of the American Medical Association, 283,* 3230–3235.

Breteler, M. M. (2000). Vascular risk factors for Alzheimer's disease: An epidemiologic perspective. *Neurobiology of Aging, 21,* 153–160.

Bynum, J. P. W., Rabins, P. V., Weller, W., Niefeld, M., Anderson, G. F., & Wu, A. W. (2004). The relationship between a dementia diagnosis, chronic illness, Medicare expenditures, and hospital use. *Journal of the American Geriatrics Society, 52,* 187–194.

Centers for Medicare and Medicaid Services. (2005). *Nursing Home Data Compendium: 2005 Edition.* Available at http://www.cms.hhs.gov/apps/files/NHDataComp2005.zip

DesRoches, C., Blendon, R., Young, J., Scoles, K., & Kim, M. (2002). Caregiving in the post-hospitalization period: Findings from a national survey. *Nursing Economics, 20,* 216–221.

Doraiswamy, P. M., Leon, J., Cummings, J. L., Marin, D., & Neumann, P. J. (2002). Prevalence and impact of medical comorbidity in Alzheimer's disease. *Journal of Gerontology: Medical Sciences, 57A,* M173–M177.

Drebing, C. E., & Harden, T. (2006). The inpatient experience from the perspective of the isolated adult with Alzheimer's disease. In N. M. Silverstein & K. Maslow (Eds.), *Improving hospital care for persons with dementia* (pp. 99–115). New York: Springer.

Eaker, E. D., Mickel, S. F., Chyou, P-H., Mueller-Rizner, N. J., & Slusser, J. P. (2002). Alzheimer's disease or other dementia and medical care utilization. *Annals of Epidemiology, 12,* 39–45.

Fick, D. M., Agostini, J. V., & Inouye, S. K. (2002). Delirium superimposed on dementia: A systematic review. *Journal of the American Geriatrics Society, 50,* 1723–1732.

Gutterman, E. M., Markowitz, J. S., Lewis, B., & Fillit, H. (1999). Cost of Alzheimer's disease and related dementia in managed-Medicare. *Journal of the American Geriatrics Society, 47,* 1065–1071.

Hill, J., Fillit, H., Shah, S. N., del Valle, M. C., & Futterman, R. (2005). Patterns of healthcare utilization and costs for vascular dementia in a community-dwelling population. *Journal of Alzheimer's Disease, 8,* 43–50.

Hill, J. W., Futterman, R., Duttagupta, S., Mastey, V., Lloyd, J. R., & Fillit, H. (2002). Alzheimer's disease and related dementias increase costs of comorbidities in managed Medicare. *Neurology, 58,* 62–70.

Hirdes, J. P., Fries, B. E., Morris, J. N., Ikegami, N., Zimmerman, D., Dalby, D. M., et al. (2004). Home care quality indicators (HCQIs) based on the MDS-HC. *Gerontologist, 44,* 665–679.

Honig, L. S., Tang, M. X., Albert, S., Costa, R., Luchsinger, J., Manly, J., et al. (2003). Stroke and the risk of Alzheimer's disease. *Archives of Neurology, 60,* 1707–1712.

Hyde, J. (2006). The hospital experience: Perspectives of assisted living providers. In N. M. Silverstein & K. Maslow (Eds.), *Improving hospital care for persons with dementia* (pp. 55–62). New York: Springer.

Inouye, S. (2006). Delirium in older persons. *New England Journal of Medicine, 354,* 1157–1165.

Insel, K., Morrow, D., Brewer, B., & Figueredo, A. (2006). Executive function, working memory, and medication adherence among older adults. *Journal of Gerontology: Psychological Sciences, 61B,* 102–107.

Luchsinger, J. A., Reitz, C., Honig, L. S., Tang, M. X., Shea, S., & Mayeux, R. (2005). Aggregation of vascular risk factors and risk of incident Alzheimer disease. *Neurology, 65,* 545–551.

Luchsinger, J. A., Tang, M. X., Stern, Y., Shea, S., & Mayeux, R. (2001). Diabetes mellitus and risk of Alzheimer's disease and dementia with stroke in a multiethnic cohort. *American Journal of Epidemiology, 154,* 635–641.

Lyketsos, C. G., Colenda, C. C., Beck, C., Blank, K., Doraiswamy, M. P., Kalunian, D. A., et al. (2006). Position statement of the American Association for Geriatric Psychiatry regarding principles of care for patients with dementia resulting from Alzheimer disease. *American Journal of Geriatric Psychiatry, 14,* 561–573.

Mahoney, D. F. (2003). Vigilance: Evolution and definition for caregivers of family members with Alzheimer's disease. *Journal of Gerontological Nursing, 29*(8), 24–30.

Mahoney, J. E., Eisner, J., Havighurst, T., Gray, S., & Palta, M. (2000). Problems of older adults living alone after hospitalization. *Journal of General Internal Medicine, 15,* 611–619.

Maslow, K. (2006). How many hospital patients have dementia? In N. M. Silverstein & K. Maslow (Eds.), *Improving hospital care for people with dementia* (pp. 3–21). New York: Springer.

Maslow, K., Skalny, M. A., Looman, W., McCarthy, K., Bass, D., & Striano, J. (2005, April). *Partners in dementia care: Final report on an innovative partnership between Veterans Integrated Service Network 2 (VISN 2) and four upstate New York Alzheimer's Association chapters.* Washington, DC: Alzheimer's Association. Available at http://www.alz.org

McKay, M. P., Farrell, S., Ennis, K., & Binstadt, E. S. (2006). The acute care experience in the emergency department. In N. M. Silverstein & K. Maslow (Eds.), *Improving hospital care for persons with dementia* (pp. 75–98). New York: Springer.

Mezey, M., & Maslow, K. (2004). *Recognition of dementia in hospitalized older adults. Try this: Best practices in nursing care for hospitalized older adults with dementia.* New York: Hartford Institute for Geriatric Nursing, New York University, Division of Nursing. Available at http://www.hartfordign.org/resources/education/tryThis. html

Michelson, S. (2006). A geriatric social worker's perspective on Alzheimer's patients in the emergency room. In N. M. Silverstein & K. Maslow (Eds.), *Improving hospital care for persons with dementia* (pp. 63–74). New York: Springer.

Mitchell, G., Salmon, J. R., Polivka, L., & Soberon-Ferrer, H. (2006). The relative benefits and cost of Medicaid home- and community-based services in Florida. *Gerontologist, 46,* 483–494.

Naylor, M. D., Stephens, C., Bowles, K. H., & Bixby, M. B. (2005). Cognitively impaired older adults: From hospital to home. *American Journal of Nursing, 105,* 52–61. Available at http://www.nursingcenter.com/library/JournalArticle.asp?Article_ID= 541520

Newcomer, R., Clay, T., Luxenberg, J. S., & Miller, R. H. (1999). Misclassification and selection bias when identifying Alzheimer's disease solely from Medicare claims records. *Journal of the American Geriatrics Society, 47,* 215–219.

Nyenhuis, D. L., & Gorelick, P. B. (1998). Vascular dementia: A contemporary review of epidemiology, diagnosis, prevention, and treatment. *Journal of the American Geriatrics Society, 46,* 1437–1448.

Partners in Caregiving. (2002). *A national study of adult day services 2001–2002.* Winston-Salem, NC: Wake Forest University School of Medicine.

Rosenblatt, A., Samus, Q. M., Steele, C. D., Baker, A. S., Harper, M. G., Brandt, J., et al. (2004). The Maryland assisted living study: Prevalence, recognition, and treatment of dementia and other psychiatric disorders in the assisted living population of central Maryland. *Journal of the American Geriatrics Society, 52,* 1618–1625.

Schubert, C. C., Boustani, M., Callahan, C. M., Perkins, A. J., Carney, C. P., Fox, C., et al. (2006). Comorbidity profile of dementia patients in primary care: Are they sicker? *Journal of the American Geriatrics Society, 54,* 104–109.

Sloane, P. D., Zimmerman, S., & Ory, M. G. (2001). Care for persons with dementia. In S. Zimmerman, P. D. Sloane, & J. K. Eckert (Eds.), *Assisted living: Needs, practices, and policies in residential care for the elderly* (pp. 242–270). Baltimore: Johns Hopkins University Press.

Travis, S. S., Bernard, M. A., McAuley, W. J., Thorton, M., & Kole, T. (2003). Development of the family caregiver medication administration hassles scale. *Gerontologist, 43,* 360–368.

U.S. Department of Health and Human Services, Centers for Medicare and Medicaid Services. (2004). Unpublished data from Rollup Summary Reports, case mix means and episode counts, national values for the 12-month period from March 2003 to February 2004, Baltimore.

Wolf-Klein, G. P., Silverstone, F. A., Brod, M. S., Levy, A., Foley, C. J., Termotto, V., et al. (1988). Are Alzheimer patients healthier? *Journal of the American Geriatrics Society, 36,* 219–224.

Zhu, C. W., Scarmeas, N., Torgan, R., Albert, M., Brandt, J., Blacker, D., et al. (2006). Clinical characteristics and longitudinal changes of informal cost of Alzheimer's disease in the community. *Journal of the American Geriatrics Society, 54,* 1596–1602.

PART II

The Early Stage and Interventions With Families

CHAPTER FIVE

The Experiences and Needs of People With Early-Stage Dementia

Lisa Snyder

A person with Alzheimer's disease is many more things than just their diagnosis. Each person is a whole human being. It's important to be both sympathetic and curious, and to have a real interest in discovery about who that person is. You have to really be willing to be present with the person who has Alzheimer's. (Snyder, 2000, p. 124)

—Betty Reichert, retired social worker diagnosed with Alzheimer's

INTRODUCTION

Betty's insightful comments provide a foundation for this chapter. As a person with Alzheimer's disease, she is more than a set of symptoms and problems to be managed; her disease exists in the context of her whole self. As a retired social worker and educator, she is addressing some of the fundamental tenets of social work practice—the establishment of a relationship based on respectful inquiry, engaged empathy, and being present, to the extent possible, in the social and psychological reality of another.

In chapter 6, Daniel Kuhn provides an overview of many practical management issues that social workers need to address with families in the early stages of dementia. This chapter introduces the social worker to the unique emotional, physical, and social issues of people in the early stages of a progressive dementia and draws on their testimony and wisdom to help enhance understanding of the direct experience of the disease. Key psychosocial issues include the experience of symptoms, responding to a diagnosis, changes in interpersonal relationships, coming to terms with losses, and finding meaningful activity and support. The role of social policy and research in shaping practice as well as the unique role people with dementia have in policy advocacy are also reviewed.

Although this chapter is based on the author's extensive experience working with people with dementia, it is critical for the social worker to recognize that these summations of symptoms and issues cannot encompass the unique complexity inherent in each person's subjective experience of the disease. Rather, this chapter serves as an overview and introduces the social worker to areas that may warrant sensitivity, exploration, or intervention when addressing the needs of people with early-stage dementia.

A SYSTEMS OVERVIEW

Recent medical advances have resulted in a strong emphasis toward earlier detection and diagnosis of Alzheimer's disease and related dementias. Most available treatment interventions, as well as those under investigation, have their highest therapeutic value in the first stages of disease. As a result, many physicians are identifying and diagnosing Alzheimer's at a much earlier stage in its progressive course, and people are living for many years with only mild symptoms of the disease.

These individuals are negotiating a world in which they may still be very active participants, but their roles are changing. Their physical appearance is preserved, yet inwardly their sense of personal identity is being threatened by disruptive shifts in memory, perception, and ability.

Social work practice is based on an acknowledgment of the interplay between human beings and their environment, and this dynamic can undergo profound changes even in the early stages of dementia. The extent to which family, social, medical, and community systems are employed to maximize functioning and coping can have significant impact on the well-being of the person with early-stage dementia.

Consistent with the concepts of systems theory is the work of Sabat and others who have employed *social constructionist* theory as a framework for understanding the enduring expression of self in people with dementia and the impact of communication and social constructs on the maintenance of or threat to selfhood (Sabat, 2001). Social constructionists argue that all reality has both subjective and relative aspects and that knowledge is formed from the views and meanings that people, situated in their own history and context, ascribe to a particular experience (Shotter & Gergen, 1989).

Common metaphors of dementia, including "losing one's mind," "becoming an empty shell," and "the loss of self," can contribute to devaluing the capacity for selfhood. It is important to understand that selfhood remains in people with dementia if they are nurtured by personally and socially supportive relationships. People with dementia can still display the ability to attend, to initiate social contact, and to exhibit self-respect, social sensitivity, creativity, helpfulness, and politeness (Sabat & Collins, 1999; Temple, Sabat, & Kroger, 1999) through various expressions of selfhood well into the advanced stages of the disease.

A systems overview or social constructionist framework must incorporate cultural influences that can affect a family's interpretation of dementia symptoms. The degree to which an individual or family is acculturated to Western medicine will also greatly impact their approach to symptoms. In intergenerational families, younger members may be more acculturated to a Western medical or help-seeking model than their elders and may be frustrated with their "old-fashioned" views (Yeo & Gallagher-Thompson, 1996). It is the social worker's responsibility to discern the interplay of culture on each person's experience of and response to a progressive dementia.

UNDERSTANDING SYMPTOMS
OF EARLY-STAGE DEMENTIA

People in the early stages of Alzheimer's or a related dementia usually have mild to moderate problems in multiple areas of cognition. Short-term memory loss is significant enough to impact on independent activities of daily living, including managing complex finances, engaging in some previously enjoyed hobbies, cooking elaborate meals, and managing appointments. Basic activities of daily living, including dressing, bathing, and toileting, are not usually affected in the early stages of the disease, and many people maintain good personal care. They may still be active socially and in the community and can utilize cuing and reminder techniques such as calendars, daily medication dispensers, or personal memos to maintain adequate functioning.

A guiding philosophy in the care of people with Alzheimer's or related dementias was articulated by Dr. William Osler, a founding father of internal medicine, who stated, "It's important to know what disease the person has, but it is more important to know what person the disease has" (Fazio, Seman, & Stansell, 1999, p. 63). As dementia progresses, shifts in thinking and behavior not only are the result of neurological changes in the brain but are sometimes the more complex expression of feelings, experiences, and personality that an individual can no longer express directly. Although a social worker should be familiar with common symptoms of dementia, it is critically important not to lose sight of the unique person experiencing these symptoms.

Memory Loss

Memory loss is the foundation of dementia and affects daily functioning, self-esteem, communication, and relationship dynamics. In her analysis of data from conversations with 13 people with early-stage dementia, Phinney (2002) reports that everyone spoke of being unable to remember certain facts such as names and recent events. Although long-term memories are usually well preserved, memory for recent events is significantly affected. Losing things, missing appointments, becoming disoriented in familiar places, and having difficulty maintaining conversations are all potentially demoralizing experiences. Such memory loss is often unpredictable and contributes to confusion for both people with dementia and their family members. Sheila (1999) writes, "I can't even say, 'Well I remember these kinds of things, but I have a hard time remembering those kinds of things.' There's no neat pattern. Today I may be fine and then tomorrow, not so fine" (p. 2). Memory may be better for things that involve greater emotion, while more mundane events or information can be retained less effectively (Fleming, Kims, Doo, Maguire, & Potkin, 2003).

Functional Loss

Much of what we may think of as habitual behaviors (dressing, washing dishes, driving, calculating change at the grocery store, or mowing the lawn) actually involve a complicated series of steps and problem solving that require considerable memory. The ability to complete these tasks is disrupted by the cognitive losses of dementia. It becomes more challenging to remember sequencing, and tasks need to be broken down into distinct steps.

Some persons also experience visual agnosia, the inability to identify what they see, and this, too, contributes to functional problems. One woman states, "Sometimes what I'm looking for will be lying right in front of me and I won't see it. I don't always misplace things; they're right there, but I just don't recognize them" (Snyder, 2000, p. 21). Depth perception can also be affected, resulting in inability to judge distance and spaces between steps or a curb and the street.

Problems with both reading (*alexia*) and writing (*agraphia*) are common and can impact on enjoyment of activities and basic functioning. For Bill, a retired editor, the experience is acutely painful: "The lunacy of this gets to me ... I read along a line but then when I go to the next line, I can't find it. It takes so long to find the next line that I have forgotten what was on the previous line ... I can read little things, but I can't read a book anymore" (Snyder, 2000, p. 49). Large-print books, short stories, or books on tape can be meaningful resources for people with dementia who can no longer read with ease.

Suspiciousness

Some people with dementia experience feelings of suspiciousness that can arise from the confusing experiences of memory loss or from a generalized decreased sense of security in the face of frightening cognitive disability. Reflecting on his paranoia about his finances and reasons why people with dementia may hoard or guard their possessions, Robert Davis (1989) writes with exceptional insight: "The loss of self, which I was experiencing, the helplessness to control this insidious thief who was little by little taking away my most valued possession, my mind, had made me especially wary of the rest of my possessions in an unreasonable way" (p. 91).

Although suspiciousness can evolve into delusions that warrant medical attention, such disturbing feelings can also be rooted in legitimate events. People with dementia are at significant risk of financial and physical abuse as well as exploitation. It is important to investigate the legitimacy of any comments that suggest abuse before concluding that they are a symptom of dementia.

Social workers must be aware that client confidentiality may need to be overridden by the responsibility of reporting suspected abuse, and this can pose ethical challenges (Bergeron & Gray, 2003). State laws differ slightly in categories of abuse and in mandatory versus voluntary reporting laws. Therefore, it is important to be familiar with the reporting laws in each state and to be acquainted with local Adult Protective Services agencies. The National Center on Elder Abuse (http://www.elderabusecenter. org) provides useful information concerning reporting instructions and requirements.

Irritability and Depression

Because caregivers often experience their own frustrations, the feelings of the person with dementia can receive less acknowledgment than the caregiver's concerns. In their interviews with 17 individuals with early-stage

Alzheimer's, Harris and Sterin report that all but one person expressed extreme frustration with trying to accomplish tasks; with forgetting people, places, or things; or with treatment by others. Sometimes these feelings were displaced onto others, as expressed by one woman: "I get so frustrated at this disease. I have had lots of successes in my life until this disease hit.... Now I do well at nothing. I get so frustrated, it comes out as steam at the people around me" (Harris & Sterin, 1999, p. 246).

Since much of the experience of early-stage dementia is a private mental process and not an outward physical one, the social worker needs to inquire about the client's feeling and experiences associated with memory loss and other cognitive changes. Although some people with dementia have limited awareness of their own losses or may be defensive when asked, others will welcome the opportunity to have their feelings acknowledged and addressed.

It is estimated that 30% to 50% of people with dementia have symptoms of depression, including sadness, pessimism, apathy, sleep disturbance, social withdrawal, and irritability (Olin, Katz, Meyers, Schneider, & Lebowitz, 2002). Given the significant losses and changes due to dementia, it is understandable that individuals could experience considerable distress. Medication cannot always remedy these feelings, but symptoms of depression warrant referral to a physician for evaluation and treatment. One man who contemplated suicide tells his support group, "I vacillate between periods of joy and hope and periods of profound sadness and resignation, and periods of being in the slough of despondency. If it were not for my wife's unflagging love and my own love for my children, I would be a lost cause" (Devine, 1999, p. 6).

Although the prevailing perception has been that people with dementia have a low incidence of suicide, more recent reports suggest that the risk of suicide may actually be increased in people with dementia relative to the general population (Arciniegas & Anderson, 2002). It is important to assess for suicidal ideation in depressed individuals with dementia and to take all references to ending one's life seriously.

Communication Challenges

Verbal expression and communication can be affected in the early stages of dementia. People commonly describe difficulty with finding words (*aphasia*) and can lose their train of thought midstream. For others, by the time they remember the word they wanted to say, they have forgotten the context and may not be able to complete their sentence or thought. One woman confides to friends in an early-stage dementia social club: "I'm aware that I'm losing larger and larger chunks of memory ... I lose one word and then I can't come up with the rest of the sentence.

I just stop talking and people think something is really wrong with me" (Trabert, 1997, p. 7).

Language comprehension can also be compromised, especially in large groups with multiple people talking at once. When talking with a person with dementia, the social worker needs to eliminate distractions, maintain eye contact, and talk directly to the person to maintain his or her attention.

OBTAINING AND RESPONDING TO THE DIAGNOSIS

People with dementia report varying experiences obtaining a diagnosis. Some have no recollection of the event but are aware that a diagnosis was made. Others may be confused or ambivalent about the information because it was never clearly presented to them. One woman states, "I'm sure almost every doctor I went to knew that Alzheimer's disease was a part of this, and they didn't want to deal with it. I'm very angry about that. I can understand that you could be cautious in some cases, but they need to give the person some idea of what they might have instead of protecting themselves" (Snyder, 2000, p. 73).

In her analysis of the comments made by people with dementia about their medical care, Young (2002) notes that individuals "complained bitterly" about many aspects of interaction and communication with physicians, including not being treated respectfully or competently. Because of the prevalence of this problem, the Alzheimer's Association (2003b) has published educational materials to teach families to advocate for the services and communication that they need with their health care providers. The social worker can be a valuable resource for families by helping them access necessary medical services in the crucial early stages of the dementia.

Although some people feel a sense of relief in obtaining a diagnosis and having an explanation for their symptoms, others respond with skepticism or denial. Denial may result from an individual's difficulty identifying with the prevailing images of people with Alzheimer's disease or related dementias. Until recently, both media coverage and written literature have focused on the devastating functional and behavioral disturbances associated with moderate to late-stage dementia. A newly diagnosed, higher-functioning person cannot identify with this stereotype and thinks, "That can't be me." Denial can also be supported by the collusion of friends or family who confirm that the person with early-stage disease "seems perfectly normal" and that "everyone forgets." Sometimes a person will acknowledge "memory loss" or "getting old" while opposing any reference to Alzheimer's disease or dementia.

Denial is not necessarily a psychological defense. As a brain disease, dementia can influence a person's capacity for insight by affecting regions of the brain responsible for memory and self-awareness. As such, some people with dementia forget that they are forgetful and have little recollection of the daily circumstances or events that reveal their disability. The social worker must appreciate the considerable amount of trust required of persons with memory impairment to concede disability or a diagnosis to a health care provider or a family member when they have little awareness or memory of their own symptoms. It is important to consider the full range of neurological, social, and psychological factors that impact on awareness and acceptance of symptoms.

Many people with dementia not only are wrestling with their own response to the diagnosis but also are concerned about responses from others. This may result in attempts to conceal symptoms from family or friends. Keady and Nolan report that some people describe a sense of personal achievement in their abilities to disguise their initial symptoms, but eventually this cover-up becomes too exhausting. One man with dementia states, "I knew that what I was doing was wrong and not like me, but I really did not want to admit it to anyone else. In the end, I had to. I couldn't go on anymore, you see. It's strange, but I also knew that others knew and it made it all ten times worse" (Keady & Nolan, 1995, p. 378).

Some people also fear that acknowledging the disease will mean a progressive loss of independence and autonomy. In his book *My Journey Into Alzheimer's,* Robert Davis (1989) writes, "I live with the imminent dread that one mistake in my daily life will mean another freedom will be taken from me" (p. 91). Many people, however, report that friends and family are supportive, and some people with dementia readily disclose their diagnosis to heighten awareness in their social circle and the public at large.

A small but growing number of people with early stage dementia present on panels at dementia conferences or fund-raisers (Kuhn, 2004). Increasing numbers of people with dementia are talking with the media to reduce stigma and to share their invaluable perspectives, while others are publishing articles and essays in professional journals or newsletters (Sterin, 2002; The Group Members, 2003).

FAMILY RELATIONSHIPS

Recurrent themes for people with dementia in family relationships include fear or recognition of becoming a burden, role changes, loss of autonomy, mutual adjustments, and increased reliance on family (Snyder,

2002). One man's statement encompasses many of these issues: "There are times when I have a difficult time doing things and I ask for her help. I guess that's different from what it used to be. Years ago, I was the macho man. I was the guy who did everything. Now she does most things and that I don't like, but it's something that has to be done.... To be truthful, the only person I really need is my wife" (Tilleli, 1996, p. 2).

Each person in a family brings preexisting relationship dynamics, strengths, and vulnerabilities to the challenge of dementia that will likely impact on the family system's adjustment and ability to cope. These dynamics are compounded by the varying effects that dementia has on each person. Some people with dementia express little understanding of the impact of their symptoms on their loved ones and are unaware of the responsibilities that they have taken on. Others are concerned about their caregivers and are deeply appreciative of their assistance and support. While relationship shifts pose challenges for many families, some families report positive changes and discuss their deeper appreciation for one another and the ways they maximize their time together.

Some people with dementia experience feelings of diminished significance in family or social relationships. Barb, interviewed in an illuminating video about the subjective experience of dementia, discusses how people defer conversations to her husband: "Some people, when my husband and I are together, they refer to me as her, not us or them or you two. It's like I'm there but they can't see me.... And it's so aggravating—I want to stick my tongue out and say, 'I have Alzheimer's but I can still comprehend and speak for myself most of the time'" (*Alzheimer's disease*, 1995).

Although grossly insensitive, it is not uncommon for health care practitioners, including social workers, to talk about the person with early-stage dementia with a caregiver in the person's presence. Social workers must make every attempt to avoid this dynamic. It is often helpful to afford each party the opportunity to talk privately with the social worker and well as in joint consult so that sensitive issues can be discussed candidly and both parties' perspectives are acknowledged. The social worker may be better able to assess an affected person's level of insight, subjective experience, and personal concerns in the absence of a caregiver. Persons with dementia are likely to defer to their more dominant or capable caregiver or may not always be candid for fear of creating discord with their loved one. Distressed caregivers often will speak for or interrupt the less verbal person with dementia. Through separate interviews, the social worker can determine the similarities and differences in their perspectives and establish the groundwork for further counseling as needed.

It is important to conduct a brief individual and relationship history assessment to better understand the adaptive and maladaptive coping styles that each family member may employ and to introduce new coping skills when possible. Because insight can be variable in both people with dementia and their caregivers throughout the course of dementia, the social worker must provide ample and ongoing opportunity for dialogue along the continuum of care.

SPECIAL NEEDS OF YOUNGER PEOPLE WITH DEMENTIA

Although aging is the greatest risk factor for dementia, approximately 6% to 8% of people with Alzheimer's develop the disease before age 65 and range in age from their late 20s to early 60s at the time of diagnosis (Mayo Foundation for Medical Education and Research, 2005). Other types of dementia may be diagnosed in younger years as well (see chapter 2 for a discussion of atypical dementias). These individuals with "early-onset" Alzheimer's or a related dementia experience the same symptoms as those who are older, but they and their loved ones often face a unique set of familial, social, and economic challenges.

In their qualitative analysis of interviews with 38 people with early-onset dementia, Harris and Keady (2004) note that common challenges for these younger individuals include obtaining a clear diagnosis, changing family roles and relationships, workforce and retirement issues, and feelings of social isolation. Early-onset individuals are often in the midst of their careers, raising families, and earning income necessary for a comfortable retirement. Their spouses may also be challenged to meet their caregiving responsibilities while also maintaining their jobs. Legal and financial planning is a priority as couples adjust to changes in income and expenses brought on by disability. Social workers can be instrumental in helping arrange consultation about medical and financial benefits due to disability as well as planning for long-term care needs.

In many families with early-onset dementia, it is not uncommon to find children or adolescents still living in the home. Children can experience varied feelings as they try to cope with the changes in their affected parent. They may need care from a parent at the same time that the affected parent is in need of more assistance. Young family members can be stressed by juggling responsibilities at school and home and need support from peers, teachers, and the family to cope (Beach, 1994; National Alliance for Caregiving, 2005). The Alzheimer's Association has educational and support materials written specifically for children and teens so that these vulnerable family members are not overlooked.

Since the great majority of people experiencing dementia are over age 65, early-onset families frequently have difficulty meeting peers and find themselves in support groups and Alzheimer's programs with participants 10 to 50 years their senior. Some communities are beginning to develop special programs for early-onset families in an attempt to build social connections and decrease the isolation experienced by many of these families (Alzheimer's Association, 2003a). Although some families can weather these challenges with flexibility and grace, most benefit from counseling or professional guidance as they attempt to adjust to these multiple stressors.

COMING TO TERMS WITH LOSSES

Self-determination is a tenet of social work practice, and social workers generally assist clients in identifying and meeting their personal goals. However, symptoms of dementia can significantly disrupt a person's ability to set or meet realistic goals. This poses a significant loss for the person with dementia while also posing ethical challenges for the social worker.

Social workers may have to evaluate a person with dementia's rights to self-determination when that person's actions threaten their own or someone else's well-being. Diminished insight about symptoms coupled with threats to autonomy can result in grief, anger, and ambivalence for many people with dementia who struggle with increased dependence on others. One woman who lives alone states, "There are a lot of people who help you in the beginning. That's their job. There are people who very early in this process said you must get someone to do your checkbook. I wasn't at that point yet. It was very insulting to me to be told, 'Never mind what you think. This is what I think you should do.' There is a lot of that attitude in these well-intentioned people. I fought like hell during every single step in getting help" (Snyder, 2000, p. 69).

Whenever possible, assistance needs to be introduced incrementally to foster trust and teamwork between the social worker and the person with dementia. In some cases when services are refused and a person's safety is at risk, a report to Adult Protective Services or community case management may be necessary.

Symptoms of dementia can also significantly diminish self-esteem and self-worth. One woman states, "I still would like to be treated like a person, you know, because I'm still a person whether I do it wrong or right ... I want to feel like I'm somebody, too, worth somebody because a lot of times with this—already with what I have ... I really don't belong any place" (Cleveland Chapter of the Alzheimer's Association, 1994). The social worker must be sensitive to the ambivalence surrounding these shifts in independence and personal autonomy and acknowledge these losses when engaging in suggested or necessary intervention.

Some persons with dementia experience the loss of driving privileges as one of the most significant and bitter losses. Although many people with mild dementia can continue to drive for a limited period of time after diagnosis, driving ultimately becomes a dangerous prospect and must be stopped. Although there are numerous logistical issues for the social worker to address (see chapter 15 on mobility), it is also important to be sensitive to the personal ramifications of losing one's driving privileges.

Many people fear the extra burden placed on their caregiver as well as the loss of independence and spontaneity that driving affords. Limited means of transportation can result in a shrinking social network and leave people with dementia at risk for isolation and withdrawal from pleasurable activities. For others, the automobile is an extension of personal identity, and the loss of driving privileges feels like a personal injury. In the automobile-driven culture that most people live in today, a car can also be equated with status or with social belonging. Reflecting on the loss of driving privileges, one woman told her support group, "It makes you feel like a second class citizen" (Snyder, Quayhagen, Shepherd, & Bower, 1995, p. 98). When counseling a person with dementia about the issue of driving, it is most helpful to determine what significance the act of driving has for that person specifically in order to help reconcile feelings and logistics surrounding this loss.

FINDING MEANINGFUL ACTIVITY AND SUPPORT

A newly diagnosed man spoke out during a local seminar and expressed the urgency some people with dementia feel in finding ways to move forward in the face of a foreboding diagnosis: "I need you to tell me how I can live with this, not just how I'm going to die from it. I need information to help me cope." With the advent of earlier diagnosis, there is a growing movement to provide educational and support programs to people with early-stage dementia. These programs include weekly support groups for people with early-stage dementia or time-limited supportive educational programs for entire families that provide an overview of dementia and methods of coping in the early stages. These programs provide an invaluable service to people with dementia and families who would otherwise be overwhelmed or discouraged by attending programs for those coping with more advanced symptoms.

In the limited research that has been done on evaluating the effectiveness of early-stage support groups, recurrent positive outcomes of program participation include the opportunity to learn more about the disease and how to cope with it and socialization with others who have similar problems (Logsdon, McCurry, Teri, & Hunter, 2005; Yale, 1995; Yale & Snyder, 2002; Zarit, Femia, Watson, Rice-Oeschger, & Kakos, 2004). Exposure to others who are living with mild impairment can help dispel the denial and fear associated with dementia and ease feelings of loneliness or isolation.

For some, the notion of a "support group" is equated with psychological problems and is threatening or unappealing. The social worker can emphasize that support groups provide a primary educational function where people with similar symptoms can solve problems and share information and methods of resourceful coping. This reframing can shift the emphasis from support to learning and make the group concept more agreeable.

An alternative to support groups is a more socially focused program that may incorporate culturally enriching outings, volunteer work, or cognitive stimulation. These programs appeal to people who do not necessarily want to talk about their symptoms but enjoy the comfort and safety afforded by being in a more structured group of their peers (Einberger, 2005; Trabert, 1997). These programs also address the need for mentally stimulating activity to fill the void left when the ability to engage in previously enjoyed hobbies is lost. Any local chapter of the Alzheimer's Association can direct the social worker and families to early-stage programs in the community. It is also important to recommend that people with dementia have access to the limited but growing number of resources written specifically for them, including newsletters, Web sites, and literature available through various national and international Alzheimer's associations and organizations.

Some people with dementia report adequate activity and social interaction, often in sharp contrast to the caregiver's report that the person is apathetic, does very little, and relies heavily on the caregiver for companionship. Memory loss, the need to feel that one is still productive, or daily fatigue from symptoms can result in people with dementia thinking that they are doing a great deal more than others observe. Moreover, many people with dementia would prefer to maintain the illusion of a normal routine for as long as possible, and attending a structured program introduces a change in routine that can feel threatening or foreign. Others are able to maintain previously enjoyed social connections, hobbies, or engagements for quite some time, and it may be premature to introduce a dementia-specific activity.

It is important to evaluate the perspective of the person with dementia as well as the caregiver and determine each person's unique needs and interests before making generalized recommendations. Some people have never been "joiners," may balk at participating in a group activity, and are content with considerable amounts of quiet time. The caregiver's need for respite may be more compelling than the affected person's need for more activity, and these needs must be clarified so that appropriate recommendations can be made.

PUBLIC POLICY AND RESEARCH

As the baby-boom generation ages and begins to show signs of Alzheimer's or related dementias, a growing number of people with mild dementia are becoming powerful spokespersons and advocates at local and federal government levels. The Alzheimer's Association conducts an annual Public Policy Forum in Washington, D.C., and in recent years individuals with dementia have been invited to provide testimony at advocacy hearings before Congress (Knauss & Moyer, 2006).

In January 2006, the Alzheimer's Association created a national Advisory Group of People with Dementia to consult with association leaders on best practices and important policy issues related to the disease. Such advisory groups have been established in other regions of the world and are evidence of a growing movement to partner with people with dementia in the development of public awareness, programs, and education to meet the needs of families in the early stages.

The earlier diagnosis of dementia allows for a growing number of people around the world to network online while their symptoms are still mild. The Dementia Advocacy and Support Network International was founded in 2000 by a group of people with dementia and has grown to include interested professionals and care partners. Their mission is to promote respect and dignity for persons with dementia as well as to provide a forum for the exchange of information, support, and resources (see their Web site at http://www.dasninternational.org/). Members with dementia post news of their advocacy work as well as personal essays. They frequently attend national and international conferences and are now represented on the board of Alzheimer's Disease International (Truscott, 2004). Thus, people with dementia are having a growing and powerful influence in creating a climate in which, ultimately, knowledge, awareness, advocacy, and compassion can grow to override this devastating disease. Whenever possible, social workers must facilitate opportunities for their voices to be heard.

Cotrell and Shultz (1993) noted that in the majority of research on Alzheimer's, the person with the disease is viewed as a disease entity to be studied rather than a human being who can have an active role in helping us understand the illness and its course. Fortunately, since that time, a growing number of researchers have advocated for or begun to include the perspective of the person in research concerning clinical drug trials, service delivery, and values, preferences, and decision making for daily care situations (Feinberg, Whitlatch, & Tucke, 2000; Traynor, Pritchard, & Dewing, 2004). These efforts need to be reinforced so that, to the extent possible, research is conducted *with* rather than *on* persons with dementia. Helpful guidelines have been outlined to conduct meaningful and sensitive research on the perspectives of people with dementia and on the ethical issues surrounding their involvement in research (McKillop & Wilkinson, 2004; Wilkinson, 2002).

CONCLUSION

Betty's opening words to this chapter call on social workers and others to acknowledge the "whole human being" and to embrace a sense of discovery in this process. As social workers strive to address the needs of people with dementia, it is also imperative to address the common ground that unites us with those we serve. If we see primarily our distinctions from people with Alzheimer's or a related dementia, we deny our common ground and our shared humanity. It is quite likely that at some point in our lives, we will be faced with a temporary, progressive, or permanent condition that will threaten our autonomy, capacity, and functioning. We may become dependent, disabled, or separated from mainstream society. We will rely on others to build bridges that connect us to one another and to meaningful activity.

As social workers and as a society, we must examine our approach to the care of people with dementia because our common needs far outweigh our differences. People with dementia experience the hope for continuing pleasurable experiences in life, the hope that they will be treated with dignity and care, the hope for meaningful relationships with others, and the hope that we listen when they try to communicate. These hopes are consistent with the core values of the social work profession and are the foundation for humane and effective practice.

REFERENCES

Alzheimer's Association. (2003a). Early-onset Alzheimer's brings special challenges. *Advances—Progress in Alzheimer Research and Care, 22*(4), 1, 11.

Alzheimer's Association. (2003b). *Partnering with your doctor—A guide for persons with memory problems and their care partners.* Chicago: Alzheimer's Disease and Related Disorders Association.

Alzheimer's disease: Inside looking out. (1995). Chicago: Terra Nova Films.

Arciniegas, D. B., & Anderson, A. (2002). Suicide in neurologic illness. *Current Treatment Options in Neurology, 4,* 457–468.

Beach, D. (1994, January/February). Family care of Alzheimer victims—An analysis of the adolescent experience. *American Journal of Alzheimer's Care and Related Disorders and Research,* 12–19.

Bergeron, L., & Gray, B. (2003). Ethical dilemmas of reporting suspected elder abuse. *Social Work, 48,* 96–105.

Cotrell, V., & Shultz, R. (1993). The perspective of the patient with Alzheimer's disease: A neglected dimension of dementia research. *The Gerontologist, 33,* 205–211.

Davis, R. (1989). *My journey into Alzheimer's disease.* Wheaton, IL: Tyndale House.

Devine, W. (1999). The group. In I. Gatz (Ed.), *Early Alzheimer's* 1(3), 6–9.

Einberger, K. (2005). Mind boosters. *Perspectives—A Newsletter for Individuals with Alzheimer's or a Related Disorder, 10*(3), 6.

Fazio, S., Seman, D., & Stansell, J. (1999). *Rethinking Alzheimer's care.* Baltimore: Health Professions Press.

Feinberg, L. F., Whitlatch, C., & Tucke, S. (2000). *Making hard choices: Respecting both voices.* Final Report. San Francisco: Family Caregiver Alliance.

Fleming, K., Kims, S. H., Doo, M., Maguire, G., & Potkin, S. G. (2003). Memory for emotional stimuli in patients with Alzheimer's disease. *American Journal of Alzheimer's Disease and Other Dementias, 18,* 340–342.

Harris, P. B., & Keady, J. (2004). Living with early on-set dementia: Exploring the experience and developing evidence-based guidelines for practice. *Alzheimer's Care Quarterly, 5,* 111–122.

Harris, P. B., & Sterin, G. J. (1999). Insider's perspective: Defining and preserving the self in dementia. *Journal of Mental Health and Aging, 5,* 241–256.

Keady, J., & Nolan, M. (1995). IMMEL 2: Working to augment coping responses in early dementia. *British Journal of Nursing, 4,* 377–380.

Knauss, J., & Moyer, D. (2006). The role of advocacy in our adventure with Alzheimer's. *Dementia: The International Journal of Social Research and Practice, 5,* 67–72.

Kuhn, D. (2004). The voices of Alzheimer's disease. *Alzheimer's Care Quarterly, 5,* 265–273.

Logsdon, R. G., McCurry, S. M., Teri, L., & Hunter, P. (2005, November 21). Benefits of early-stage Alzheimer's support groups. Poster presented at the annual conference of the Gerontological Society of America, Miami, FL.

Mayo Foundation for Medical Education and Research. (2005, February 28). Early-onset Alzheimer's: An interview with a Mayo Clinic specialist. Available at http://www.cnn.com/HEALTH/library/AZ/00009.html

McKillop, J., & Wilkinson, H. (2004). Make it easy on yourself! Advice to researchers from someone with dementia on being interviewed. *Dementia, 3,* 117–125.

National Alliance for Caregiving. (2005). Young caregivers in the U.S.: Findings from a national survey. Retrieved March 24, 2006, from http://www.caregiving.org/data/youngcaregivers.pdf

Olin, J. T., Katz, I. R., Meyers, B. S., Schneider, L. S., & Lebowitz, B. D. (2002). Provisional diagnostic criteria for depression of Alzheimer disease. *American Journal of Geriatric Psychiatry, 10,* 129–141.

Phinney, A. (2002). Living with the symptoms of Alzheimer's disease. In P. Harris (Ed.), *The person with Alzheimer's disease: Pathways to understanding the experience* (pp. 49–74). Baltimore: Johns Hopkins University Press.

Sabat, S. (2001). *The experience of Alzheimer's—Life through a tangled veil.* Oxford: Blackwell.

Sabat, S., & Collins, M. (1999). Intact social, cognitive ability, and selfhood: A case study of Alzheimer's disease. *American Journal of Alzheimer's Disease, 14,* 11–19.

Sheila. (1999). What it's like to live with Alzheimer's. *Perspectives—A Newsletter for Individuals with Alzheimer's Disease, 4*(3), 2.

Shotter, J., & Gergen, K. J. (1989). *Texts of identity*. London: Sage.

Snyder, L. (2000). *Speaking our minds—Personal reflections from individuals with Alzheimer's*. New York: W. H. Freeman.

Snyder, L. (2002). Social and family relationships—Establishing and maintaining connections. In P. Harris (Ed.), *The person with Alzheimer's disease: Pathways to understanding the experience* (pp. 112–133). Baltimore: Johns Hopkins University Press.

Snyder, L., Quayhagen, M. P., Shepherd, S., & Bower, D. (1995). Supportive seminar groups: An intervention for early stage dementia patients. *The Gerontologist, 35*, 691–695.

Sterin, G. (2002). Essay on a word: A lived experience of Alzheimer's disease. *Dementia, 1*(1), 7–10.

Temple, V., Sabat, S., & Kroger, R. (1999). Intact use of politeness in the discourse of Alzheimer's sufferers. *Language and Communication, 19*, 163–180.

The Group Members. (2003). Reflections of an early-stage support group for persons with Alzheimer's and their family members. *Alzheimer's Care Quarterly, 4*, 185–188.

Tilleli, D. (1996). Reflections. *Perspectives—A Newsletter for Individuals with Alzheimer's Disease, 2*(2), 1–3.

Trabert, M. (1997). The DRC Club. *Perspectives—A Newsletter for Individuals with Alzheimer's Disease, 2*(3), 7.

Traynor, V., Pritchard, E., & Dewing, J. (2004). Illustrating the importance of including the views and experiences of users and carers in evaluating the effectiveness of drug treatments for dementia. *Dementia, 3*, 145–159.

Truscott, M. (2004). Alzheimer's disease international 18th annual conference, Barcelona, Spain. *Dementia, 3*, 233–239.

Wilkinson, H. (2002). *The perspectives of people with dementia—Research methods and motivations*. London: Jessica Kingsley.

Yale, R. (1995). *Developing support groups for individuals with early-stage Alzheimer's disease: Planning, implementation, and evaluation*. Baltimore: Health Professions Press.

Yale, R., & Snyder, L. (2002). The experience of support groups for persons with early-stage Alzheimer's disease and their families. In P. Harris (Ed.), *The person with Alzheimer's disease: Pathways to understanding the experience* (pp. 228–245). Baltimore: Johns Hopkins University Press.

Yeo, G., & Gallagher-Thompson, D. (Eds.). (1996). *Ethnicity and the dementias*. Washington, DC: Taylor & Francis.

Young, R. (2002). Medical experiences and concerns of people with Alzheimer's disease. In P. Harris (Ed.), *The person with Alzheimer's disease: Pathways to understanding the experience* (pp. 29–46). Baltimore: Johns Hopkins University Press.

Zarit, S. H., Femia, E. E., Watson, J., Rice-Oeschger, L., & Kakos, B. (2004). Memory club: A group intervention for people with early-stage dementia and their care partners. *The Gerontologist, 44*, 262–269.

CHAPTER SIX

Helping Families Face the Early Stages of Dementia

Daniel Kuhn

When Mrs. Chatham's husband was diagnosed with cancer, she did not respond as expected according to her daughter, one of four children in the family. Mrs. Chatham, age 80, seemed overwhelmed by her husband's illness despite her customary problem solving approach to life. She could not recall details about her husband's medical treatment. She occasionally repeated herself in conversations and no longer seemed comfortable in social situations. She got lost while driving her car on a few occasions too. Mr. Chatham privately shared with the children that "mother seems to be slipping." The daughter, who visited several times weekly, believed that depression was the cause. Mrs. Chatham agreed to a trial of antidepressant medication but showed no improvement. Then the family's attention shifted exclusively to Mr. Chatham as his illness worsened. On his death, Mrs. Chatham grieved appropriately but showed increasing signs of cognitive impairment. At the insistence of her daughter, Mrs. Chatham was referred to a neurologist who determined that she was in early stages of Alzheimer's disease.

INTRODUCTION

Families like Mrs. Chatham's are often puzzled by the initial changes observed in a loved one with dementia and do not know where to turn for help. Most people with Alzheimer's disease (AD) or a related dementia live alone or with relatives for the major part of the illness. Since dementia ultimately results in disability and dependency, the lives of the affected person and his or her family are inextricably linked.

Social workers in a variety of settings can play vital roles in preserving the independence of individuals with dementia, minimizing the disabling effects of dementia, and helping family members adjust to their role as providers of care throughout its course. However, there is probably no more critical time for intervention than the early stages, when affected individuals and their families face much uncertainty and fear.

While chapter 5 focused on individuals in the early stages of dementia, this chapter focuses on the challenges facing their families and how social workers may be helpful. Specifically, this chapter describes key issues that are often stressful for families with a relative in the early stages of dementia: (a) obtaining a diagnosis, (b) protecting income and assets, (c) making decisions regarding the patient's driving, and (d) creating a safe living situation. Finally, this chapter addresses some social policies and research relevant to families affected by dementia.

From the outset, it is important to understand that families are complex and heterogeneous in response to the demands of caregiving. Coping with dementia is highly individualized, and thus caution must be exercised in generalizing how families and individuals manage the series of challenges encountered over the course of dementia. Although an ecological perspective is useful, each family and person appraises the caregiving situation from a unique perspective.

AN ECOLOGICAL PERSPECTIVE

Social work's traditional commitment to understanding the person within his or her environment, often referred to in terms of several ecological/systems models, is well suited to understanding the challenges of dementia. Social workers are able to intervene at the level of dyadic relationships, social networks, bureaucratic institutions, and other social systems. In an ecological perspective, people and their environments are viewed as interdependent, complementary parts of a whole in which both are constantly changing and shaping each other. The dynamic and complex nature of dementia results in the affected individual becoming dependent on his or her family and others. Thus, social workers must address various systems in which people with dementia interact with their families and other providers of care. These interpersonal relationships are also shaped by societal norms and expectations in the forms of attitudes, beliefs, customs, policies, and laws, particularly in regard to health care and social services.

Beyond interpersonal relationships, the larger social context is a major concern of social workers interested in promoting the well-being of individuals with dementia and their families. Social change through advocacy is paramount in light of the burgeoning population of people with dementia and the inadequate patchwork of private and public services in the United States known as long-term care.

THE EARLY STAGES OF DEMENTIA

At present, AD and related dementias rob nearly 5 million Americans of their memory, thinking, language, and other intellectual functions, and that number is projected to increase to 13.2 million by 2040 (Hebert, Scherr, Bienias, Bennett, & Evans, 2003). Dementia is a relatively rare condition among persons younger than 65 years of age, but the risk doubles roughly every 5 years after age 65 (Hebert, Beckett, Scherr, & Evans, 2001). About 10% of all persons age 65 and older have dementia, and nearly half the population age 85 and older has dementia. Almost a quarter of older persons living at home with dementia are in the mild/early stages (Evans et al., 1989). Unfortunately, most people in the early stages of dementia do not seek a diagnosis, so they and their families have no context for understanding or coping with symptoms and the social and psychological fallout.

First, it is useful to consider what is meant by *early-stage dementia.* There are no strict criteria to define stages of dementia, but the early stages can be described in general terms that are important for distinguishing them from the caregiving challenges of more advanced stages.

Initial presenting symptoms of common types of dementia such as AD include mild forgetfulness about recent events, losing or misplacing things, difficulty with complex tasks, inability to use reasoning strategies, problems with word finding, loss of initiative, and disorientation regarding time and place. The hallmark of dementia is memory loss, while rare types of dementia may be characterized by personality disturbances (as seen in frontotemporal dementia) or language problems (as seen in primary progressive aphasia). The early stages of major types of dementia include changes in many other cognitive, behavioral, and functional abilities:

- Gradual withdrawal from activities
- Inconsistent performance of instrumental activities of daily living

- Deterioration of abstract thought processing
- Depression or anxiety
- Sexual dysfunction, loss of desire or ability
- Weight loss
- Decreased tolerance of new ideas or changes in routine

Despite some common symptoms, there is much variability among people in the early stages of dementia. Each individual experiences a unique progression and severity of impairments. For example, one person may be unable to identify his grandchildren but still able to drive a car safely, while another may no longer be able to cook a meal but can still identify her grandchildren.

The onset of dementia is insidious and symptoms slowly worsen over a period of many years. Pathologic changes in the brain occur long before symptoms are manifested. *Mild cognitive impairment* (MCI) represents a cognitive state between normal cognitive aging and the early stages of dementia (Petersen et al., 2001). People with MCI generally exhibit mild memory loss without other cognitive impairments. The prevalence of MCI is even higher than that of dementia (Purser, Fillenbaum, Pieper, & Wallace, 2005; Unverzagt et al., 2001). In addition to its common occurrence, MCI is significant because those with the condition are at an increased risk for dementia, especially AD, and indeed it has been argued that MCI represents the very earliest manifestations of dementia (Morris et al., 2001).

During MCI and the early stages of dementia, people who frequently interact with the affected individual may notice signs of mild impairment, but people who interact less frequently may overlook symptoms. The person with dementia is often aware of changes in memory and thinking but may downplay their significance or cover them up. Sometimes an individual with dementia appears unaware of his or her impairments, which in itself may be a manifestation of the condition. A series of incidents or a dramatic event may eventually force the symptomatic person or the family to seek a diagnosis. On the other hand, a diagnosis evaluation may be delayed or postponed altogether, resulting in preventable problems for affected individuals and families alike. In the meantime, all parties may be puzzled and frustrated, and the quality of their mutual relationships may be threatened.

Although not considered part of normal aging, dementia is fairly common among older persons, especially among the "oldest old." Complaints by individuals with symptoms or their relatives should be taken seriously. At minimum, screening for dementia is warranted in such cases, and a full diagnostic evaluation should be considered. Social workers should be familiar with symptoms of dementia and offer families a referral to a physician who can make an accurate diagnosis. If families understand the rationale for early diagnosis and treatment, they are more likely to act on a referral instead of waiting for a crisis to occur at a later time.

OBTAINING AN ACCURATE DIAGNOSIS

Despite growing public awareness about dementia, denial and lack of awareness by both the affected person and the family are still common in the early stages of dementia. In one large study, 21% of family informants failed to recognize a problem with memory among relatives subsequently found to have early stage dementia; more than half of these informants failed to recognize a more significant memory problem (Ross et al., 1997). Cognitive impairment is frequently evident to a mild degree several years before diagnosis. In a study of 528 family caregivers, there was a delay of diagnostic assessment for an average of 22.4 months after they first noticed the symptoms (Wackerbarth & Johnson, 2002). Another study, cited in chapter 1, found even longer delays.

Social and cultural factors may also influence the recognition of dementia symptoms and the speed in obtaining a diagnosis. Recent research among ethnic groups highlights differences attached to the meaning of dementia and the need for cultural sensitivity by professionals in working with individuals and families facing dementia (Coon et al., 2004; Haley et al., 2004; Hinton, Franz, Yeo, & Levkoff, 2005; Husaini et al., 2003; Roberts et al., 2003).

Families often need encouragement to consider that symptoms may be due to a medical condition such as dementia. A great deal of fear, stigma, and negative stereotypes are still associated with dementia. It is helpful to explain why early recognition of dementia may offer substantial benefits. Beyond ruling out irreversible dementias and starting treatment with antidementia drugs, early diagnosis offers opportunities to enhance personal safety and autonomy, initiate education and support, and foster communication about present and future care (Kuhn, 2003). Social workers can explain the elements and process of outpatient testing to allay undue worry and help families see beyond the pessimism often associated with dementia.

Another barrier to early diagnosis is the failure of many primary care physicians to recognize the existence or importance of symptoms and misperceptions regarding diagnostic tests and medical treatments (Boise et al., 1999). Variability of symptoms may cloud the diagnostic picture too. Biological markers are not yet available, but a high rate of diagnostic accuracy is possible using established clinical criteria and standard tests of memory and thinking, laboratory tests, and a brain scan. However, a survey of 1,480 caregivers revealed that a correct diagnosis of AD was made in only 38% of cases at initial physician consultation (Knopman, Donohue, & Gutterman, 2000). Families need to know that they can obtain and deserve an accurate diagnosis and should seek out a second opinion if unsatisfied with a physician's diagnosis or explanation for symptoms. A consultation with a specialist such as a neurologist, geriatrician, psychiatrist, or neuropsychologist should be encouraged.

Getting Everyone on the Same Page

Although an increasing number of physicians accept responsibility for anticipatory guidance of families affected by dementia, such communication is not always effective. Families report that they often do not get enough information regarding dementia from physicians (Holroyd, Turnbull, & Wolf, 2002). Moreover, physicians and families frequently disagree about what they discussed regarding treatment and caregiving issues when dementia is diagnosed (Alzheimer's Association, 2001a). Social workers may be in a position to clarify the medical facts and offer anticipatory guidance that families need after a diagnosis. In the early stages, families typically need basic medical information and strategies for coping with their changing roles and responsibilities and for how to best communicate with their loved one with dementia (Kuhn, 1998).

Face-to-face consultation should be supplemented with reading materials available through the Alzheimer's Association (http://www.alz.org) and the Alzheimer's Disease Education and Referral Center (http://www.alzheimers.org). In addition, referrals should be made to early-stage education and support programs operated by local chapters of the Alzheimer's Association or other organizations (Kuhn & Fulton, 2004; Logsdon, McCurry, & Teri, 2005; Snyder, Jenkins, & Joosten, in press).

Disclosing the Diagnosis

It is also important for social workers to encourage families to disclose the diagnosis to others. The logical strategy is to tell other family members and friends before they notice symptoms, yet in most cases, they likely have already wondered about observable changes. Other people are typically relieved to know that action has been taken and that the dementia can now be talked about openly and constructively. Family and friends can begin to learn how to be helpful in promoting independence and minimizing the disabling effects of dementia. Engaging others from the outset makes it possible for them to learn about dementia and offer emotional support and practical assistance. For example, a friend might be told, "Betty has Alzheimer's disease, so she may repeat herself often or have difficulty keeping pace in conversation. Be patient with her and give her direction as needed."

If other family members have difficulty accepting or coping with the disease, a family meeting should be held to clarify the facts and enlist everyone's support that will be needed over the long haul. In particular, family members and friends can learn how to support the main provider of care (such as a spouse or an adult child). Primary caregivers of persons with dementia bear many burdens and are well known to be at risk for ill effects in terms of their physical, psychological, social, and financial well-being (Cuijpers, 2005; Ory, Yee, Tennstedt, & Schultz, 1999; Schultz & Beach, 1999).

The early stage is the ideal time for all concerned individuals to become knowledgeable about dementia and adopt positive coping strategies in order to minimize or prevent the negative outcomes associated with caregiving. Cognitive restructuring and reframing are successful interventions employed by social workers that enable caregivers to consider the positive aspects and manage the stressors of caregiving (Mittelman, Epstein, & Pierzchala, 2002; Mittelman, Roth, Haley, & Zarit, 2004; Noonan & Tennstedt, 1997).

PROTECTING INCOME AND ASSETS

One of the first instrumental activities of daily living affected by dementia is increased difficulty managing money. This cognitive impairment may be manifested in forgetting to pay bills, making errors in calculations, failing to monitor investments, or making poor financial decisions. People in the early stages of dementia are often relieved to give up the complex tasks of financial management. On the other hand, some individuals with dementia insist on exercising autonomy and refuse to relinquish control over their finances. At the same time, their families may wish to protect them from financial mismanagement or exploitation due to impairments in memory or judgment. Social workers should encourage families to initiate conversations and make decisions aimed at protecting income and assets while preserving the autonomy of the person with dementia to the greatest extent possible.

Persons in the early stages of dementia are often quite capable of expressing their preferences (Feinberg & Whitlach, 2001; Whitlach, Feinberg, & Tucker, 2005). They and trusted family members should discuss finances in light of the likely need for long-term care, either at home or in a residential care facility. Social workers should explain this need in realistic terms while trying to achieve a consensus among all stakeholders, particularly the person with dementia. Families will benefit by consulting with an attorney and financial planner who specialize in planning for disability. If such arrangements are already in place, revisiting such specialists will be helpful in light of the diagnosis of dementia.

Advance directives, such as powers of attorney for property and health care, should be executed so that a surrogate decision can ensure that medical and finance decisions are made in accord with the patient's preferences. It is essential for all concerned parties to be proactive and complete financial and legal arrangements as soon as possible. Waiting until later means risking the chance that the person with dementia may no longer be capable of participating in decisions affecting his or her care.

People with dementia are at risk of being persuaded to give money or property to others and then forget about such "gifts" or "investments." Thus, they are at risk for serious harm if they or others do not take steps to protect their income and assets. Self-neglect and exploitation by unscrupulous relatives, friends, brokers, telemarketers, and other salespeople can result in financial ruin. Con artists use countless fraudulent schemes to take advantage of vulnerable people. Unfortunately, family members are the main perpetrators of financial exploitation (Lachs & Pillemer, 2004; Nerenberg, 1996). They are often in a position of trust and opportunity to take advantage of a relative's memory and cognitive problems and steal money and other assets.

Laws vary from state to state regarding professional responsibility for reporting alleged financial exploitation to government authorities for investigation by Adult Protective Services. Current estimates put the overall reporting of financial exploitation at only 1 in 25 cases (National Center on Elder Abuse, 2005). Any allegation of illegal taking, misusing, or concealing funds, property, or assets deserves to be taken seriously. Absolute proof is not needed to report a suspected case of financial exploitation. In many states, social workers are mandated to report suspected cases of financial exploitation and other forms of abuse against vulnerable adults. Social workers should be aware of their legal rights and responsibilities. The National Center on Elder Abuse (202-898-2586), funded by the U.S. Administration on Aging, is an excellent resource for social workers and others about financial exploitation and other forms of abuse against vulnerable adults. See http://www.elderabusecenter.org.

The value of putting financial and legal safeguards in place cannot be overstated. Trying to manage the affairs of someone with dementia, even when done with the best intentions, can be difficult if plans have not been made. Financial mismanagement or exploitation cannot be prevented if a trusted family member has not been authorized to act in behalf of the person with dementia. Thus, families should be given permission to assume leadership and become proactive participants in protecting income and assets. They should not hesitate to become involved if the person with dementia asks for help with handling finances. Even if not asked, assistance should be offered in a nonthreatening manner to ensure that bills are paid and assets are properly managed. If inadvertent mismanagement or exploitation has occurred, corrective action can be initiated with legal authorities.

Above all, social workers should encourage family members to execute legal and financial plans. This important step can result in achieving the twin goals of preserving personal autonomy while meeting the dependency needs of the person with dementia. Social workers can counsel families on how to best achieve these goals while enabling them to resolve their differences regarding preferences and desirable outcomes.

TO DRIVE OR NOT TO DRIVE?

The issue of dementia and driving has engendered much private and public debate. There are no consistent public policies or laws that address this important matter of both personal autonomy and public safety. Driving is more than a means of transportation and staying connected to other people and places. It is also a symbol of individual freedom. As a result, driving has practical and emotional implications. Although some people may consider driving to be a personal right, it is essentially a privilege bestowed by society to those who can demonstrate competence to safely operate a motor vehicle. Driving safely requires a complex set of abilities, including coordination, orientation, concentration, perception, memory, and processing a lot of information quickly. Impairment of any of these abilities due to dementia may affect driving skills and lead to traffic violations and accidents resulting in injury and death.

Unfortunately, the ability to drive safely is often compromised in the early stages of dementia. However, some people retain good driving skills for months, even years, in spite of their symptoms. Therefore, a diagnosis of dementia alone is not sufficient for cessation of driving. In fact, some studies indicate that some persons in the early stages of dementia may cease driving prematurely (Carr, Shead, & Storandt, 2005; Hunt et al., 1997). At present, there are no simple ways to identify or assess whether someone in the early stages of dementia is too impaired to drive safely. Consequently, the individual's personal desire to continue driving may conflict with the public's need for safety. On the other hand, families may press the person with dementia to stop driving despite intact driving skills.

A number of organizations, including the American Academy of Neurology (Dubinsky, Stein, & Lyons, 2000), the American Medical

Association (2003), and the Alzheimer's Association (2001b), have formulated consensus statements on the issue of driving and dementia. Such documents are aimed primarily at providing physicians with guidelines concerning the assessment of cognitive status in relation to driving. In general, these statements recognize that dementia in the middle to late stages precludes safe driving but that certain individuals with early-stage dementia should be assessed for their driving competence. Performance tests have been effective in determining driving fitness among drivers with dementia (Hunt et al., 1997) but have not been adopted into routine practice because of costs and other practical issues. See chapter 15 for a complete discussion of driving and related mobility issues.

The Need for Family Participation

If a driver with dementia is no longer safe on the road and does not readily recognize the risks, others need to point them out. According to a study by O'Neill and Dobbs (2004), as many as 20% of people with dementia referred to memory disorder clinics are actively driving. The decision whether to impose driving restriction or a ban should depend on a careful assessment of a driver's ability. However, this assessment is often made by family members with opportunities to witness firsthand the driving performance of someone with dementia. Voicing their concerns about safety may be enough to convince the person to reconsider driving. Social workers can direct families to Web-based information developed by the Hartford Financial Services Group, Inc., and the MIT AgeLab (2004) so that they may initiate productive and caring conversations about driving safety.

A frank yet diplomatic approach is recommended in which concerns are expressed yet self-esteem is supported. Sometimes family members hesitate to intervene, rationalizing that the benefits of driving outweigh the risks. For example, a spouse who relies on the person with dementia for transportation may see no alternative and deny the growing danger. In such cases, social workers should initiate discussions about the pros and cons of driving and recommend a discussion with one's physician or a formal assessment of driving skills. Driver evaluation programs are usually operated by hospitals specializing in rehabilitation. An expert, typically an occupational therapist with expertise in this area, will assess the person's driving skills using a variety of vision and cognitive tests as well as a road test.

Sometimes people with dementia refuse to give up driving although their driving skills are obviously impaired to others. Continued resistance by an unsafe driver who has little or no insight requires intervention. Every state empowers physicians with some measures to curb driving by their patients because of medical conditions, and this legal authority should be invoked if necessary. Social workers should instruct families to first privately share concerns about driving with the physician. Such firsthand reports are crucial in helping physicians to decide whether a driving ban or restriction is necessary or if further assessment is warranted. At any rate, the physician should take responsibility for telling an uncooperative person to stop driving. In this way, family members avoid becoming the focus of anger or resentment and can play a supportive role to the person who is deemed no longer able to drive safely.

For the most part, neither laws nor medical guidelines are clear about driving and dementia. Therefore, families are ultimately responsible for ensuring the safety of the person with dementia as well as the safety of the public. Their cooperation is often necessary to encourage cessation of driving and provide transportation alternatives. Social workers can counsel them to accept this leadership role and take active steps so that the person with dementia remains as independent and active as possible.

MAXIMIZING INDEPENDENCE AND MINIMIZING RISK AT HOME

People in the early stages of dementia deserve to be as independent as possible in order to enjoy living in the community, yet the risks posed by their cognitive impairments may impose constraints. Social workers may enable families to assess their strengths and weakness and help balance the needs of all stakeholders. Personal, environmental, social, and financial resources must be carefully assessed and mobilized in behalf of those who provide care and receive care at home.

An estimated one-third of all people with dementia residing in the community live alone (Ebly, Hogan, & Rockwood, 1999), and only half of them have caregivers (Prescop et al., 1999). Those in the early stages of dementia who live alone are even more likely to be without formal or informal services than persons with more advanced dementia (Webber, Fox, & Burnette, 1994). They are often at risk for safety problems due to self-neglect and other difficulties related to their dementia. Numerous problems may arise stemming from inabilities to follow a medication regime, buy and cook nutritious food, and use household appliances safely. Malnutrition is particularly problematic among those with dementia who live alone (Nourhashemi et al., 2005). In a study of 131 people with dementia who lived alone, 21% experienced an incident of harm resulting in physical injury or property loss or damage and required emergency community interventions over a period of 18 months (Tierney et al., 2004).

Unless those at risk are identified early and given informal or formal services, those living alone are at risk for hospitalization and premature placement in residential care facilities. Social workers may be in a position to ask families and significant others to intervene and ward off a crisis. Likewise, social workers may refer cases of self-neglect to Adult Protective Services, although states vary in terms of mandatory reporting and mechanisms to provide safety.

Related to the challenges of living alone is the fact that contemporary families are highly mobile and may live long distances from a relative with dementia. A national survey found that 15% of caregivers live more than an hour away from their care recipients (National Alliance for Caregiving & AARP, 2004). Social workers can make families aware of the services of geriatric care managers who typically have backgrounds in social work or nursing. For a fee, these professionals can assess and manage needs of people with dementia on behalf of those who are long-distance caregivers. It is essential that families investigate the credentials of care managers since it an unregulated profession at this time. The specialty credentials of the National Association of Social Workers in either gerontology or case management may be helpful in this regard. In addition, the National Association of Professional Geriatric Care Managers (520-881-8008) offers referrals to its members throughout the United States (http://www.caremanager. org). For those who lack financial resources to hire such help, the Eldercare Locator (800-677-1116), funded by the U.S. Administration on Aging, directs families to local area agencies on aging and other nonprofit organizations that offer services (http://www.eldercare.gov).

Someone with dementia who resides with others may require more help than families are aware of at first. The extent of one's need for assistance with personal or instrumental activities of daily living, for example, may be underestimated. Social workers may help families understand these needs and offer recommendations for meeting them with formal and informal supports. Again, the goal should be to minimize risks while enabling the highest possible level of independence.

Assistance from relatives, neighbors, and friends may leave gaps in the support required. Even with full-time help from informal sources, respite care may be needed. Therefore, hiring someone to assist the person or moving the person into a relative's home or a formal care setting may be desirable. Many families are unaware of home and community-based options such as paid companions and adult day services. Families are even more perplexed by residential care options and paying for such care. Social workers can provide information and referral and help families weigh the advantages and disadvantages of choices for care. Clearly, the person with dementia will be unable to live alone indefinitely without increasing levels of help as the dementia progresses.

The time line for implementing changes in the living situation, however, depends on each person's unique needs and resources. If a family has the foresight to plan ahead and make adjustments in care arrangements as necessary, the need to make decisions in a crisis can be avoided. In the early stages of dementia, social workers can direct families to organize how and when decisions will be made in the best interests of all concerned. Convening family conferences for periodic assessments of care plans may be invaluable in keeping everyone abreast of changing needs and how to best address them.

SOCIAL POLICY AND RESEARCH

Dementia is a large and growing concern for families as well as society. There is ample evidence that dementia exacts an enormous toll on families who are the main providers of care. It is also well known that Medicare expenditures for people with dementia are higher than the average for all other beneficiaries (Bynum et al., 2004; Kane & Atherly, 2000). Even prior to diagnosis, when people with dementia are likely to be in the early stages, they are more likely to use Medicare outpatient and ambulatory care (Albert et al., 2002). Medicare is in need of modernization so that dementia is recognized as a chronic condition that is treated primarily by families who work hard with few public resources to prevent or delay health care crises, excess disabilities, and institutionalization. As is true in treating any chronic medical condition, early intervention in dementia can benefit persons with dementia as well as their families.

In order to overhaul Medicare and provide chronic care through home and community-based services, a universal long-term care system must be created, as seen in other developed countries. Social workers must advocate for such sweeping policy changes and must make a case for their roles in implementing a long-term care system that takes into account the complex medical and psychosocial needs of families affected by dementia. Rather than an ancillary role in providing services through Medicare, social workers could assume a leadership role in a public system in which health and social services are blended to suit the diverse needs of individuals and families. Case management would enable families to better care for their relatives from the onset of dementia to the end of life.

In addition to reform of laws and entitlement programs, the American workplace must become more supportive of employees who care for relatives with dementia. A study commissioned by the Alzheimer's Association estimated that the costs of dementia caregiving to U.S. businesses is $61 billion annually in terms of lost productivity, turnover, and other direct and indirect costs (Koppel, 2002). Employers must be willing to invest in programs and services so that employees who are caregivers can achieve a work–life balance. Social workers, particularly in employee assistance programs, can potentially develop, test, and disseminate innovative practices that are mutually beneficial to employers and employees who are caregivers. For example, a consortium of large companies known as the American Business Collaboration for Quality Dependent Care funded the development of a successful Web-based course about self-care for employees (Kuhn et al., in press), and other Internet-based courses about dementia.

Supporting caregivers through simple interventions such as respite, counseling, and other services can have a major impact on health care costs, economic well-being, and quality of life. Social work research must focus on evaluating early intervention with families in an effort to document such outcomes. For example, a study by Gaugler, Kane, Kane, & Newcomer (2005) demonstrates that families who utilize in-home help services earlier in their dementia caregiving careers are more likely to delay institutionalization. Such cost-effective interventions benefit individuals, families, and society.

CONCLUSION

Social workers are well suited to address the practical concerns of individuals and families coping with the early stages of dementia. Thus far, the social work profession in the United States has generally not addressed dementia specifically as a focus for public policy or research. The increasing number of people with dementia presents enormous challenges to society that will intensify in the coming decades. Social workers must become more engaged in efforts to shape social policies and improve practice through applied research, particularly in relation to the early stages of dementia.

REFERENCES

Albert, S. M. et al. (2002). Primary care expenditures before the onset of Alzheimer's disease. *Neurology, 59,* 573–578.

Alzheimer's Association. (2001a). *Alzheimer's disease report: Communication gaps between primary care physicians and caregivers.* Retrieved November 24, 2006, from http://www.alz.org/Media/newsreleases/2003/alzheimerreport.pdf

Alzheimer's Association. (2001b). *Alzheimer's Association and driving.* Retrieved November 24, 2006, from http://www.alz.org/AboutUs/PositionStatements/overview.asp#driving

American Medical Association. (2003). *Physician's guide to assessing and counseling older drivers.* Washington, DC: National Highway Traffic Safety Administration.

Boise, L. et al. (1999). Diagnosing dementia: Perspectives of primary care physicians. *The Gerontologist, 39,* 457–464.

Bynum, J. P., Rabins, P. V., Weller, W., Niefeld, M., Anderson, G. F., & Wu, A. W. (2004). The relationship between a dementia diagnosis, chronic illness, Medicare expenditures, and hospital use. *Journal of the American Geriatrics Society, 52,* 187–194.

Carr, D. B., Shead, V., & Storandt, M. (2005). Driving cessation in older adults with dementia of the Alzheimer's type. *The Gerontologist, 45,* 824–827.

Coon, D. W., Rubert, M., Solano, N., Mausbach, B., Kraemer, H., Arguelles, T., et al. (2004). Well-being, appraisal, and coping in Latino and Caucasian female dementia caregivers: Findings from the REACH study. *Aging and Mental Health, 8,* 330–345.

Cuijpers, P. (2005). Depressive disorders in caregivers of dementia patients: A systematic review. *Aging and Mental Health, 9,* 325–330.

Dubinsky, R. M., Stein, A. C., & Lyons, K. (2000). Practice parameter: Risk of driving and Alzheimer's disease (an evidence-based review): Report of the quality standards subcommittee of the American Academy of Neurology. *Neurology, 54,* 2205–2211.

Ebly, E. M., Hogan, D. B., & Rockwood, K. (1999). Living alone with dementia. *Dementia and Geriatric Cognitive Disorders, 10,* 541–548.

Evans, D. A., Funkenstein, H. H., Albert, M. S., Scherr, P. A., Cook, N. R., Chown, M. J., et al. (1989). Prevalence of Alzheimer's disease in a community population of older persons higher than previously reported. *Journal of the American Medical Association, 262,* 2551–2556.

Feinberg, L. F., & Whitlatch, C. J. (2001). Are persons with cognitive impairment able to state consistent choices? *The Gerontologist, 41,* 374–382.

Gaugler, J. E., Kane, R. L., Kane, R. A., & Newcomer, R. (2005). Early community-based service utilization and its effects on institutionalization in dementia caregiving. *The Gerontologist, 45,* 177–185.

Haley, W. E., Gitlin, L. N., Wisniewski, S. R., Mahoney, D. F., Coon, D. W., Winter, L., et al. (2004). Well-being, appraisal, and coping in African-American and Caucasian dementia caregivers: Findings from the REACH study. *Aging and Mental Health, 8,* 316–329.

Hartford Financial Services Group, Inc., & the MIT AgeLab. (2004). *Family Conversations with Older Drivers.* Retrieved November 24, 2006, from http://www.thehartford.com/talkwitholderdrivers (see also http://www.thehartford.com/alzheimers/)

Hebert, L. E., Beckett, L. A., Scherr, P. A., & Evans, D. A. (2001). Annual incidence of Alzheimer disease in the United States projected to the years 2000 through 2050. *Alzheimer Disease & Associated Disorders, 15,* 169–173.

Hebert, L. E., Scherr, P. A., Bienias, J. L., Bennett, D. A., & Evans, D. A. (2003). Alzheimer disease in the US population: Prevalence estimates using the 2000 census. *Archives of Neurology, 60,* 1119–1122.

Hinton, L., Franz, C. E., Yeo, G., & Levkoff, S. E. (2005). Conceptions of dementia in a multiethnic sample of family caregivers. *Journal of the American Geriatrics Society, 53,* 1405–1410.

Holroyd, S., Turnbull, Q., & Wolf, A. M. (2002). What are patients and their families told about the diagnosis of dementia? Results of a family survey. *International Journal of Geriatric Psychiatry, 17,* 218–221.

Hunt, L. A., Murphy, C. F., Carr, D., Duchek, J. M., Buckles, V., & Morris, J. C. (1997). Reliability of the Washington University Road Test: A performance-based assessment for drivers with dementia of the Alzheimer's type. *Archives of Neurology, 54,* 707–712.

Husaini, B. A., Sherkat, D. E., Moonis, M., Levine, R., Holzer, C., & Cain, V. A. (2003). Racial differences in the diagnosis of dementia and in its effects on the use and costs of health care services. *Psychiatric Services, 54,* 92–96.

Kane, R. L., & Atherly, A. (2000). Medicare expenditures associated with Alzheimer disease. *Alzheimer Disease and Associated Disorders, 14,* 187–195.

Knopman, D., Donohue, J. A., & Gutterman, E. M. (2000). Patterns of care in the early stages of Alzheimer's disease: Impediments to timely diagnosis. *Journal of the American Geriatrics Society, 48,* 300–304.

Koppel, R. (2002). *Alzheimer's disease: The costs to U.S. businesses in 2002.* Washington, DC: Alzheimer's Association. Retrieved November 24, 2006, from http://www.alz.org/Media/newsreleases/2002/062602ADCosts.pdf

Kuhn, D. (1998). Caring for relatives in the early stage of Alzheimer's disease. *American Journal of Alzheimer's Disease, 10,* 189–196.

Kuhn, D. (2003). *Alzheimer's early stages: First steps for family, friends and caregivers* (2nd ed.). Alameda, CA: Hunter House.

Kuhn, D., & Fulton, B. R. (2004). Efficacy of an educational program for relatives of persons in the early stages of Alzheimer's disease. *Journal of Gerontological Social Work, 42,* 109–123.

Kuhn, D., Hollinger-Smith, L., Presser, J., Civian, J., & Batsch, N. (in press). Powerful tools for caregivers online: An innovative approach to support employees. *Journal of Workplace Behavioral Health.*

Lachs, M. S., & Pillemer, K. (2004). Elder abuse. *Lancet, 364,* 1263–1272.

Logsdon, R. G., McCurry, S. M., & Teri, L. (2005). Time limited support groups for individuals with early stage dementia and their care partners. *Clinical Gerontologist, 30,* 5–19.

Mittelman, M. S., Epstein, C., & Pierzchala, A. (2002). *Counseling the Alzheimer's caregiver: A resource for health care professionals.* Chicago: American Medical Association.

Mittelman, M. S., Roth, D. L., Haley, W. E., & Zarit, S. H. (2004). Effects of a caregiver intervention on negative caregiver appraisals of behavior problems in patients with Alzheimer's disease: results of a randomized trial. *Journals of Gerontology B: Psychological Sciences and Social Sciences, 59,* P27–P34.

Morris, J. C., Storandt, M., Miller, J. P., McKeel, D. W., Price, J. L., Rubin, E. H., et al. (2001). Mild cognitive impairment represents early-stage Alzheimer disease. *Archives of Neurology, 58,* 397–405.

National Alliance for Caregiving & AARP. (2004). *Family caregiving in the U.S.: Findings from a national survey.* Bethesda, MD: National Alliance for Caregiving; Washington, DC: American Association of Retired Persons.

National Center on Elder Abuse. (2005). *NCEA fact sheet: Elder abuse prevalence and incidence.* Retrieved November 24, 2006, from http://www.elderabusecenter.org/pdf/publication/FinalStatistics050331.pdf

Nerenberg, L. (1996). *Financial abuse of the elderly.* Washington, DC: National Center on Elder Abuse.

Noonan, A. E., & Tennstedt, S. L. (1997). Positive aspects of caregiving and its contribution to caregiver well-being. *The Gerontologist, 37,* 785–794.

Nourhashemi, F., Amouyal-Barkate, K., Gillette-Guyonnet, S., Cantet, C., Vellas, B., & REAL.FR Group. (2005). Living alone with Alzheimer's disease: Cross-sectional and longitudinal analysis in the REAL.FR Study. *Journal of Nutrition Health and Aging, 9,* 117–120.

O'Neill, D., & Dobbs, B. M. (2004). Age-related disease, mobility, and driving. In Transportation Research Board (Ed.), *Transportation in an aging society: A decade of experience* (pp. 56–68). Washington, DC: Transportation Research Board. Retrieved November 24, 2006, from http://onlinepubs.trb.org/onlinepubs/conf/reports/cp_27.pdf

Ory, M., Yee, J., Tennstedt, S., & Schulz, R. (1999). Prevalence and impact of caregiving: A detailed comparison between dementia and nondementia caregivers. *The Gerontologist, 39,* 177–185.

Petersen, R. C., Stevens, J. C., Ganguli, M., Tangalos, E. G., Cummings, J. L., & DeKosky, S. T. (2001). Practice parameter: Early detection of dementia: Mild cognitive impairment (an evidence-based review): Report of the Quality Standards Subcommittee of the American Academy of Neurology. *Neurology, 56,* 1133–1142.

Prescop, K. L. et al. (1999). Elders with dementia living in the community with and without caregivers: An epidemiological study. *International Psychogeriatrics, 11,* 235–250.

Purser, J. L., Fillenbaum, G. G., Pieper, C. F., & Wallace, R. B. (2005). Mild cognitive impairment and 10-year trajectories of disability in the Iowa Established Populations for Epidemiologic Studies of the Elderly cohort. *Journal of the American Geriatrics Society, 53,* 1966–1972.

Roberts, J. S., Connell, C. M., Cisewski, D., Hipps, Y. G., Demissie, S., & Green, R. C. (2003). Differences between African Americans and whites in their perceptions of Alzheimer disease. *Alzheimer Disease and Associated Disorders, 17,* 19–26.

Ross, G. W., Abbott, R. D., Petrovitch, H., Masaki, K. H., Murdaugh, C., Trockman, C., et al. (1997). Frequency and characteristics of silent dementia among elderly Japanese-American men: The Honolulu-Asia Aging Study. *Journal of the American Medical Association, 277,* 800–805.

Schultz, R., & Beach, S. R. (1999). Caregiving as a risk factor for mortality. *Journal of the American Medical Association, 282,* 2215–2219.

Snyder, L., Jenkins, C., & Joosten, L. (in press). The effectiveness of support groups for people with mild-to-moderate Alzheimer's disease—An evaluative survey. *American Journal of Alzheimer's Disease and Other Dementias.*

Tierney, M. C., Charles, J., Naglie, G., Jaglal, S., Kiss, A., & Fisher, R. H. (2004). Risk factors for harm in cognitively impaired seniors who live alone: A prospective study. *Journal of the American Geriatrics Society, 52,* 1435–1441.

Unverzagt, F. W., Gao, S., Baiyewu, O., Ogunniyi, A. O., Gureje, O., Perkins, A., et al. (2001). Prevalence of cognitive impairment: Data from the Indianapolis Study of Health and Aging. *Neurology, 7,* 1655–1662.

Wackerbarth, S. B., & Johnson, M. M. (2002). The carrot and the stick: Benefits and barriers in getting a diagnosis. *Alzheimer Disease and Associated Disorders, 16,* 213–220.

Webber, P. A., Fox, P., & Burnette, D. (1994). Living alone with Alzheimer's disease: Effects on health and social service utilization patterns. *The Gerontologist, 34,* 8–14.

Whitlatch, C. J., Feinberg, L. F., & Tucker, S. (2005). Accuracy and consistency of responses from persons with cognitive impairment. *Dementia: The International Journal of Social Research and Practice, 4,* 171–184.

CHAPTER SEVEN

Family Care and Decision Making

Carol J. Whitlatch and Lynn Friss Feinberg

INTRODUCTION

Providing assistance or care to persons with chronic illnesses or disabilities, including those with dementia, takes many forms. This assistance can be instrumental, personal (i.e., hands-on), affective, financial, or otherwise of value or necessity to the person who needs it. It can be provided by family members, friends, or service providers, and it can vary in its intensity and duration. Caregiving can last for 1 hour per day, 1 weekend per year, or 24 hours a day for years at a time. Caregiving can occur within a community or home setting, in an institutional or assisted living setting, or from a distance.

In general, the provision of care or assistance involves making difficult decisions that can affect the quality of life of both caregiver and care receiver. Yet the assistance typically has the purpose of allowing the care recipient to maintain an optimal level of independence and autonomy with dignity and comfort. Providing care can be stressful to both caregivers and care recipients, and its effects can last for many years after care responsibilities have ended.

The number of research studies on informal and formal caregivers of persons with chronic conditions, including dementia, has grown dramatically in both quality and quantity over the past decades. Caregiving research is currently characterized by its continued advances in theory, methodology, intervention development, and application for public policy development. To appreciate the growing significance of caregiving research and its impact on intervention development and family decision making, it is important to understand the prevalence and impact of caregiving and the specific nature and challenges of caring for persons with dementia.

WHO ARE FAMILY CAREGIVERS, AND WHAT DO THEY DO?

The number of adults in the United States aged 65 and older (and particularly those over the age of 85) has grown dramatically and, in turn, had a significant impact on the prevalence of caregiving. Families and friends provide the majority of assistance with hands-on care as well as emotional and financial support to the over 7 million adults in the United States age 65 and older who require assistance with personal care or daily activities (e.g., bathing, dressing, and housekeeping). Most older people (65 and older) with a disability living in the community rely entirely on family and friends for support and assistance. Another 26% of older people supplement their informal care by formal care, and 9% utilize paid care only (Spillman & Black, 2005).

By 2007, households that care for persons aged 50 and over could reach 39 million (National Alliance for Caregiving & American Association of Retired Persons, 1997). Although informal care (i.e., care provided by unpaid family or friends) is the most preferred and frequently used source of assistance, formal care services also supply a great deal of support, especially for the millions of older adults who live alone or have no family or friends available to assist. Older adults who have a choice, however, prefer that family and friends are the providers of assistance once it becomes necessary.

Families often go through a period of reorganization as they restructure their lives in order to provide care to an impaired family member. A naturally occurring hierarchy often exists within families that leads one person to take on the role of primary caregiver. For care recipients who are married, spouses will most likely become the primary caregiver. Adult daughters are also likely candidates. According to Spector, Fleishman, Pezzin, and Spillman (2000), approximately 13.4% of family caregivers are wives, 10% are husbands, 26.6% are adult daughters, 14.7% are sons, and another 17.5% and 8.6% are "other" female or male relatives, respectively.

The primary caregiver's main responsibility, although rarely specified, is to be the direct provider and/or manager of the elder's care. The stressful and long-term nature of providing care causes many primary caregivers to seek assistance from other family members, friends, or service providers. Within most families there is often the understanding (though this understanding is not necessarily made explicit) that the primary caregiver is the main person in charge of managing, arranging, and/or providing the relative's care.

Social network characteristics, household income, and access to community services also affect provision of care. While it is often true that many families use formal services only after they have exhausted all sources of informal assistance, use of services is also linked to factors related to social network characteristics (e.g., size and proximity of network members and their knowledge of community resources). Moreover, income level is associated with use of formal services because most community-based long-term care is paid out of pocket. Thus, income and network characteristics are interrelated and instrumental to the accessibility of services.

The type of assistance caregivers provide varies depending on characteristics of both the caregiver and the care receiver (e.g., type of functional impairment and the nature of the disease). One factor influencing the type of care required is presence of dementia because these adults have care needs that differ from the care needs of physically impaired adults who are cognitively intact. For example, caregivers of adults with physical impairments (e.g., stroke, multiple sclerosis) report providing substantial assistance with self-care activities such as bathing, dressing, and walking. In addition to assisting with self-care activities, caregivers of adults with dementia and other cognitive impairments (e.g., stroke, Parkinson's disease) report spending a great deal of time and energy dealing with their relative's problem behaviors, such as agitation, memory loss, and wandering. These varying care needs have a differential impact on caregiver stress and well-being (Pearlin, Aneshensel, Mullan, & Whitlatch, 1995).

A final consideration concerns the roles and responsibilities of family caregivers who continue to provide care to relatives in institutional settings including assisted living. A move from home to an institutional setting often becomes necessary when the demands of providing care in the home become too stressful for a family caregiver or if their relative's symptoms and needs dramatically worsen. In other situations, a specific crisis such as illness and/or hospitalization of the caregiver or their relative precipitates such a move. Yet the responsibilities of family caregivers do not end once their relative enters an institutional setting. Caregivers continue to remain active in the lives of their impaired family members visiting nearly 4 days per week, traveling great distances, and spending about 10 hours per week at the facility (Zarit & Whitlatch, 1992). These family caregivers perform many of the same tasks they did while caring at home, including assistance with eating, personal care, and walking.

The continued involvement of family caregivers following placement may result in additional or new sources of distress. Once their relative is institutionalized, caregivers must restructure their lives and adjust to their new role. Recent research indicates that the stresses of caregiving are not alleviated by placement. Although these caregivers are relieved of the day-to-day demands of caregiving, many continue to feel distress and some exhibit symptoms well above their preplacement levels of distress. Placement appears to alter rather than eliminate caregiver stress.

These findings have important implications for practitioners and other professionals who may advocate for caregivers to place their relatives because it is assumed to alleviate the stressors of caregiving. Although some caregivers experience relief soon after their relative has moved, most caregivers continue to be vulnerable to stress, which may continue for many years after the initial placement. In general, caregivers who continue to provide substantial assistance to their institutionalized relatives risk compromised emotional outcomes. Yet, as time passes, caregivers are more likely to adjust well at work and in their emotional well-being (Aneshensel, Pearlin, Mullan, Zarit, & Whitlatch, 1995).

Social workers, counselors, and other professionals must be aware that placement is not a panacea for the short- and long-term stress of providing care. Placement does not eliminate the "commitment, caring, involvement, or the pain associated with seeing a loved one go through a long period of decline" (Aneshensel et al., 1995, pp. 250–251).

HOW DOES PROVIDING CARE AFFECT FAMILY CAREGIVERS?

Providing in-home care over the long term affects a family caregiver's mental and physical health. For example, caregivers of persons with dementia are more depressed than age-matched controls; exhibit deficits in physical health and depressed immunologic functioning; use prescription drugs for depression, anxiety, and insomnia two to three times as often as the rest of the population; have higher rates of comorbid health conditions and mortality; and report increased financial strain (Haley, Levine, Brown, Berry, & Hughes, 1987; Schulz, O'Brien, Bookwala, & Fleissner, 1995). Another potential consequence of caregiving is its negative effects on the caregiver's relationships with family members, friends, and leisure and social activities (Aneshensel et al., 1995). Family caregivers often reveal that they have no personal or leisure time. Hence, their participation in social and recreational activities declines, as does their ability to travel and take vacations, which can lead to social isolation and loneliness, missed medical appointments, and lack of exercise.

Studies of caregiving families suggest that women experience greater distress than men regardless of the care receiver's diagnosis and level of impairment and the caregiver's employment status. Caregiving wives have been found to experience greater health strain and stress and be more depressed than caregiving husbands (Ingersoll-Dayton & Raschick, 2004; Miller, 1990; Yee & Schulz, 2000). Studies that compare adult daughter and wife caregivers suggest mixed results: some studies find daughters to be more distressed, while other studies report the reverse or find no differences by kinship tie.

One explanation for these differences draws on studies of health and well-being in the general population indicating that women commonly score higher than men on indicators of stress, suggesting that women may be more comfortable than men expressing feelings of stress. It has also been suggested that the nurturant role developed by men in later life may be rewarding or act as a form of repayment for the care they received in the past, which in turn helps counteract the otherwise negative effects of caregiving.

The effects of caregiver age are also indicated in studies of caregiver stress, yet the effects of age are nearly impossible to disentangle from the effects of other caregiver and care receiver characteristics. For example, age and kinship tie are confounded for spouse caregivers who are significantly older than other groups of caregivers. There is conflicting evidence about the relationship between caregiver age and distress; some studies find older caregivers to be the most distressed, while other studies find younger caregivers to be the most stressed. However, among employed caregivers, especially those with both child and adult care responsibilities, younger caregivers are more likely to experience greater distress as well as absenteeism, interruptions at work, and difficulty in combining work and family.

A growing body of research focuses on how the caregiving experience varies in relation to cultural and ethnic identity (Dilworth-Anderson, Williams, & Gibson, 2002; Foley, Tung, & Mutran, 2002). Across all ethnic groups, family care is the most preferred and relied-on source of assistance. Yet for family members in the United States who care for relatives with a variety of disabilities, there is no clear relationship between the caregivers' ethnicity and the amount of stress they experience. Extensive and supportive kin networks have been documented in Americans of all ethnic backgrounds, including Mexican Americans, African Americans, Asian Americans, and Euro-Americans (e.g., Greek, Italian, Polish, Irish).

An extensive literature has documented the adverse effects of long-term caregiving for persons with chronic conditions and dementia. Yet there is increasing evidence that the provision of care is also associated with positive effects, benefits, and rewards (Bearon, 2004; Donelan et al., 2002; Farran, Miller, Kaufman, Donner, & Fogg, 1999; Kramer, 1997). Family members often report that caregiving is satisfying, gives meaning to their lives, and provides a sense of personal mastery or self-efficacy. It is important to gain more knowledge about caregiving's benefits in order to have a more balanced perspective on the caregiving experience. A more comprehensive view will help clinicians and service providers use a strength-based approach to service plans that capitalize on and enhance caregivers' capabilities.

The consequences and benefits that family caregivers experience as a result of providing care vary slightly depending on the symptoms and care needs of the relatives for whom they provide care. Research suggests that family caregivers of persons with functional losses (e.g., declining ability to feed or dress themselves or prepare meals) or behavioral difficulties (e.g., wandering, agitation, inappropriate verbal and/or physical behaviors) often report feelings of role overload, that is, being completely overwhelmed by the responsibilities of providing care (Pearlin et al., 1995). Caring for a loved one with dementia, on the other hand, has the effect of causing caregivers to feel a deep sense of loss over the person they are caring for. In other words, persons experiencing dementia gradually lose their ability to contribute and participate in their normal routines. Although they maintain their familiar outward appearance, they behave and react much differently than they did before they became cognitively impaired. In turn, caregivers feel they have lost the person they once knew. This sense of loss is more acute for family caregivers of persons with dementia than for caregivers of persons with physical and behavioral difficulties.

The varying care needs of persons with memory and/or physical conditions are considered primary stressors of caregiving. These stressors are not primary in importance but rather are primary because they are based on the behaviors and resulting care needs of persons with chronic conditions. These primary stressors lead to secondary stressors related to role and intrapersonal consequences including work strain, financial strain, and family conflict as well as mastery, competency, and self-esteem (Pearlin, Mullan, Semple, & Skaff, 1990). Primary and secondary stressors are associated with caregiver outcomes such as depression and physical health consequences (for a full description of the stress process model of family caregiving, see Aneshensel et al., 1995). Within the stress process are numerous points and junctures that are amenable to the buffering or moderating effects of intervention and prevention programs. These potential interventions are increasingly available to caregiving families as part of local, state, and federal initiatives.

FEDERAL AND STATE-LEVEL FAMILY CARE
PROGRAMS AND POLICIES

Family members and other informal caregivers may have different needs and preferences at different times during their caregiving experience. A variety of support services can bolster them in providing care to a loved one. However, services specific to dementia caregivers are a relatively small part of the publicly funded home and community-based services (HCBS) system, and patterns of service use among caregivers of persons with dementia living in the community are comparatively unknown.

Given the many stressors that caregivers experience as a result of their long-term role, it is surprising that until recently there were relatively few publicly funded programs that targeted family caregivers as the identified client. More common are programs that support family caregivers as part of a larger care plan directed to bring in support and services for persons with disabilities. Before passage of the National Family Caregiver Support Program in 2000, state general revenues financed most publicly funded caregiver services. However, some states have covered respite care, an important benefit for family caregivers, under their Medicaid HCBS waiver programs. Today, the National Family Caregiver Support Program, state-funded programs, Medicaid waivers, and some federal demonstration grants (e.g., Alzheimer's Disease Demonstration Grants to the States) provide the bulk of public financing for family caregivers. In the next section, we provide a brief overview of public programs that support family caregivers of persons with chronic conditions and dementia.

The National Family Caregiver Support Program

The National Family Caregiver Support Program (NFCSP) is the most comprehensive federal legislation that supports caregivers of older relatives (age 60 and older), grandparents, and other relatives who care for children 18 years of age and younger and older adults caring for persons with developmental disabilities (Fox-Grage, Coleman, & Blancato, 2001). Funded through the Older Americans Act (OAA) reauthorization in 2000, the NFCSP provides funds to states to work with area agencies on aging and local service providers to develop multifaceted systems of caregiver support in five areas: (a) information about available caregiver services, (b) assistance in gaining access to services, (c) counseling and the organization of support groups and caregiver training, (d) respite care, and (e) other services that complement the care provided by caregivers.

All income groups are eligible for NFCSP services, but states must give priority to those providing care to older individuals in the greatest social or economic need with particular attention to low-income individuals. Functional eligibility criteria vary by type of service: individuals 60 years and older must have two or more limitations in activities of daily living (e.g., bathing, dressing) or a cognitive impairment for the caregiver to be eligible for respite or supplemental services. Other service categories (e.g., counseling, support groups) are available to family caregivers regardless of the care recipient's functional status.

All states now provide some explicit caregiver support services as a result of the passage of the NFCSP in 2000. Yet the modest level of NFCSP funding to the states ($138.7 million in 2003) leaves gaps in caregiver support services that vary substantially from state to state. Similar to HCBS in general, the availability of caregiver support services varies greatly across the United States because of differences in philosophy, program eligibility criteria, funding, and approaches to design and administration of the services (Feinberg, Newman, Gray, Kolb, & Fox-Grage, 2004).

In the relatively few states that have state-funded respite care programs for dementia caregivers only (i.e., California, Connecticut, Kentucky, Maine, New Jersey, Ohio, and Pennsylvania), the NFCSP has been used to develop caregiver support services beyond a focus on respite care only and to reach a population broader than dementia caregivers alone (Feinberg, Newman, & Van Steenberg, 2002). In most other states, however, caregiver support services under the NFCSP serve family and informal caregivers of older persons with a range of diseases/disabilities, including but not limited to dementia caregivers.

Medicaid

Medicaid, the major public funder for HCBS, is financed by the federal government and the states. As an entitlement program, Medicaid has a large impact on state budgets, with substantial implications for state policy overall and for family caregivers in particular. While the Medicaid program is an entitlement, the HCBS waiver program is not. The Medicaid HCBS waiver program plays an important role in strengthening family caregiving. Waiver programs offer services that Medicaid traditionally does not provide under the regular program, such as respite care or caregiver education and training. Total national respite expenditures for Medicaid HCBS waiver programs in fiscal year 2002 (the most recent year for which these data are available) were about $101 million (Feinberg et al., 2004).

To qualify for a waiver program, beneficiaries must meet an institutional level of care and meet state residency and financial requirements. Each state has its own guidelines in determining whether a person is nursing home eligible, using, for example, medical diagnosis or number of limitations in activities of daily living. Medicaid HCBS waiver programs allow beneficiaries to have somewhat higher incomes than permitted for Medicaid eligibility, generally incomes at or below 300% of the federal Supplemental Security Income level.

State-Funded Programs

State funds generally pay for the HCBS that have the most flexible eligibility criteria. These programs usually offer services that Medicaid will not cover or are more liberal and expand eligibility to people who do not qualify for Medicaid HCBS waivers, OAA services, or other programs (Summer, 2003). Not bound by federal Medicaid or OAA regulations, state-funded programs can provide specific services (e.g., respite care) to distinct populations (e.g., family members of persons with dementia). State funding may also be used to augment services available under federally funded programs. One example is Connecticut's state-funded Alzheimer's Respite Care Program. Its eligibility requirements focus on the income and assets of the care receiver, who can be of any age; income cannot exceed $30,000 per year, and assets cannot total more than $80,000.

State-administered programs offer an array of services to support family and informal caregivers. Respite care is the service strategy most commonly offered to caregivers and is available in all 50 states, although the amount of respite to family caregivers varies substantially from state to state and program to program within states. In a 50-state study of caregiving programs, only nine states (Alaska, California, Florida, Kentucky, Maine, New Jersey, Ohio, Pennsylvania, and Texas) were identified as having any state-funded programs intended solely for persons with dementia and their caregivers (Feinberg et al., 2004).

Access to program information or services varies by type of program. Even within the same state, caregivers typically do not find the same range of services to be available. At a practical level, such service gaps and variations can pose challenges for caregivers by limiting choices for needed support services that may not be available where they live. Service inequities may also place more pressure on already strained caregiving families and compromise the caregivers' abilities to care for their relative (Feinberg et al., 2004).

Alzheimer's Disease Demonstration Grants

To improve services to persons with Alzheimer's disease, Congress established the Alzheimer's Disease Demonstration Grants to States (ADDGS) program under section 398 of the Public Health Service Act as amended by the Health Professions Education Partnerships Act of 1998 and administered by the U.S. Administration on Aging. Since 1992 when the first state demonstration grants were awarded, the program's goal has been to expand support services for persons with Alzheimer's disease and their family caregivers, including a focus on serving the hard-to-reach and underserved population. In fiscal year 2005, 38 state government agencies were awarded demonstration grants totaling $12 million. Unlike many federal programs, this demonstration has been characterized by regional differences in program development and implementation. The ADDGS program has also expanded the range of respite care options available for dementia caregivers in many of the states funded under this program (Montgomery, 2002).

Consumer Direction and Decision Making

In its broadest sense, consumer direction enables people to make meaningful choices regarding their care or the care they are providing (Sciegaj, 2001). Although some older people as well as younger adults with disabilities insist on self-direction and person-centered care, family and informal caregivers are often key partners in consumer-directed programs. Within consumer-directed programs, family members can assume a variety of roles: from information gather and coordinator of care to representative or surrogate decision maker for persons with dementia to the person paid to provide care. Many policymakers and program administrators are increasingly viewing the "consumer" in consumer-directed care not as the individual with the disability but rather as the dyad—that is, the care receiver *and* his or her family (Ditto, 2004; Doty, 2004; Feinberg, Whitlatch, & Tucke, 2000).

The NFCSP, Medicaid HCBS waivers, and some state-funded programs permit consumer-directed approaches depending on each state's rules and regulations. For example, under the NFCSP, states may make direct payments to family caregivers or provide a voucher or budget for goods and services (e.g., grab bars, respite care) to meet their needs and those of the care receiver. Although the trend toward consumer direction is increasing, the availability of these options for family caregivers varies by state and also by programs within states (Feinberg et al., 2004).

Programs that strive to be truly consumer directed have the challenge of designing services that are responsive to the needs and preferences of both members of the care dyad, that is, family caregivers and the persons with dementia. Balancing the needs of both care partners is often difficult, especially as dementia progresses, affecting a person's ability to communicate and function. Yet early and more accurate diagnosis has created an opportunity for involving persons with dementia in decision making earlier and more actively than in the past. A growing body of research indicates that persons with mild to moderate dementia are able to answer questions about their preferences for daily care and to choose a person to make decisions on their behalf (Feinberg & Whitlatch, 2002; Whitlatch, Feinberg, & Tucke, 2005b). Including persons with dementia in decision making about current and future care needs is beneficial to both care partners and may alleviate distress for caregivers over the long term. For example, an intervention that facilitates structured discussions between care partners and a trained professional has shown positive effects for both caregivers and persons with dementia (Whitlatch, Judge, Zarit, & Femia, 2006). These promising findings reflect the growing trend to develop interventions that empower and meet the needs of both care partners.

INTERVENTIONS AND SERVICES FOR FAMILY CAREGIVERS

Over the past 20 years, assessment, services, and interventions targeted to family caregivers have become more widely available, in large part because of expectations that these programs will help ameliorate the stressful effects of long-term caregiving. These services include respite care, peer-led and professionally led support groups, education programs in care-related skills, training in problem solving skills and behavioral techniques for patient management, and counseling and psychotherapy. Evaluations of these interventions have yielded mixed results, and a number have been compromised by sampling and other methodological limitations (Sörensen, Pinquart, & Duberstein, 2002). In the next sections, we describe the challenges to assessing, designing, and evaluating effective interventions for family caregivers of persons with dementia.

Assessing Specific Needs of Family Caregivers

The value of systematic assessment of family caregivers' needs in health care and in long-term care has gained increased attention in recent years. This interest stems, in part, from the recognition of the fundamental need to improve direct supports for family caregivers and to focus on outcomes and quality of care. Indeed, the well-being of the caregiver is often the deciding factor in determining whether a frail elder can remain at home or must move to an institutional setting.

Caregiver assessment is generally used to describe a systematic process of gathering information about a caregiving situation and identifying the particular problems, needs, resources, and strengths of the family caregiver. It approaches issues from the caregiver's perspective and culture, focuses on what assistance the caregiver may need, and seeks to maintain the caregiver's own health and well-being. The goal of the caregiver assessment is to develop a plan of care that indicates appropriate provision of services and supports for the family caregiver and any measurable outcomes of such services.

In practice settings, social workers have the opportunity to work with the person with dementia *and* the family caregiver and promote family-centered care and interventions. Effective caregiver assessment requires social workers to have specialized knowledge and skills, such as understanding of the caregiving process and its impacts as well as the benefits and elements of an effective caregiver assessment. As the population ages, social workers and other practitioners will become critically important to assess and address the complex needs of people with dementia and their family caregivers.

Because family caregivers are a core part of health care and long-term care, it is important to recognize, respect, assess, and address their needs. Caregiver assessment should embrace a family-centered perspective, inclusive of the needs and preferences of both the person with dementia and the family caregiver. Indeed, assessment of the needs of the family is the beginning of the intervention process itself and helps families decide on needed services and supports and to make appropriate decisions about care. Caregiver assessment should be multidisciplinary in approach, reflect culturally competent practice, and be periodically updated by reassessing the family caregiver's needs and situation (Family Caregiver Alliance, 2006).

Anecdotal reports from California's state-funded Caregiver Resource Centers—a program that has uniformly assessed the needs of family caregivers since 1988—suggest that family clients appreciate the assessment process because they gain a sense that their situations are taken seriously. The information collected during the assessment and reassessment process not only helps families with decision making but also acknowledges their strengths and the effectiveness of their care plans (Ellano, 1997).

Even though understanding the role, multiple stressors, and particular situation of the family caregiver is viewed as essential to any care plan developed for the care receiver, few federal and state HCBS programs uniformly assess the family caregiver's well-being and needs for support. Nonetheless, state officials who administer these programs recognize the value of uniformly assessing caregiver needs, using the information to inform policy and practice, and the importance of practice guidelines and training in this area (Feinberg et al., 2004). As states pursue making their long-term care systems more receptive to the needs of different consumer populations and their families, the concept of assessing the needs of family caregivers, as well as the care recipient, is taking hold.

Which Interventions Work Best?

When developing and/or evaluating interventions for family caregivers, it is important to determine (a) what would be the most effective intervention for a specific type of caregiver, (b) the most effective timing of the intervention, and (c) the most appropriate duration of use. As noted, there is great heterogeneity across groups of and individual caregivers; thus, there is no one caregiving intervention that fits every caregiver at every stage of their caregiving career. Interventions must be targeted to the caregiver's specific needs and stressors and be available and structured in a manner so that the caregiver is receptive to and accepting of the program.

In order to target specific caregiver needs, a systematic assessment must be administered that is sensitive to varying care circumstances (Bass, 2001; Feinberg, 2004). A caregiving wife may have different concerns and needs than an adult daughter caring for her father. A caregiving husband may need an intervention to lessen his anger, resentment, and overload, while a caregiving son may need help providing hands-on care for his mother. These scenarios illustrate the great diversity of caregiver stressors and needs. For an intervention to be successful, it must be sensitive or targeted to treat diverse stressors. Thus, a psychoeducational intervention would be useless to or even add stress to a caregiver who is overwhelmed by the daily care needs of his or her family member. Instead, an intervention that addresses care needs and/or behavioral difficulties would most likely be an effective method for treating the caregiver's stress.

The timing of the intervention is also critical to its success. Family members in the early stages of enacting their role as caregiver have very different needs and expectations than caregivers who have provided care for many years. A caregiver new to the role is often best helped by information and educational materials about his or her relative's condition; knowing what to expect and/or what might help the impaired relative can be valuable to many caregivers. But as the loved one's condition worsens, the caregiver's stress is exacerbated so that an effective intervention and/or service must address these new stressors, including feelings of overload, isolation, family conflict, and work strain.

Likewise, caregivers involved in moving a loved one to an institutional setting (e.g., assisted living or nursing home care) or dealing with the death of their relative may be best helped by support groups or counseling. It is also important to provide supervision (if needed) for the caregiver's loved one so that the caregiver is able to participate fully in the intervention rather than be distracted by or concerned about their relative. Finally, the duration, intensity, and accessibility of the intervention is critical to its effectiveness. For some caregivers, a focused individual intervention may be more effective than a group design, and some caregivers may prefer to attend programs with their relative, while others may wish to attend independently of their relative.

Taken together, it becomes clear that the effectiveness of a caregiver intervention is driven by the needs, stressors, stage, and availability of the caregiver seeking treatment. Also relevant but less widely examined are factors surrounding the care receiver and how his or her experience and expectations play a role in the caregiver's stress. Moreover, determining effectiveness depends on enrolling sufficient numbers of caregivers in study samples, even when the service is provided free of charge (see Lawton, Brody, & Saperstein, 1989).

Various explanations offered for the apparent underutilization of care-related services include unfamiliarity with the service, lack of perceived need, reliance on informal helpers for care-related assistance, absence of culturally relevant services, and barriers to the service system and the delivery of services. To date, relatively little empirical attention has been given to the prevalence, sources, and predictors of care-related service use. In general, however, the predictors of caregiver service use are kinship tie (adult child), living with the care receiver, being employed, more perceived care-related stress, and more informal and formal assistance provided to the care receiver.

The many challenges that arise when evaluating an intervention's effectiveness are not insurmountable. Briefly, research indicates that a variety of interventions and services are modestly effective in ameliorating the stress of providing long-term care in the home. Family caregivers often indicate a great need for respite (i.e., time away from their caregiving responsibilities), but its use is not uniformly associated with less caregiver distress (Lawton et al., 1989).

Adult day care is one form of respite that shows promise for reducing the deleterious effects of providing care (Gaugler & Zarit, 2001; Zarit, Stephens, Townsend, & Greene, 1998), although its usefulness may depend on how long the caregiver uses the program and what stressors are measured. Psychoeducational programs may be of subjective interest to family caregivers, but the subjective and positive effects of these programs are not universally found. Individual and family counseling has been found to be more effective than support groups in lessening the consequences of caregiving (Whitlatch, Zarit, & von Eye, 1991), but again these findings are not universal (Sörensen et al., 2002). In general, many interventions show promise in alleviating the negative consequences and enhancing the positive aspects of providing care to a relative with dementia. While these interventions vary in their strength, duration, and goals, their primary objective is typically to meet the needs of the family caregiver with less attention paid to the person with dementia.

Decision-Making Interventions

A relatively recent development in research and intervention design is the emphasis on working simultaneously with both the family caregiver and the care recipient (i.e., the care dyad). These research studies and interventions most typically focus on care dyads that include persons with early-stage dementia (Lyons, Zarit, Sayer, & Whitlatch, 2002; Yale, 1999) or cognitively intact care recipients with varying degrees of physical conditions (Horowitz, Silverstone, & Reinhardt, 1991). The impetus for this growing body of dyadic work is based on evidence that both care partners (e.g., caregiver and care recipient) experience stress and negative consequences as well as positive gains and that care partners are concerned with each other's well-being. Unfortunately, fragmented service delivery models typically serve either the caregiver or the impaired relative (rarely serving both), making it nearly impossible to design and conduct dyadic interventions.

Drawing on research using the stress process model of family caregiving (SPM; Aneshensel et al., 1995) and based on discussions with social workers and counselors, our research team expanded the SPM to include stressors associated with the caregiver's knowledge and understanding of their relative's values, preferences, and involvement in care (Feinberg & Whitlatch, 2001; Whitlatch, Feinberg, & Tucke, 2005b). Our findings indicated that caregivers were fairly accurate in their perceptions of their relative's care preferences. However, caregivers were not always accurate in their perceptions of just how important certain preferences were to their relatives, and caregivers sometimes disagreed with their relative's preferences.

To illustrate, let's take the case of a caregiving wife who accurately believes that her husband prefers to maintain his autonomy but does not realize that autonomy is extremely important to her husband. In fact, her husband reports that maintaining his autonomy is more important than feeling safe in his home even if it restricts his activity. The wife, who disagrees with her husband's preference and is getting overwhelmed with his increasing care needs, may decide to hire a home care aide to help her husband dress and bathe. The wife may become increasingly distressed if she knows hiring an aide is in opposition to her husband's preferences. Does her need for help outweigh his preference for autonomy? How can the needs of both care partners be balanced? These questions face families and service providers every day as they try to balance the needs and preferences of both caregivers and care recipients.

Balancing the needs and preferences of both care partners is especially challenging when dementia is involved. Divergent opinions, life histories, and care preferences become more difficult to resolve when one member of the dyad has dementia. As described earlier, research indicates that both caregivers and care recipients prefer family and friends to provide care and assistance and that the primary caregiver is the most preferred person within the informal network. Yet having one person provide the majority of care presents a huge challenge for families as the chronic condition worsens and the burden of care increases. Findings from our longitudinal research with care dyads indicate great variety in the amount of discussion between care partners about care preferences. The amount of discussion was only slightly related to knowledge about and agreement on specific care preferences (Clark, Whitlatch, & Tucke, 2005) and related care outcomes. We wondered if structured discussions with trained clinicians would have a positive impact on outcomes for care dyads. Thus, our research team designed and evaluated a dyadic intervention for caregivers and persons with early-stage dementia: early diagnosis dyadic intervention (EDDI; Whitlatch et al., 2006).

The EDDI program uses the opportunity afforded by early diagnosis to help both the caregiver and the person with dementia express their preferences and concerns about their care situation. As a result of their participation in EDDI, the dyad is expected to develop a stronger relationship bond (whether spousal or parent–child) through improved communication and problem solving. EDDI views both members of the dyad as partners rather than as a "giver" and a "receiver" of care and spends considerable time on dementia-specific care issues. Ultimately, dyads work together to develop a mutual plan for coping with the disease over the long term. The EDDI program is designed to be reassuring to caregivers and care receivers in the present and provide caregivers with a blueprint for how to approach difficult decisions in the future when the care receiver is no longer able to participate actively in the decision-making process (Whitlatch et al., 2006).

Briefly, EDDI consists of up to nine sessions and includes time for care partners to meet together and separately with the intervention specialist. Session 1 provides dyads with information about Alzheimer's disease and other dementias, memory loss, the implications of diagnosis, and available resources and introduces communication skills. Sessions 2 and 3 directs care partners to assess, prioritize, and compare their care values and preferences so that the dyad leaves session 3 with a "Shared Care Values" worksheet. In sessions 4 through 6, care partners examine where and how to find services or support that could be useful and discuss other topics that facilitate open communication between care partners. For sessions 7 and 8, the dyad discusses future challenges and the barriers for utilizing help and elicits possible solutions for overcoming these barriers. In session 9, the final session, the interventions specialist provides a final review to assess the progress made, identify unresolved issues, and review where one can go to get help.

Preliminary evaluation of the EDDI program indicates its feasibility and acceptability to both care partners and to the counselors who delivered the intervention (Whitlatch et al., 2006). EDDI's impact on care outcomes and well-being is also promising with preliminary evidence suggesting that both care partners benefit from their participation. The EDDI program as well as other early intervention and dyadic programs (see Clare, 2002; Yale, 1999) show promise for alleviating some of the stress and concerns experienced by both care partners.

CONCLUSION

This chapter has provided an overview of the issues, programs, and services specific to family caregivers who provide care for relatives with dementia. This overview illustrates that the experience of providing care and assistance to an older relative with dementia can be both stressful and rewarding. Professionals working with these families must have a thorough understanding of the nature and scope of these care stressors and rewards in order to provide care partners with effective services and interventions. Rather than working with one or the other of the care partners, it may be most effective to intervene with both care partners in a therapeutic environment that is compassionate and structured. Meeting and working with both the caregiver and the care recipient empowers both members of the care dyad and gives them the tools to make difficult care decisions throughout their care experience and as the dementia progresses.

REFERENCES

Aneshensel, C. S., Pearlin, L. I., Mullan, J. T., Zarit, S. H., & Whitlatch, C. J. (1995). *Profiles in caregiving: The unexpected career.* New York: Academic.

Bass, D. (2001). *Content and implementation of a caregiver assessment* (NFCSP Issue Brief). Washington, DC: U.S. Administration on Aging.

Bearon, L. B. (2004). *The burdens and blessings of family caregiving.* North Carolina Cooperative Extension Service.

Clare, L. (2002). We'll fight it as long as we can: Coping with the onset of Alzheimer's disease. *Aging and Mental Health, 6,* 139–148.

Clark, P. A., Whitlatch, C. J., & Tucke, S. S. (2005, November). *Knowledge and agreement of care preferences and dyadic well-being.* Paper presented at the annual meeting of the Gerontological Society of America, Orlando, Florida.

Dilworth-Anderson, P., Williams, I. C., & Gibson, B. E. (2002). Issues of race, ethnicity, and culture in caregiving research: A 20-year review (1980–2000). *The Gerontologist, 42,* 237–272.

Ditto, W. (2004). Lessons from cash and counseling. In *Innovations in Personal Assistance Services.* Symposium conducted at the annual meeting of the American Society on Aging and the National Council on the Aging, San Francisco, CA.

Donelan, K., Hill, C. A., Hofman, C., Scoles, K., Feldman, P. H., Levine, C., et al. (2002). Challenged to care: Informal caregivers in a changing health system. *Health Affairs, 21,* 222–231.

Doty, P. (2004). *Consumer-directed home care: Effects on family caregivers.* San Francisco: Family Caregiver Alliance.

Ellano, C. (1997, December). California CRC Assessment Tool training: Presentation to clinical staff. San Francisco, CA.

Family Caregiver Alliance. (2006). *Caregiver assessment: Principles, guidelines and strategies for change* (Report from a National Consensus Development Conference, Vol. 1). San Francisco: Author.

Farran, C. J., Miller, B. H., Kaufman, J. E., Donner, E., & Fogg, L. (1999). Finding meaning through caregiving: Development of an instrument for family caregivers of persons with Alzheimer's disease. *Journal of Clinical Psychology, 55,* 1107–1125.

Feinberg, L. F. (2004). The state of the art of caregiver assessment. *Generations, 27,* 24–32.

Feinberg, L. F., Newman, S. L., Gray, L., Kolb, K. N., & Fox-Grage, W. (2004). *The state of the states in family caregiver support: A 50-state study.* San Francisco: Family Caregiver Alliance.

Feinberg, L. F., Newman, S. L., & Van Steenberg, C. (2002). *Family caregiver support: Policies, perceptions, and practices in 10 states since passage of the National Family Caregiver Support Program.* San Francisco: Family Caregiver Alliance.

Feinberg, L. F., & Whitlatch, C. J. (2001). Are cognitively impaired adults able to state consistent choices? *The Gerontologist, 41,* 1–9.

Feinberg, L. F., & Whitlatch, C. J. (2002). Decision-making for persons with cognitive impairment and their family caregivers. *American Journal of Alzheimer's Disease and Other Dementias, 17,* 237–244.

Feinberg, L. F., Whitlatch, C. W., & Tucke, S. (2000). *Making hard choices: Respecting both voices* (Final Report to the Robert Wood Johnson Foundation). San Francisco: Family Caregiver Alliance.

Foley, K. L., Tung, H., & Mutran, E. J. (2002). Self gain and self-loss among African American and White caregivers. *Journal of Gerontology: Social Sciences, 57B,* S14–S22.

Fox-Grage, W., Coleman, B., & Blancato, R. B. (2001). *Federal and state policy in family caregiving: Recent victories but uncertain future.* San Francisco: Family Caregiver Alliance.

Gaugler, J. E., & Zarit, S. H. (2001). The effectiveness of adult day services for disabled older people. *Journal of Aging and Social Policy, 12*(2), 23–47.

Haley, W. E., Levine, E. G., Brown, S. L., Berry, J. W., & Hughes, G. H. (1987). Psychological, social and health consequences of caring for a relative with senile dementia. *Journal of the American Geriatrics Society, 35,* 405–411.

Horowitz, A., Silverstone, B. M., & Reinhardt, J. P. (1991). A conceptual and empirical exploration of personal autonomy issues within family caregiving relationships. *The Gerontologist, 31,* 23–31.

Ingersoll-Dayton, B., & Raschick, M. (2004). The relationship between care-recipient behaviors and spousal caregiving stress. *The Gerontologist, 44,* 318–327.

Kramer, B. J. (1997). Gain in the caregiving experience: Where are we? What next? *The Gerontologist, 37,* 218–232.

Lawton, M. P., Brody, E. M., & Saperstein, A. R. (1989). A controlled study of respite service for caregivers of Alzheimer's patients. *The Gerontologist, 29,* 8–16.

Lyons, K. S., Zarit, S. H., Sayer, A. G., & Whitlatch, C. J. (2002). Caregiving as a dyadic process: Perspectives from caregiver and receiver. *Journals of Gerontology: Psychological Sciences, 57B,* P195–P204.

Miller, B. (1990). Gender differences in spouse caregiver strain: Socialization and role explanations. *Journal of Marriage and the Family, 52,* 311–321.

Montgomery, R. J. V. (2002). In R. J. V. Montgomery (Ed.), *A new look at community-based respite programs: Utilization, satisfaction and development.* New York: Hawthorne.

National Alliance for Caregiving & American Association of Retired Persons. (1997, June). *Family caregiving in the U.S.: Findings from a national survey.* Bethesda, MD: National Alliance for Caregiving; Washington, DC: American Association of Retired Persons.

Pearlin, L. I., Aneshensel, C. S., Mullan, J. T., & Whitlatch, C. J. (1995). Caregiving and its social support. In L. K. George & R. H. Binstock (Eds.), *Handbook of aging and the social sciences* (4th ed., pp. 283–302). New York: Academic.

Pearlin, L. I., Mullan, J. T., Semple, S. J., & Skaff, M. M. (1990). Caregiving and the stress process: An overview of concepts and their measures. *The Gerontologist, 30,* 583–594.

Schulz, R., O'Brien, A. T., Bookwala, J., & Fleissner, K. (1995). Psychiatric and physical morbidity effects of dementia caregiving: Prevalence, correlates, and causes. *The Gerontologist, 35,* 771–791.

Sciegaj, M. (2001, October 18). Elder preferences for consumer direction. Paper presented at "Consumer Voice and Choice" conference, Scripps Gerontology Center, 4th Conference on Long-Term Care, Columbus, OH.

Sörensen, S., Pinquart, M., & Duberstein, P. (2002). How effective are interventions with caregivers? An updated meta-analysis. *The Gerontologist, 42,* 356–372.

Spector, W. D., Fleishman, J. A., Pezzin, L. E., & Spillman, B. C. (2000, September). *The characteristics of long-term care users* (AHRQ Publication No. 00–0049). Rockville, MD: Agency for Healthcare Research and Policy.

Spillman, B. C., & Black, K. J. (2005). *Staying the course: Trends in family caregiving* (Issue Paper No. 2005–17). Washington, DC: AARP Public Policy Institute.

Summer, L. (2003). *Choices and consequences: The availability of community-based long-term care services to the low-income population.* Washington, DC: Georgetown University, Long-Term Care Financing Project.

Whitlatch, C. J., Feinberg, L. F., & Tucke, S. T. (2005a). Accuracy and consistency of responses from persons with dementia. *Dementia: The International Journal of Social Research and Practice, 4,* 171–183.

Whitlatch, C. J., Feinberg, L. F., & Tucke, S. T. (2005b). Measuring the values and preferences for everyday care of persons with cognitive impairment and their family caregivers. *The Gerontologist, 45,* 370–380.

Whitlatch, C. J., Judge, K., Zarit, S. H., & Femia, E. (2006). Dyadic counseling for family caregivers and care receivers in early stage dementia. *The Gerontologist, 46,* 688–694.

Whitlatch, C. J., Zarit, S. H., & von Eye, A. (1991). Efficacy of interventions with caregivers: A reanalysis. *The Gerontologist, 31,* 9–14.

Yale, R. (1999). Support groups and other services for individuals with early-stage Alzheimer's disease. *Generations, 23,* 57–61.

Yee, J. L., & Schulz, R. (2000). Gender differences in psychiatric morbidity among family caregivers: A review and analysis. *The Gerontologist, 40,* 147–164.

Zarit, S. H., Stephens, M. A. P., Townsend, A., & Greene, R. (1998). Stress reduction for family caregivers: Effects of day care use. *Journal of Gerontology: Social Sciences, 53B,* S267–S277.

Zarit, S. H., & Whitlatch, C. J. (1992). Institutional placement: Phases of the transition. *The Gerontologist, 32,* 665–672.

CHAPTER EIGHT

Coping With Alzheimer's Disease: Clinical Interventions With Families

Cynthia Epstein

INTRODUCTION

Dementia has been characterized by Kahn (Groves et al., 1984) as a bio-psychosocial phenomenon. According to Roth and his colleagues, "50% of the behavior associated with Alzheimer's disease is not accounted for by loss of brain cells" but primarily by "the individual's personality, personal history, and current life situation" (Groves et al., 1984, p. 40). The needs of caregivers can be similarly understood. Social workers, committed by training and mind-set to the dignity, autonomy, and self-actualization of each client within the framework of a biopsychosocial understanding, are particularly suited to respond to families caring for a relative with Alzheimer's disease (AD), the most common form of dementia, and to the people with AD who rely on their support. The synergy speaks for itself.

This chapter describes the well-documented effects of caregiving for a family member with AD and some of the interventions tested in research studies that have proven helpful. It will also offer clinical impressions gathered from working with people with AD, their primary caregiver, and their family members at the New York University (NYU) Aging and Dementia Research Center in New York City and in private practice. My role in the NYU Spouse-Caregiver Study, described here, offered me a unique opportunity to provide counseling and support within the context of rigorous research protocol over the course of many years. It is hoped that information from this study and other sources, presented here in a question-and-answer format, will provide a supportive base from which social work clinicians can expand their skills and knowledge.

THE NYU SPOUSE-CAREGIVER STUDY

The NYU Longitudinal Spouse-Caregiver Study is an example of an intervention to enhance caregiver well-being and is comprised of several components. It provides individualized counseling and support over the entire course of the illness, whether the ill person lives at home or is transferred to a nursing home, and continues 2 years after the death of the person with AD. More than 406 spouse-caregivers have been followed since 1987. Those in the treatment group receive individual and family counseling and are encouraged to participate in a weekly support group, with counselors readily available to the caregiver and family members. The control caregivers are interviewed on the same schedule as treatment group members and receive information and help whenever it is asked for. Important outcomes of this study include the findings that treatment caregivers delay nursing home placement of their spouses by 329 days and do not show increases in depression compared to the control group (Mittelman, 2003).

"Progressive dementia is more disruptive of family life, more likely to have negative mental health outcomes for family caregivers (especially women), and more likely to limit the patient's capacity to live alone when compared to family care for other chronic conditions of late life" (Gwyther, 2000, p. 999). Dementia caregivers have been found to suffer disproportionately from depression, anxiety, stress, burden, and isolation. Physical and emotional well-being frequently decline. Contact with friends, as well as time spent on hobbies, travel, and other pleasurable activities, is reduced, and the conflict between work and family responsibilities increases. Ultimately, even premature mortality has been associated with caregiver strain among AD spouses (Gwyther, 2000). The toll on the caregiver may have serious consequences for the person with AD, causing the quality of home care to suffer and/or the person to be transferred to a nursing home.

Unfortunately, counselors at NYU and other researchers have found that even when the difficult decision to place a family member has been made for good reasons, new and different kinds of problems may arise.

Family members have to deal with their relative's and their own reaction to the new setting as well as to new people and systems. While there may eventually be a satisfactory adjustment for the resident and the family members, the distress is sometimes ongoing. "Every time I go to the nursing home I die a little," said a 92-year-old husband of his visits to his wife of 67 years. "I see her in that chair trying to get out, and I am sick in my heart." Congregate care can rarely match the standard of good in-home care. Residents may not receive enough individual attention, and their freedoms and activities may be limited by the availability of staff to keep them safe and occupied. Often families are not aware that they can hire additional help to personally attend to their relative. Counselors at NYU routinely offer this information when nursing home placement is considered, and many families provide their relatives with this service despite its considerable cost.

Research on Coping and Clinical Practice With Caregivers

Even when the decline of the person with AD does not result in transfer to a nursing home or other care facility (in the absence of medical illness, people with AD do not decline precipitously), caregivers experience repeated cycles of upset. "You get used to the way it is and even let yourself believe that things won't change" is a feeling expressed by many caregivers. Then something does change, and it is necessary for the caregiver to readjust and establish "a new normal" (Gwyther, 2000) until, as is inevitable, the cycle is repeated.

The clinician's knowledge of the progression of the illness can help caregivers anticipate the next likely change and prepare for the "here we go again" moment, allowing them to feel more empowered to carry on. This proactive stance, called *problem focused* or *instrumental,* is a kind of coping strategy that research has identified as constructive (leading to lower levels of depressive symptoms). It is distinct from *avoidance coping*—refusal to believe the situation exists, wishfulness, or emotional discharge—which is associated with depressive symptoms (Powers, Gallagher-Thompson, & Kraemer, 2002). Wishing does not make it so. Addressing the issue does.

What Can Help

The protocol of the NYU Spouse-Caregiver Study requires that clinicians contact participants on a regular basis, although they are permitted to (and frequently do) initiate additional contacts on the basis of their assessment of possible need. The clinician, by checking in with caregiving clients who do not reach out for help, do not acknowledge that they are having a problem, or are too overwhelmed to remember to call, serves as a model for taking a proactive stance. Incipient problems and high levels of stress can be picked up before a crisis develops. At such strategic moments, caregivers may be receptive to suggestions to exercise, meditate, or make changes in their caregiving plan or style. In almost all cases, these calls are really appreciated. Over time, caregivers may "catch on" to the clinician's approach and become more self-aware and "on top" of their caregiving needs. Participants enrolled in the Spouse-Caregiver Study repeatedly cited the counselors' reliable availability as the service that was most beneficial and comforting to them. "Even if I didn't call, I knew that I could and that someone would be there for me, and that made all the difference" was a comment by a study participant that expresses the sentiments of many (Mittelman, 2003).

Acceptance is another coping strategy that is associated with decreases in negative affect in caregivers. Thought of as a bridging concept with elements of both emotional and instrumental modes of coping, it represents an active stance in which the caregiver chooses to bring acceptance to the painful emotions of helplessness, grief, and sorrow; and then, no longer depleted by the struggle to avoid them, is able to take steps to ameliorate the situation. These actions may include joining a support group or exercise program, cultivating a hobby, going back to a project that has been deferred or neglected, or just allowing oneself to "be" and not "do." They might also include making changes in the home that enable the person with AD to get around more easily or have more emotionally satisfying experiences, such as listening to music or exercising together.

Responding creatively to the changes in function or cognition of the person with AD can be a gratifying and empowering experience. Acceptance is a realistic stance, neither morbid nor euphoric. It is a solid platform from which the caregiver can take care of him- or herself and consequently the person with AD.

The Mediators of Research Outcomes: How Are the Findings Explained?

Stress and coping theories have been the basis of research efforts to identify the mediators—those variables that most strongly account for study outcomes, whether positive or negative. The experience of stress is generally understood as dependent on the individual's appraisal of both the situation and his or her perceived ability to cope (Neundorfer, 1991). Interventions directed toward modifying these variables have been designed and tested and can provide direction to clinical work.

Social Support

The stress/coping perspective is supported by the findings of the NYU study, which showed that both appraisal of the difficult behaviors of AD and feelings of depression are mediated by social support. Social support is a buttress against the potential emotional and physical drain of caregiving, thereby enhancing feelings of well-being and, both directly and indirectly, the ability to cope with caregiving (Roth, Mittelman, Clay, Madan, & Haley, 2005).

Although the design and intention of the study was carefully explained at the time of enrollment, many of the participating spouse-caregivers had mixed feelings about seeking emotional and concrete support for themselves. Thus, the counselor's first step in implementing the protocol was to explain the potential benefits of help and then to encourage each caregiver to use the family sessions to ask for the kind of help he or she wanted (rather than resentfully wait for it to be offered) and ultimately to accept help when offered. It was also important to teach the caregiver how to let go of expectations from relatives who had been persistently disappointing and focus on those that had been more satisfying. In our research, we found that negative interactions with a family member from whom help was anticipated increases the stress on the caregiver—sometimes, ironically, to a greater degree than positive ones help.

In the first of two individual sessions, spouses identified potential attendees for four family sessions, and despite the parent's fears, no adult child failed to respond to a request to attend during the course of the study, even when there was a history of family acrimony, busy schedules, or other commitments. Some alienated children welcomed the opportunity to reconnect with their family. If the parent feels unable to contact the children or other potential attendees, the counselor might take the initiative so that the collaborative process can get underway.

The sessions sought to identify areas in which the caregiver needed support, such as staying with the ill person, accompanying him or her to visit a friend, filing documents, communicating with lawyers, mowing the lawn, doing household repairs, or speaking more often on the telephone. Tasks were allocated according to the willingness and abilities of different family members to fulfill them. Since planning for the future involves decisions that may affect all members of the family, it is be best if they can work together to address them (Mittelman, Epstein, & Pierzchala, 2003). With this in mind, the counselor focused the discussion on the issues at hand (rather than the settling of old scores) and provided education, resources, and referrals as needed.

Appraisal

Change in a caregiver's *appraisal* (the personal meaning attributed to an event) of his or her situation or of the behavior of his or her relative with AD, can have a significant impact on reactivity and subsequent feelings of anxiety and depression. The NYU Spouse-Caregiver Study has shown that caregivers can learn to become less reactive to dementia-related behaviors, such as becoming distressed when the person continues to ask the same question over and over. The difference in reaction might result from shifting the appraisal from "He is doing this to annoy me" or "She could do better if she tried" to "I guess this is really a symptom of the cognitive loss of AD" or "It must be really frightening when he doesn't remember where we need to go." From this perspective there is no victim and no victimizer—just two people trying to cope as best they can.

To the degree that caregivers remain unrealistic about their relatives' intentions or capacities—whether because of denial of the illness, reactivation of past issues, paranoia, or other personality problems—both are in jeopardy. There is a risk of abuse and neglect of the person with the illness and of emotional deterioration of the caregiver. Based on the assessment of the caregiver's capacity to care for his or her relative with dementia, extensive supportive counseling or referral for more intensive treatment may be indicated as well as, in some instances, institutional placement of the person with AD.

OTHER STUDIES

There are literally hundreds (maybe thousands) of studies that have tested various protocols, such as providing skills training for caregivers to enhance their response to difficult behaviors, helping them appreciate and assume a more clinical belief set about caregiving, and increasing their awareness of pleasant activities they might engage in while encouraging them to exercise, modify the home, and utilize available services (Hepburn, Tornatore, Center, & Ostwald, 2001). Some of these interventions are offered in the home to the caregiver and care recipient; others are group interventions in which participants share common concerns. Some are more didactic; others are more interactive. They can take place in community centers, AD centers, churches, libraries, or other accessible settings. Interventions that contain many different elements that can be individualized generally have the best outcomes, although teasing out the "active" (element of the program responsible for the results) ingredient in them remains a research challenge (Schulz et al., 2002).

Clinicians working with family caregivers will want to be up to date on the latest research findings. However, the translation of these findings into acceptable and workable solutions that affect changes in caregiver behavior is a clinical task that will be as difficult or as easy as helping any other client grow and change.

What Research Doesn't Tell Us About Coping

Researchers have not yet definitively determined whether individuals will use the same coping strategies over time regardless of their effectiveness or whether they will flexibly adopt the most effective methods to fit the situation. For instance, a wife who is trying to deal with her husband's confusion in new places may become overprotective—preventing him from going to the corner newsstand, for instance, which he is still able to find—as an expression of her own limited anxiety tolerance. "You know I am a worrier," says the wife, who is rarely free of concern about her husband. "Will you please leave dad alone, he'll be all right," replies the son, who can tolerate more risk.

However, those who deny the dangers may not be adequately protective, thereby placing the person with AD at risk of getting lost, taking the wrong medication, being exploited, or mismanaging resources that may endanger him or her or the well-being of the family. Clinicians therefore need to be mindful of each client's coping repertoire and help him or her compensate for ineffective methods or develop the confidence to try new approaches.

What Can Help

Some caregivers may gain a more objective view of their own reactions by reviewing research studies. It may also help them to be more compassionate toward themselves if they have an idea of how many studies it has taken for researchers to begin to understand the complex experience of caring for a person with AD. Role playing can also be an effective tool for helping caregivers try out and practice new behaviors.

ISSUES FAMILIES FACE UPON A DIAGNOSIS OF AD

Once a diagnosis of AD is made, families face a number of issues, including concerns about the accuracy of the diagnosis, deciding when and how to discuss the diagnosis with others, and discussing their own feelings about the situation. They will need to understand the medical, legal, and financial decisions involved in caring for someone with AD. They may also worry about where the family member with AD will ultimately live and how their own lives will change as a result.

Is the Diagnosis Correct?

According to Rabins (2006), physicians are typically 90% accurate in diagnosing the cause of dementia. However, it is sometimes necessary and even sound medical thinking to get second and third opinions before accepting a diagnosis of AD. At the same time, repeated searching for a different diagnosis may also be an expression of an inability to accept the reality of the illness and what it entails.

What Can Help

Clinicians should explore prior experiences that may explain the client's help-seeking behavior and reaction to the diagnosis of AD. Have mistakes been made in the past? Is AD too upsetting to contemplate? What is the prior experience with the illness? The question "What would it feel like to let yourself know that your husband/wife (or father/mother, etc.) has AD?" can be a starting point for understanding reactions to the diagnosis.

Who Should Be Told of the Diagnosis?

Families sometimes request that their relative not be told they have AD. They also wonder if other family members or friends should be told. Those who feel that their relative is still able to carry on social interactions fairly normally or are particularly upset by the inappropriate social behaviors may be afraid of the rejection that their relative and they themselves will experience if the diagnosis is known. While there may be some validity in their concern, they are putting themselves and their relative under the additional pressure of trying to conceal and control something that cannot be controlled and that will inevitably be revealed. Eventually, the symptoms will be undeniable. Consequently, it is best to clarify the nature of the problem so that open communication can be maintained.

What Can Help

The practitioner should explore what family members are afraid of—the reaction of their relative, of others, or of their own feelings. Families need to know that on many occasions when the diagnosis is presented, the person who receives it appears not to hear it and does not seem to come away from the interview upset. Sometimes the person acknowledges the diagnosis but without the expected reaction of sadness and worry. These responses may represent a self-protective defense that should not be challenged at the time or maybe ever.

If the person is in the early stage of the illness and understands and accepts the diagnosis, he or she may welcome the opportunity to talk about it and to participate in making plans for care and other necessary financial, legal, and medical arrangements. Such a person might want to join a support group for people in the early stage. The diagnosis may even come as a relief and make sense of the changes that have been noticed but not understood.

However, even when the diagnosis is entirely expected or has been given before, the person with the illness, as well as the family members, may experience shock. It is helpful to normalize this response. Coming to true acceptance is a process that takes time. In many cases, disclosure can be made over time, on an as-needed basis. Unfortunately, since extensive and persistent denial can put the person with the illness and others at risk, the clinician must challenge such denial.

Who Must Be Told About the Diagnosis?

Doctors must be informed that their patient has been diagnosed with dementia and may not be able to provide reliable medical information, take medications, or follow a prescribed regime or diet. Such failures can be life threatening.

What Can Help

It is essential that persons with dementia are accompanied to medical appointments and procedures. It is also potentially dangerous to leave a person with AD unsupervised in a hospital. The combination of a medical illness, a strange environment, and unfamiliar people and procedures can put a person with AD, even in the early stage, at high risk for an extended stay and a poor outcome. Sometimes family members think that a hospitalization can provide a respite opportunity for them since the hospital staff is responsible for the care of the patient. However, staff is usually stressed to the limit and may lack the capacity to meet the needs of a person with cognitive impairment.

As soon as the diagnosis is known, families should be encouraged to find a doctor who understands dementia and is responsive to their needs. The doctor should be prepared to work collaboratively with the family and other medical providers and be alert to illness and depression in the caregiver. A supportive doctor can greatly ease the task of providing preventive and acute care for the person with AD. Such care will in turn ease the stress and burden of the caregiver.

In addition to their doctors, other professionals such as lawyers and accountants who provide services to the person with dementia should be made aware of the diagnosis. With their guidance, the need to inform institutions such as banks can be determined. However, a diagnosis of dementia does not mean that a person cannot continue to make decisions regarding his or her life and care. Even if the person does not remember what he or she has decided, the ability to express an opinion can still inform the decision-making process.

Sharing Feelings About the Illness

When a person is diagnosed with AD, everyone in the family—particularly spouses and adult children—will have different responses and feelings about the illness.

Spouses

In the early stages of AD, subtle differences in a patient's functioning may not be easily noticed by others, yet the husband or wife may already be compensating for them by providing reminders and cues and keeping an eye open for potential problems. The spouse may not yet be aware of his or her need for emotional or practical support or, if he or she is, may not be sure how much distress to share with friends and adult children and how much help can be realistically expected. "Close friends or family may not recognize the losses in intimacy and companionship they may be experiencing, intensifying their feelings of loss, isolation, and abandonment" (Rankin, Haunt, & Keefover, 2001, p. 30). Throughout the course of the illness, spouses constantly have to readjust their expectations of their partner and redesign the landscape of their marriage as well as virtually all other aspects of their life.

What Can Help

A new intervention for couples, one of whom is in the early stage of AD, is currently being tested at the NYU Aging and Dementia Center. Counseling shows promise of facilitating constructive discussion of reactions to the diagnosis and its effect on each person individually as well as on the relationship. The experience of openly expressing feelings to each other may support the couple's bond and mitigate some of the losses resulting from the illness.

When the identity of the well spouse is deeply dependent on the declining partner, the progressive loss of a sense of self and internal stability can put such a spouse in what may feel like a continuing struggle for survival as a person, similar to that of the partner with AD. It takes considerable effort and therapeutic support for such a spouse to fill in what is experienced as missing pieces of him- or herself and to feel whole again.

Counselors should be aware that when couples have been experiencing marital difficulties before the onset of dementia, the spouse-caregiver is more vulnerable to the negative effects of caregiving. Providing care out of a sense of obligation puts him or her at increased risk of depression (Morris, Morris, & Britton, 1989).

Spouses should be encouraged to join support groups to increase their understanding of the illness and contact with others who are dealing with similar issues. In some settings, there may also be activity groups that people with dementia and their family members can attend together, thereby maintaining a sense of social connectedness.

Adult Children

In my experience, adult children are generally less reluctant than spouses to reveal a diagnosis of AD. They generally attach less stigma to the illness and often find that their peers are dealing with similar issues. However, the demands that caregiving places on adult children may exceed those on spouses.

In general, adult children are juggling more roles and complex caregiving situations than caregiving spouses. Those who live with their ill parent often seem a lot like spouses in their caregiving style. They are often reluctant to hire help, suffer from social isolation, and compromise their financial well-being to attend to their parent. Sometimes both parents require care, and the one caring for the person with dementia may be frail or ill him- or herself. This parent may want and need the support of adult children but have different ideas about the nature of that support that frustrate family members' efforts to help.

An example of such a situation involved an alcoholic husband who made what seemed like excessive demands on his children to care for their mother while retaining control over her medications, which he altered at will, and supporting her resistance to attend a day care center, which might have been beneficial to her. The counselor's observation to the son that his feelings of powerlessness in ensuring better care for his mother was causing him pain came as a surprise to him. He then reflected how his father's irrational behavior had for years left him feeling helpless when taking essential steps in his life.

What Can Help

This son is like a lot of other adult children who need help identifying and prioritizing the needs of their parent or parents and balancing them with their own. When there is more than one sibling, they often need help in working together as a team, although it is also common for one to become the primary caregiver, with the other(s) feeling either resentful or relieved. If it is at all possible to bring the family together, many of these issues can at least be addressed and workable arrangements developed. It is becoming more common for grandchildren, out of respect for and attachment to their grandparent, to share in the caregiving and help their caregiving parents. Their presence at a family meeting can enliven the energy and manifest the continuity of the generations.

Even adult children who are keeping their distance from their parents are usually willing to come for one counseling meeting when it is made clear that this is not an effort to recruit them into active service but rather to maintain open communication. Whether an adult child lives near the parent with dementia, with the parent, or at a distance from the parent, he or she is more often than not painfully aware of the changes in the parent and in need of his or her own support.

Family members can benefit by joining support groups and attending conferences and lectures that will help them see how others are coping. Enrolling in a clinical trial is another resource that can provide added support and access to the newest medications and clinical interventions as well as the opportunity to contribute to the understanding of AD and caregiving. Both NYU and the University of Minnesota are currently enrolling adult children who are primary caregivers for a parent with dementia in a replication of the intervention that has proven so helpful to spouse-caregivers. There is never a cost to participate; sometimes compensation is offered, and strict oversight by institutional review boards ensures that no harm will come to study subjects. Studies can be located at http://www.clinicaltrials.gov.

Where Should the Person With AD Live?

The question of relocation—should the ill parent move in with or closer to the children or to a care facility or remain in place?—should be examined in detail, ideally in a family meeting since individual members frequently do not have adequate information about the implications of each option and make impulsive, if well-intentioned, decisions.

What Can Help

Encourage family members to verbalize in detail the reasons they are advocating for a certain living arrangement. Too often adult children have unrealistic images of how it will be to have their parent live with them or in a care facility and need help in evaluating their options and doing extensive research about the decisions they will make. Elderly people are generally reluctant to relocate, and their wish to stay in familiar surroundings should always be appreciated. When such a move is unavoidable, every effort should be made to re-create the comforts of home.

How Will Roles in the Family Change?

When a relative is diagnosed with AD, family members are frequently referred to by professionals as caregivers and the person with AD as their loved one. These terms represent assumptions and expectations that may not accurately reflect how family members view and feel about each other and should not be used automatically. Family members may not think of themselves as caregivers, certainly not when their relative is in the early stage of the illness, and people with AD may not view their relatives as their caregivers. Family members generally continue to refer to each other in terms of their relationships—my mother, my husband, and so on—and clinicians should be aware of the power of language to communicate recognition of the person's continued role in the family. Of a dying old woman in the late stage of the illness, a middle-aged daughter said, "She is still my mother, even though she hasn't recognized me in years."

In families where the roles are clearly defined and any changes in them a threat to the existing structure, it may feel frightening and even disrespectful to assume tasks formerly performed by the now ill person. A wife, for example, who may not have been informed about family finances, may find herself having to prepare the income taxes or deal with insurance companies for the first time. A husband may need to shop for food, household goods, and personal products and have no idea about brands and sizes. Adult children may be reluctant to ask parents about their resources or to take on roles they have always performed. However, in order to maintain the integrity of the family system, be it that of a couple or an extended family, tasks will have to be reallocated.

What Can Help

It may take an outsider to articulate the difficulty family members are experiencing. Fear of being accused of usurping the position of the ill relative, metaphorically killing him or her off, may leave family members immobilized. It is of course realistic to be concerned about one's ability to perform certain tasks, but it is possible for relatives to set about learning what to do and/or how to get help. It obviously requires a sufficient degree of awareness and acceptance of the effects of the illness on the family member to move ahead. Each family member's knowledge and understanding of AD can be a natural place to start the discussion.

Medical, Legal, and Financial Issues

There are important issues that should be addressed while the person with AD is still able to participate in the process and express his or her point of view. These issues can be highly charged and may evoke conflict between the person with AD and the spouse or adult child closely involved in care but may also reverberate throughout the family.

Medical Issues

Many medical settings request that patients complete advance directives indicating their wishes for care or appoint a proxy should they become unable to express themselves. While everyone should complete these documents, they are especially relevant to people with dementia because their inability to express themselves can be anticipated. Caregivers who know their relative's wishes, even if they do not agree with them, are obligated to fulfill them. This situation is preferable to not knowing what the patient would have wanted and always wondering whether the decisions made were in the best interests of the patient. A residue of guilt for treatments given or withheld can be a tragic legacy of caregiving. Clinicians should therefore take the initiative in raising the issues of medical and end-of-life care.

Legal/Financial Issues

Powers of attorney should be executed as soon as possible to enable the person with AD to play a part in the designation. The use of funds for care, the kind of care the person with AD wants, and how such decisions will be made can be a source of family conflict. It is common for each family member to envision these choices playing out differently and to have different agendas and needs. The steps that must be taken to access entitlements may be stressful, and the absence of mutual trust may prevent parents and children from taking them.

What Can Help

Family members can attend seminars at the Alzheimer's Association or other such reliable sources to get basic information about these difficult issues. The decisions they will need to make can be complex and confusing and entwined with feelings about who should care for the person with AD, who should help, what kind of care is required, and how resources should be allocated and preserved. Again, family meetings (with a lawyer, an accountant, and a social worker present) may be the most efficient venue for addressing these questions.

When Should a Person With AD Stop Driving?

Determining when a person with AD can no longer drive safely is one of the most difficult decisions families face early in the disease process and often triggers a call for help. Even those who no longer feel safe in the car with their relative are reluctant to address this issue. Sometimes the person with AD is the only one who knows how to drive, and public transportation is not easily available. More often it is the reluctance to inflict further emotional pain that prevents family members from acting.

What Can Help

Knowing what to look for. Family members should be aware of the following warning signs: braking often for no apparent reason, missing signs and signals, getting angry easily, swerving in and out of lanes, and getting lost in familiar places ("The Driving Decision," 2006). Fender benders or other minor accidents that may be rationalized as someone else's fault still pose a risk of serious injury to the person with AD and others. The possibility that the insurance company may not cover such accidents if the diagnosis becomes known can provide further leverage that allows the person with AD to relinquish the wheel. When rational entreaties fail, it may be necessary to resort to such strategies as disabling the car, hiding the keys, or getting rid of the car altogether. In spite of their protests, some seniors are actually grateful to be relieved of the burden of driving. Access-a-ride and similar programs may be acceptable if not entirely satisfactory substitutes for the loss of the independence of driving a car. For further discussion, see chapter 15.

WHEN FAMILIES MAY NEED TO HIRE HELP

Most likely, families will not need to hire help during early stage AD. As it progresses, however, help may be needed.

Early-Stage Issues

It is difficult and not usually necessary to introduce formal or paid help at this time. If friends and relatives are available to accompany the person with AD to activities or appointments, it will ease the role of the primary caregiver and can provide a pleasant social occasion for both parties. In addition, the responsibilities of people who are already in the system, such as a housekeeper, bookkeeper, or teenager who mows the lawn, can be unobtrusively extended to be more available to the person with AD. Volunteers, students, and aspiring actors who often need temporary employment and have the right temperament for the job can also be suitable companions for people in the early stage.

It is wise to enroll people in the early stage in the Safe Return Program, a nationwide registry maintained by the Alzheimer's Association that enables the police to identify a person with AD who has become lost and to locate his or her family. Family members and the person with AD often protest that it is too soon to take this step, but the clinician should be persistent and insistent. The potential danger to the person with AD and the distress the family will experience may not be fully grasped until it is too late. To enroll, a family member can call toll-free 800-272-3900.

Middle-Stage Issues

Caring for a person in the middle stage of AD can be very demanding of a caregiver's time, energy, and creativity. The person needs help with the activities of daily living and almost constant supervision. The behavioral symptoms such as agitation, wandering, aggressiveness, incontinence, delusions, and hallucinations also emerge at this point in the illness. Some people are placed in nursing homes because of incontinence and aggression during this stage, although most continue to be cared for at home.

If family and friends have not yet developed a support network and the person with AD is to remain at home, it is time to discuss involving others in his or her care. In our experience at NYU, wives were generally more reluctant than husbands (or adult children) to involve an outsider in the care of their spouse. Some adult children, especially daughters, may feel a cultural imperative to provide all the care. It is essential to work with and around this expectation before the caregiver emotionally or physically breaks down. Caregivers may need help in engaging and developing a working relationship with a professional caregiver. An experienced home health aide can take over many of the personal care tasks performed by the family, thereby providing physical and emotional relief. Sometimes financial constraints are a factor in limiting the option of paid help.

Family caregivers may need special skills and benefit from training to help them respond to the demands of this stage without getting injured or allowing the interactions with their relative to escalate into a confrontation. While it may not be possible to eliminate behaviors that can be troubling to the person with AD as well as the caregiver, it is certainly possible to avoid exacerbating them, and in some situations, when the need behind the behavior is understood and satisfied, the behavior may remit.

Caregivers need to know the cardinal rule that a person with AD should never be forced or hurried. They should also understand the concept of the *progressively lowered stress threshold,* which explains that the person with dementia can tolerate less and less stimuli before feeling overwhelmed, especially as the illness progresses (Richards & Beck, 2004).

Sensitivity to the perspective of the person with AD who may be confused, frightened, and experiencing a loss of control and subsequent embarrassment can help caregivers assume a gentle, nonthreatening approach that will enable their relative to cooperate with care and often diffuse tense situations. The daily schedule and environment should be geared to meet the person at his or her comfort level. The proper use of incontinence products and initiation of a toileting schedule can reduce the practical concerns around incontinence. To their surprise, many family caregivers get over their initial reaction to incontinence, and spouses may continue to share a bed long after it emerges.

There are numerous articles and Web sites that offer information about coping with the middle stage. They address creating an AD-friendly environment (consistent, well lit, engaging, but not overstimulating), suitable activities that preserve involvement and maintain self-esteem, and effective communication techniques, all of which can do much to mitigate the symptoms of this stage. I have listed many of these Web sites in the resource section at the back of this book.

Sometimes medications are necessary to reduce anxiety, hallucinations, delusions (only if they are disturbing to the person with AD), and sleep problems when other options have not been successful. However, medicating an elderly person who has dementia requires specific knowledge and sensitivity and is probably best handled by a geriatric psychiatrist or neurologist. The side effects of medications and their interactions are always a concern, and caregivers need to be taught what to look for and how to respond.

People in the middle stage frequently suffer from what has been called the "empty day syndrome," which results from their inability to initiate and follow through on an activity. Attending a day care center may be a very practical and constructive response that alleviates the situation and provides respite for the caregiver.

What Can Help

Entitlements and community resources that offer scholarships or low-cost help may be available and not known to the caregiver. The local Alzheimer's Association may be aware of aides trained in dementia care who are looking for work as well as other resources. Even so, language and cultural differences can make finding a compatible fit among the person with AD, family members, and a home health aide an extended process in which the social worker can play a mediating and interpretive role. However, relationships with paid and unpaid help can be a source of support as well as disappointment. When a trusted aide leaves, the caregiver suffers yet another loss and may need counseling to regroup emotionally in order to initiate and have trust in a new relationship.

Late-Stage Issues

By the end of this stage, people with AD need to be fed, bathed, changed, comforted, and attended to in every way. This does not mean that it is not important to speak to the person, touch and massage him or her, play music, and create a comfortable physical and emotional environment. As questions around such medical and end-of-life care as the use of feeding tubes emerge, the issues caregivers face are literally awesome. Ideally, the family has discussed end-of-life issues in the past, and the wishes of the person are known. Even when this is the case and there are no family conflicts, implementing the directives and living through the dying process with their relative can be very stressful.

What Can Help

The stages of AD may unfold over as many as 20 years, with the final stage lasting for months or even years. The family caregiver will need support for staying the physical and emotional course that is leading to the inevitable death of the person with AD. Home health care as well as ongoing participation in a support group or counseling are needed. Families usually have little information about the implications of the use of a feeding tube with people who have late-stage dementia. They may have fantasies about the suffering a person would experience if he or she were not fed or hydrated but little understanding of the consequences of using these measures when the body is shutting down.

Helping family members meet with medical personnel who can explain what is understood about how the body dies may allow them to feel more comfortable with their decision not to use extraordinary measures if, as the proxy, they have this option. Enrolling the ill person in hospice, a program dedicated to providing comfort, support, and relief of suffering while preserving the patient's dignity, can be a great help during this difficult time. Services for the patient include home care, medication, and medical supplies, nurse and doctor visits, and provision to transport the body when the person dies without having to call 911. Hospice also reaches out to family members with a range of services such as counseling, support groups, massage, and a 24-hour hotline.

Whether offered at home or in a hospital, nursing home, or inpatient hospice unit, hospice is available to all AD patients who are in the very latest stage of the illness and is covered by both Medicare and Medicaid. When the decision has been made to stop aggressive treatment, family members need to be educated about hospice and have myths about the service and its meaning dispelled. Family members who fear that they are withholding treatment can view hospice care as an opportunity to give their family member the best possible care until the last moment of life. In some cases they may need help advocating for this decision with the patient's doctors (Mittelman & Epstein, 2002).

If the patient has asked that all means be used to preserve life, the family may be spared the decision-making process. As much as information, families need emotional support to face end-of-life care issues, a forum to resolve conflicts among themselves, and a holding environment in which to express and explore their feelings. If the patient is in a hospital, it may be necessary to convene the ethics committee when conflicts among family members cannot be resolved. Representatives of the clergy may offer comfort and support, and the clinician should reach out for these and any other available supports on behalf of the family.

The Death of the Person With AD

It is not unusual for family members to have both wished for and feared the death of the person with AD and to have experienced these mixed feelings over the course of the illness. When death finally comes, especially if the person is not in the late stage, both guilt and sorrow may be expressed. These feelings need to be met with acceptance by professional caregivers to help family members accept them within themselves.

The death of a person, even when viewed as a relief of suffering, remains a profound event and should be respected as such. Family members sometimes say that the person they knew died a long time ago, but the actual death that brings an end to caregiving alters the day-to-day life of the caregiver and can leave a void and a sense of loss when the activities that have organized his or her time for years are no longer needed.

There is some evidence that dementia caregivers experience two kinds of grief. Initially, it is for the person as he or she was at death. In time, grief for the person as he or she was before the dementia may emerge, and the mourning process may be experienced again. Some caregiver support groups expect a member to leave at a predetermined time after the death. A caregiver may experience this as yet another loss and feel angry and rejected. Even when this ending does not seem to be premature, individual sessions may still be useful at this time. After the acute grief response remits, a bereavement group may provide ongoing support and community.

Keeping the Big Picture in Mind

Alzheimer's is often not the only issue family members are dealing with, and their reactions to it may be influenced by other concerns, such as an ill child or grandchild, a recent relocation, financial concerns, or the poor health of the well spouse or the person with AD. All these concerns need to be taken into account in creating a care plan for coping with the AD.

IS THERE AN UPSIDE TO CAREGIVING?

The positive effects of caregiving are now receiving more attention from researchers and service providers. This perspective may have been fueled by the current focus on positive psychology, the recognition of potential benefits of alternative therapies, mind–body practices, and an appreciation of the spiritual components of the caregiving experience. Efforts to develop measures for capturing the positive elements—frequently defined as "satisfaction" but also as "pleasures and rewards, enjoyment of caregiving"—and the variables that account for them are underway (Tarlow et al., 2004).

CONCLUSION

Across the spectrum of caregiving, families need support to cope with the ongoing practical and emotional challenges they face. There is probably no substitute for a caring therapeutic relationship and alliance to facilitate changes and growth, to enable caregivers to integrate new learning, to use resources effectively, and to fully experience the sorrows, losses, and gratifications of caregiving. Clinicians who share this journey will undoubtedly be altered by it as well. The opportunity and responsibility of relieving the suffering of a fellow human being may indeed be a spiritual experience and the unintended gift of AD to us all. The need for the person with AD to find meaning in life and maintain a positive sense of self deserves the same support and access to resources as other family members. More than anyone else, this is the person who must cope with AD; the social worker can be a great help in this coping process.

REFERENCES

The driving decision: Time to give up the keys? (2006, March). *The Johns Hopkins Medical Letter: Health After 50, 18,* 6–7.

Groves, L., Lazarus, L. W., Newton, N., Frankel, R., Gutmann, D. L., & Ripeckyi, A. (1984). Brief psychotherapy with spouses of patients with Alzheimer's disease: Relief of the psychological burden. In L. W. Lazarus (Ed.), *Clinical approaches to psychotherapy with the elderly* (pp. 38–53). Washington, DC: American Psychiatric Press.

Gwyther, L. P. (2000). Family issues in dementia: Finding a new normal. *Neurologic Clinics, 18*(4), 993–1010.

Hepburn, K. W., Tornatore, J., Center, B., & Ostwald, S. W. (2001). Dementia family caregiver training: Affecting beliefs about caregiving and caregiver outcomes. *Journal of the American Geriatrics Society, 49,* 450–457.

Mittelman, M. S. (2003). Psychosocial intervention for dementia caregivers: What can it accomplish? *International Psychogeriatrics, 15*(Suppl. 1), 243–249.

Mittelman, M. S., & Epstein, C. (2002). *The Alzheimer's health care handbook: How to get the best medical care for your relative with Alzheimer's disease, in and out of the hospital.* New York: Marlowe.

Mittelman, M. S., Epstein, C., & Pierzchala, A. (2003). *Counseling the Alzheimer's caregiver: A resource for health care professionals.* Chicago: AMA Press.

Morris, L. W., Morris, R. G., & Britton, P. G. (1989). The relationship between marital intimacy, perceived strain and depression in spouse caregivers of dementia sufferers. *British Journal of Medical Psychology, 61,* 231–236.

Neundorfer, M. M. (1991). Coping and health outcomes in spouse caregivers of persons with dementia. *Nursing Research, 40,* 260–265.

Powers, D. V., Gallagher-Thompson, D., & Kraemer, H. C. (2002). Coping and depression in Alzheimer's caregivers: Longitudinal evidence of stability. *Journal of Gerontology: Psychological Sciences, 57B,* P205–P211.

Rabins, P. (2006, March). When is dementia reversible? *The Johns Hopkins Medical Letter: Health After 50, 18,* 1–5.

Rankin, E. D., Haut, M. W., & Keefover, R. W. (2001). Current marital functioning as a mediating factor in depression among spouse caregivers in dementia. *Clinical Gerontologist, 23,* 27–44.

Richards, K. C., & Beck, C. K. (2004). Progressively lowered stress threshold model: Understanding behavioral symptoms of dementia. *Journal of the American Geriatrics Society, 52,* 1774–1775.

Roth, D. R., Mittelman, M. S., Clay, O. J., Madan, A., & Haley, W. E. (2005). Changes in social support as mediators of the impact of a psychosocial intervention for spouse caregivers of persons with Alzheimer's disease. *Psychology and Aging, 20,* 634–644.

Schulz, R., O'Brien, A., Czaja, S., Ory, M., Norris, R., Martire, L. M., et al. (2002). Dementia caregiver intervention research: In search of clinical significance. *The Gerontologist, 42,* 589–602.

Tarlow, B. J., Wisniewski, S. R., Belle, S. H., Rubert, M., Ory, M. G., & Gallagher-Thompson, D. (2004). Positive aspects of caregiving. *Research on Aging, 26,* 429–453.

PART III

Diversity and Dementia

CHAPTER NINE

Culture and Dementia

Carole B. Cox

INTRODUCTION

As culture shapes perceptions and behaviors, it also shapes responses to cognitive impairment and dementia. Cultural belief systems are influential in the ways that symptoms such as wandering, confusion, or forgetfulness are perceived, whether they are indicative of disease, a punishment, or accepted as a normal part of aging. Consequently, culture impacts on the actions that persons take in regard to the symptoms and the treatment they seek. In addition, the very roles that caregivers play are influenced to a great extent by cultural values and beliefs. Thus, as society is increasingly diverse, effective social work practice necessitates understanding cultural differences and the ways in which they affect the experience of dementia. This chapter provides an overview of culture and describes the experience of dementia among four major groups: African Americans, Hispanics, Asian Americans, and Native Americans.

CULTURE

Culture involves values, norms, and beliefs shared by a particular group. Ethnic groups are often defined as belonging to a specific culture, which

173

distinguishes them from others in society and binds them together through common symbols and traditions. It is through culture that persons learn their roles and expected ways of interacting. Cultural expectations are conveyed through norms that govern behaviors and that are often most apparent in the ways social roles are enacted. Thus, men may be expected to be the main providers in the family, to make the decisions, and to discipline the children, while women are expected to adhere to these decisions and to focus on the home.

However, ethnicity is not a constant, and ties to cultural values and norms alter with generations, acculturation, and assimilation. First-generation immigrants are usually more closely tied to traditional values and norms of behavior than their children or grandchildren. Older persons may expect their children to provide all needed assistance, while adult children who have become acculturated to the new society may feel less obligated as their adherence to such norms have weakened. These differences can create stress and conflict within families and within the children themselves as they find that they are torn between traditional expectations and the demands of their new roles.

The Perception of Dementia

As culture can influence our views of the world, it may also influence the way in which dementia is perceived. Consequently, these perceptions are often influential in the responses to the symptoms. As an example, a study of Asian and Pacific Islanders found that spiritual possession was often thought to be the cause of dementia, and therefore persons turned toward prayer and faith healing to ward off the evil spirits believed to be causing the illness (Braun & Browne, 1998). Among some ethnic groups, folk models are used to interpret dementia that attribute it to stress, losses, worries, or normal aging; moreover, persons often combine such beliefs with Western biomedical knowledge (Hinton, Franz, Yeo, & Ledkoff, 2005). As long as traditional beliefs prevail, it is difficult to engage persons in treatment.

When mental health problems are perceived as a stigma reflecting on the family or group, persons may be extremely reluctant to seek care. Among ultraorthodox Jews, mental illness within a family is viewed as a disgrace and can also be an impediment to arranged marriages. Such feelings can impede treatment and even act as barriers to caregivers using supports. If feelings of shame occur in conjunction with beliefs that dictate filial support, persons will be extremely reluctant to seek assistance either for the relative or for themselves (Elliott, DiMinno, & Lam, 1996).

Ethnicity and Assessment

When families do seek medical care, ethnicity can impact the diagnosis itself. Traditional screening measures for cognitive impairment rely on a specific degree of literacy or knowledge that may not be relevant for those who were not educated in the United States or whose formal education was limited or nonexistent. Valle and Lee (2002) caution about the accuracy and conclusions based on these instruments, noting that there continues to be confusion between lower rates of literacy and higher rates of cognitive impairment.

False positives on literacy-based standard cognitive and psychological tests of functioning place many ethnically diverse persons at a higher risk of Alzheimer's disease (AD) and related dementias. It is not unusual for low-literate persons who do poorly on tests measuring cognitive functioning have been shown to demonstrate appropriate cognitive activity for everyday functioning. Consequently, instruments assessing dementia must be sensitive to the variations that may be associated with ethnicity, history, and education, which can in themselves affect the scores that individuals receive and, consequently, their diagnosis.

Ethnicity and Caregiving

As discussed previously, ethnicity affects caregiving as it influences values and norms associated with providing assistance to family members. It is important to note that in many cultures, familial assistance is so normative that the concept of "caregiver" does not exist. Relatives are simply doing their expected tasks associated with their traditional roles and do not identify it with caregiving.

Research studies on caregiving among ethnic groups range from studies of cultural norms to studies on variations in stress and burden among caregivers and the involvement of informal and formal supports, and the use of services. Many studies compare and contrast the experiences among ethnic groups, often comparing them with those of White caregivers coping with dementia. The studies tend to show differences among groups, but the reasons for such differences and the extent to which they are generalizable beyond the actual samples used in the research is not clear (Janevic & Connell, 2001).

Ethnicity can also affect caregivers' use of services as well as their satisfaction with such services. Many studies have compared the need for and use of services among groups of caregivers, and most tend to indicate greater unmet needs among ethnic groups. As an example, Latino caregivers, in comparison to other ethnic groups, have been found to have greater unmet social needs (Ho, Weitzman, Cui, & Leukoff, 2000).

Others have found that Asian caregivers frequently feel that existing services do not meet their needs (Li, 2004).

Barriers to service use among ethnic groups include language, knowledge and understanding of services, and limited finances. Even the way in which a program is defined may act as a barrier to utilization. Thus, a program that defines itself as promoting well-being and harmony in older persons may be more acceptable than one that describes itself as a mental health agency. Likewise, a service that stresses the health of the person with dementia may be more acceptable than one that focuses on the needs of the caregiver.

Social workers can be instrumental in ensuring that barriers to service utilization are eliminated. Because the majority of care for persons with dementia is provided by relatives within the community, ensuring their access to services is essential. African Americans and Latinos with AD spend longer times in the community without any formal assistance than do their White counterparts (Harwood et al., 1998; Miller & Mukherjee, 1999). But, as suggested, this lack of assistance does not mean a lack of need. Consequently, social work outreach and skills can be critical in helping to link persons to appropriate services.

The following discussion of dementia among the major ethnic groups in the United States is intended to show only how diversity may impact the illness. Moreover, the descriptions indicate how concepts and measures developed for the majority population may not apply to specific subgroups. Finally, it is essential to recognize the heterogeneity that exists within the four ethnic groups and that a multitude of factors will influence responses of anyone individual or family.

DEMENTIA AND AFRICAN AMERICANS

Studies indicate that African Americans in the United States have higher rates of dementia than Whites (Husaini et al., 2003). By the age of 90, they have four times the risk of developing dementia than Whites (Tang et al., 2001). Explanations for this difference include social deprivation early in life (Sachs-Erisson & Blazer, 2005) as well as variations in clinical and molecular causes (Floehlich, Bogardus, & Inouye, 2001). In addition, as stated earlier, it is important to recognize the role that education and literacy can have in the diagnosis of dementia, which may be partially reflected in the higher rates of the illness (Whitfield, 2002).

African Americans are predisposed to higher rates of multi-infarct dementia (Yeo, 1996) and are at higher risk of developing AD (Tang et al., 2001). They have high rates of high cholesterol, diabetes, and hypertension, all potential risk factors for both AD and vascular dementia. In addition, studies suggest a higher familial risk among African Americans, as first-degree relatives of a person with AD have a higher cumulative risk of developing the illness than do Whites with the same relation (Greene et al., 2002).

The prevalence of dementia among African Americans has caused the Alzheimer's Association (2004) to refer to it as the "silent epidemic of Alzheimer's disease." Particularly alarming is that as the African American population continues to age, the numbers of persons with the illness will continue to increase. Among the recommendations given to combat this epidemic are more culturally sensitive screening tools; reaching persons in an earlier stage of the illness, which can augment treatment effectiveness; and increasing the numbers of African Americans in clinical trials of potential treatments.

Because of beliefs that memory loss is a normal part of aging and thus not something requiring medical intervention, families may delay seeking care (Jett, 2006). Moreover, when they go to physicians, they are at risk of having the symptoms treated as a normal part of old age (Mahoney, Cloutterbuck, Neary, & Zhan, 2005). Disparities in care have also been found in hospitals as African American caregivers of relatives with dementia have been found to be more dissatisfied than Whites with the discharge planning process and their own involvement in it (Cox, 1996).

Compared with White caregivers, African American caregivers experience more health problems, have higher mortality rates, and underutilize formal support services (Dilworth-Anderson & Gibson, 1999). They also use fewer psychotropic drugs and rely more on religion to assist them with coping (Haley et al., 2004).

However, studies on their mental well-being show varying results. Some have found them to be less depressed than Whites (Farran, Miller, Kaufman, & Davis, 1997; Haley et al., 1996) and less burdened (Knight, Silverstein, McCallum, & Fox, 2000), while others show African American and White caregivers equally burdened and depressed (Cox, 1999; Knight & McCullum, 1998). Studies also find they report less anxiety and stress associated with caregiving than Whites even though their supports are not any greater (Janevic & Connell, 2001).

Concomitantly, some research indicates that African American caregivers may have greater expectations from their support systems and may be more vulnerable to disappointment when these expectations are not met (Cox, 1995). However, regardless of the patient's symptoms or their own levels of stress, caregivers delay nursing home placement longer than their White counterparts (Stevens et al., 2004).

Research on service use among African Americans shows caregivers less likely to use formal supports than White caregivers (Miller & Guo,

2000). A study comparing interest in specific services found African Americans more likely to desire day care and home help than White caregivers, who were more interested in information on the illness or support groups (Cox, 1999). Research also indicates that if African Americans do use services, they are more likely to be dissatisfied as a result of cultural misunderstandings (Levkoff, Levy, & Weitzman, 1999).

DEMENTIA AND HISPANICS

It is estimated that by 2050, there will be 1.3 million people of Hispanic-Latino origins with AD in the United States (Alzheimer's Association, 2004). Hispanics in the United States are extremely diverse, coming from North America, South America, the Caribbean, Central America, and Spain. Although they share a common language, there is much heterogeneity among the groups with regard to socioeconomic class, immigration histories, and even traditions. Such factors can be influential in responses to dementia and to the use of services.

Hispanics have many risk factors that can predispose them toward dementia, including an increasing life expectancy, few years of formal education, and a high incidence of diabetes, stroke, and hypertension. One study of Mexican Americans found that 43% of those with dementia had type 2 diabetes or stroke or both (Haan, 2003). Caribbean Hispanics in northern Manhattan have been found to have higher rates of AD regardless of educational level or other comorbidities (Tang et al., 2001) while Central Americans and Mexicans in California have been found to have similar rates of AD as non-Hispanics but higher rates of vascular dementia (Fitten, Ortiz, & Fonton, 2001). Among certain Hispanic subgroups, there also appears to be an increased genetic risk for AD.

As prevalent as dementia may be among older Hispanics, persons are not seeking care until the later stages of the illness. Barriers to care include personal beliefs, language, economic status, and a mistrust of the health care system. In some Hispanic groups, dementia may be attributed to "el mal de ojo" (the evil eye) or "nervosa" (nerves). It may also be viewed as punishment for past sins, further deterring families from seeking care because of the shame that may be associated with it.

Structural barriers, including a lack of health insurance and ineligibility for programs such as Medicaid, impede many older Hispanics from medical care. Culturally insensitive staff and a lack of bilingual professionals who can assist them in navigating through the systems may also impede access. An absence of information and materials in Spanish can further deter persons from services.

As found with the African American caregivers, even when medical care is sought, persons may not receive appropriate referrals from their primary care physicians. Latino and other primary care physicians often do not recognize cognitive impairment and thus do not refer persons for further diagnostic evaluations and treatment (Mahoney et al., 2005).

The majority of care is provided by the family, particularly adult daughters, and the family often accepts dementia as part of the normal course of aging. Hispanics continue to provide care at home and do so for a long period of time, delaying institutionalization in comparison to non-Hispanics (Mausbach et al., 2004). Research indicates that among Hispanics over the age of 50, it is considered crucial to avoid using a nursing home (Duffy, Jackson, Schim, Ronis, & Fowler, 2006).

Hispanic caregivers are not immune to strain and exhaustion and may be particularly vulnerable as they attempt to balance many roles (Cox & Monk, 1996). The introduction of formal services to help with the caregiving may in some instances increase feelings of distress as caregivers feel that are not competently fulfilling their expected obligations. In a study of Hispanic caregivers, the use of home care, rather than relieving caregivers, contributed to their feelings of guilt and decreased self-esteem (Cox & Monk, 1996). The stronger that caregivers adhered to feelings of filial support, the greater was their stress.

Research also finds Hispanic caregivers are less likely to seek help than non-Hispanics, even from those within their social networks. Thus, although they may be experiencing high levels of distress, they are often unwilling to turn to others for support or assistance (Valle, Yamada, & Barrio, 2004).

DEMENTIA AND ASIAN AMERICANS

There exists little data on the extent of dementia among Asian Americans. Its prevalence among these populations in the United States is drawn from diagnoses made in primary care settings that show it to be about 9% in comparison to the 16% prevalence rate found in Whites and African Americans (Valcour, Masaki, & Blanchette, 2000). The scarcity of data is a direct result of difficulties that may be attributed to a cultural reluctance of families and patients to report symptoms as well as an absence of appropriate screening tools.

A study of Chinese, Japanese, Filipino, and Vietnamese families found that they all shared many common beliefs that have effects on caregiving and help seeking. These include that dementia is a common part of aging, dementia cannot be cured, children are obligated to care for their parents, problems should remain within the family, and it is shameful to talk about senile problems in a family (Braun & Browne, 1998). Among most groups, it is looked on as a stigma that reflects on the entire family. Consequently, cognitive impairment is rarely discussed outside the family.

Among Chinese, dementia may be perceived as an imbalance in the yin and yang forms of energy or as retribution for the sins of one's ancestors. Symptoms may also be viewed as resulting from cultural shock and the stress associated with immigration. A study of Vietnamese conceptions of dementia found that they integrated many influences in their definitions, including Western biomedical explanations, normal aging, spiritual causality, health beliefs, and even ideas such as the brain becoming flat or wearing out (Yeo, Tran, Hikoyeda, & Hinton, 2001).

Asian family caregivers are less likely than either African American or White caregivers to report that the person they care for has AD or any mental confusion while they are also less likely to report feeling any stress (National Alliance for Caregiving & American Association of Retired Persons, 2004). Families are expected to play traditional roles of providing care to the elderly and tend to view dementia care as part of this process. As an example, among Korean families, daughters-in-law are expected to serve as caregivers to older parents regardless of the quality of their relationships (Youn, Knight, Jeong, & Bengston, 1999). Not fulfilling such a role implies ignoring important familial and moral obligations and jeopardizes family coherence.

A series of focus groups held by the Alzheimer's Association in northern California found Asian American caregivers confused over the causes of dementia; that they preferred to use terms such as "forgetfulness" and "dementia" rather than AD, implying shame and mental illness; and that they felt physically exhausted as well as financially burdened because of constant caregiving (Alzheimer's Association of Los Angeles, Riverside, and San Bernardino Counties, 2002). The caregivers also expressed needs for home health care, persons to assist with chores in the homes, culturally sensitive services, and training for themselves.

Finally, even if dementia symptoms are recognized, there is a lack of appropriate screening instruments for Asian populations (Chen, Foo, & Ury, 2002). Instruments that were developed in the West do not necessarily accurately assess cognitive status in Asian populations, even when translated. Part of the reason for this is the multitude of languages and dialects spoken by the many Asian groups in this country. Thus, without an accurate cross-cultural instrument that can precisely evaluate an individual, diagnoses are difficult to make.

DEMENTIA AND NATIVE AMERICANS

According to the U.S. Census, there are 4.4 million American Indians with about 550,000 living on reservations or other trust lands. The Cherokee and the Navaho are the largest tribes with more than 200,000 members each. Other tribes with more than 50,000 include the Apache, Chippewa, Choctaw, Lumbee, Pueblo, and Sioux. In comparison to the rest of the population, American Indians and Alaskan Natives are relatively young with only 7% over the age of 65 in comparison to 12.5% of the population at large.

There are few data on the prevalence of AD or other dementias among Native Americans and Alaskan Natives, but it is believed to be rare. As the populations tend to die young, the risk of AD may be decreased. At the same time, the risk for vascular dementia may be increased because of high rates of stroke, diabetes, and alcohol addiction (John, Hennessey, & Roy, 1996).

Cognitive changes and dementia are typically viewed as a part of normal aging. Spirituality is also reflected in the perception of the illness as typically Native American culture views an interconnectedness between man, the creator, and nature. In some tribes, illness is viewed as an imbalance between the spiritual, mental, physical, and social interactions of the individual and his or her family or clan (Bennahum, 1998). Thus, hallucinations may be perceived as communications with the spirit world rather than as symptoms of pathology (Henderson & Traphagan, 2005). Consequently, healing is considered sacred work and includes spirituality.

Because of an absence of measures of cognitive functioning that are culturally appropriate for many Native groups, accurate assessments and diagnoses are particularly difficult to obtain (Jervis & Manson, 2002). It is difficult to translate existing instruments into the different languages and dialects without changing their meanings. A decline in social and occupational functioning, which, according to the *Diagnostic and Statistical Manual of Mental Disorders,* is associated with dementia, does not necessarily apply to those who remain active in subsistence and craft activities (Hendrie, Hall, & Pillay, 1993).

Among the cultural values shared by many Native Americans are a focus on group harmony, cooperation, emotional control, patience, and a family orientation. Such values can be influential in the caregiving experience as well as in the construct of dementia and its treatment.

Data on caregiving for dementia among Native Americans are scarce. A large study of caregiving among Native Americans in North Dakota found that the most common practice for caregivers was to take the elder into their home. In examining difficulties associated with caregiving, persons on the reservation reported a low sense of burden although they received less informal support in their caregiving than other caregivers in the general population. Formal services that could assist them were also less available (Center for Rural Health, 2003).

A study of caregiving among Pueblo Indians found complaints of role strain, interpersonal tensions, feelings of apprehension, and self-perceived detrimental health effects (Hennesey & John, 1996). Often, these feelings were associated with the problematic behaviors of the elder. At the same time, caregivers did not express resentment toward the older person, feeling constrained, or embarrassed. Caregivers provided a high level of care to cognitively impaired elders and experienced substantial levels of burden and role strain.

These limited studies suggest that further research regarding the prevalence and experience of dementia among Native Americans is needed. Such efforts must be taken in order to develop programs, services, and interventions that meet the needs of their populations.

SOCIAL WORK INVOLVEMENT

As reflected in these four groups, responses to dementia are very much influenced by the cultural, values, beliefs, and traditions of the persons affected. Culture can be a major force from the very recognition of symptoms through the care that is received.

Social workers must ensure that the significance of culture is recognized by medical care and service providers. Thus, with some groups, it may be necessary to integrate the medical model that focuses on diagnoses, treatment, and cure with a more holistic approach that incorporates a recognition of spiritual beliefs if persons are to accept treatment.

Culturally competent services acknowledge and integrate the importance of culture; the values, beliefs, and traditions of groups; and the ways that they influence needs, behaviors, and even outcomes of care. These services are sensitive to ethnic diversity and to factors that can act as barriers to access. Culturally competent systems value diversity, have the capacity for cultural self-assessment, are conscious of the dynamics that occur when cultures interact, institutionalize cultural knowledge, and reflect an understanding of diversity (National Association of Social Workers, 2001).

Social workers can play key roles in working toward culturally competent dementia care. At the program level, they can work toward reducing structural barriers that can deter ethnic groups from using services. With communication playing such a vital role in the care of diverse groups, efforts must be made to have bilingual practitioners available.

Moreover, these interpreters must be skilled and trained regarding the terms and issues associated with dementia.

Assessment and diagnoses are dependent largely on accurate measurement instruments. As discussed previously, there remain major concerns about such accuracy with many groups, as terms and concepts used to determine impairment in the majority population may be meaningless for others. Social workers can be proactive in addressing these discrepancies by helping to ensure that terms and concepts are clearly understood by both patients and their caregivers.

Because education and information regarding dementia are critical in the course of its care, materials and brochures must be available in the languages of the groups being served. Moreover, such information should be transmitted throughout the communities to ensure that all professionals are knowledgeable about the illness and referral mechanisms.

An important part of service delivery is the specific knowledge that can be obtained only from persons of the ethnic groups being served. These persons can provide insight into the values, traditions, and norms that may influence the ways in which groups perceive and care for dementia. Including these individuals as program advisers and involving them in the development of programs and services is important in developing community relationships and programs that are sensitive to community needs and preferences.

Even though ethnic caregivers may report less stress, burden, and depression than other groups, their high rates of health problems such as hypertension and heart disease indicate that they may be susceptible to the same strains as other caregivers. Understanding the factors that can inhibit persons from admitting to such difficulties and stress is essential if interventions are to be made acceptable. Incorporating beliefs, values, and traditions is basic to assuring that caregivers both receive and accept needed assistance. At the same time, interventions must reflect and build on the groups' strengths, such as spirituality and community, which are often primary sources of support.

Social workers must also be cautious with regard to assumptions about the viability and extensiveness of informal support systems. Although they may use less formal services, caregiver needs are not necessarily being met. For many caregivers, particularly those with fewer resources, informal supports and thus assistances may be limited. Competing demands associated with child rearing and employment may severely restrict the relatives' involvement with the caregiver. In addition, the increasing incapacity and escalating needs of the impaired relative may supersede the assistance that others can offer, causing the primary caregiver to feel dissatisfied with the support that is given (Cox, 1995). Such feelings can further stress these important relationships.

In working with caregivers, social workers must help them clarify their needs and expectations. It is essential that caregivers understand the illness and its progression so that they may become more accepting of interventions that can support them. Helping them accept their own limitations, as well as those of their support systems, can further encourage their acceptance of formal interventions.

As effective programs are developed, they must be used as models for service delivery. An example is that of El Portal, which was developed by the Los Angeles Alzheimer's Association and serves as a model for service delivery for the Hispanic population. The program's development has been carefully documented, services have been evaluated, and a protocol has been created so that the model can be used for the development of programs in other communities and with other ethnic groups (Alzheimer's Association, 2004). By staying informed about new and innovative systems of care, social workers can further their adoption.

CONCLUSION

The increasing diversity of the population necessitates that social workers involved with persons with dementia and their caregivers are knowledgeable about the ways in which culture, with its beliefs, values, and norms, affect the "dementia experience." Understanding the role that culture can play is critical for the development of effective services and relationships. At the same time, it is equally important to be aware of the heterogeneity within ethnic populations. Social class, education, income, gender, age, immigration, religion, literacy, and geographic location can create much intragroup diversity that can affect responses to symptoms and the illness (Hinton et al., 2005).

Moreover, a reluctance to use medical care or other social services may reflect years of poor care, long waits, and insensitive service providers, resulting in disappointment in and a mistrust of formal services. Consequently, although persons are in need of assistance, they may resist going to formal services. Thus, social workers will need to establish their credibility and competence before any interventions and services will be accepted.

Social workers can play major roles in ensuring that the needs of ethnic persons with dementia and their caregivers are adequately addressed. As practitioners, they must ensure that interventions are appropriate and acceptable to specific groups. As researchers, they must use their skills to ensure that needs and concerns particular to specific groups are identified and understood, while as advocates, they must work for the development of sensitive and responsive systems to meet these diverse needs.

REFERENCES

Alzheimer's Association. (2004). *Hispanics/Latinos and Alzheimer's disease*. Chicago: Author.

Alzheimer's Association of Los Angeles, Riverside, and San Bernardino Counties. (2002). *Asian and Pacific Islander Dementia Care Network Project*. Los Angeles: Author.

Bennahum, D. (1998, February). Navajo beliefs and end-of-life issues. In New Mexico Geriatric Education Center (Ed.), *Indian elder caregiver* (pp. 3–5). Albuquerque: New Mexico Geriatric Education Center.

Braun, K., & Browne, C. (1998). Perceptions of dementia, caregiving, and help seeking among Asian and Pacific Islander Americans. *Health and Social Work, 23,* 262–274.

Center for Rural Health, University of North Dakota School of Medicine and Health Sciences. (2003). *National Family Caregiver Support Program: North America's Indian caregivers*. Grand Forks, ND: Author.

Chen, H., Foo, S., & Ury, W. (2002). Recognizing dementia. *Western Journal of Medicine, 176,* 267–270.

Cox, C. (1995). Comparing the experiences of Black and White caregivers of dementia patients. *Social Work, 40,* 343–349.

Cox, C. (1996). Outcomes of hospitalization: Factors influencing the discharges of African American and white dementia patients. *Social Work in Health Care, 23,* 23–38.

Cox, C. (1999). Service needs and use: A further look at the experiences of African American and White caregivers seeking Alzheimer's assistance. *American Journal of Alzheimer's Disease, 13,* 93–101.

Cox, C., & Monk, A. (1996). Strain among caregivers: Comparing the experiences of African American and Hispanic caregivers of Alzheimer's relatives. *International Journal of Aging, 32,* 93–105.

Dilworth-Anderson, P., & Gibson, B. (1999). Ethnic minority perspectives on dementia, caregiving, and interventions. *Generations, 23,* 40–45.

Duffy, F., Jackson, F., Schim, S., Ronis, D., & Fowler, K. (2006). Racial/ethnic preferences, gender preferences and perceived discrimination in end-of-life care. *Journal of the American Geriatrics Society, 54,* 1236–1244.

Elliott, K., DiMinno, M., & Lam, D. (1996). Working with Chinese families in the context of dementia. In G. Yeo & D. Gallagher-Thompson (Eds.), *Ethnicity and dementia* (pp. 89–108). Washington, DC: Taylor & Francis.

Farran, C., Miller, B., Kaufman, J., & Davis, L. (1997). Race, finding meaning and caregiver distress. *Journal of Aging and Health, 9,* 316–333.

Fitten, L., Ortiz, F., & Fonton, M. (2001). Frequency of Alzheimer's disease and other dementias in a community outreach sample of Hispanics. *Journal of the American Geriatrics Society, 49,* 1301–1308.

Floehlich, T., Bogardus, S., & Inouye, S. (2001). Dementia and race: Are their differences between African Americans and Caucasians? *Journal of the American Geriatrics Society, 46,* 490.

Greene, R., Cupples, L., Go, R., Benke, K., Edeki, T., Griffith, P., et al. (2002). Risk of dementia among White and African American relatives of patients with Alzheimer's disease. *Journal of the American Medical Association, 287,* 329–336.

Haan, M. (2003). Prevalence of dementia in older Latinos: The influence of diabetes mellitus, stroke, and genetic factors. *Journal of the American Geriatrics Society, 52,* 169–177.

Haley, W., Gitlin, L., Wisniewski, S., Mahoney, D., Coon, D., Winter, L., et al. (2004). Well-being, appraisal, and coping in African American and Caucasian caregivers: Findings from the REACH study. *Aging and Mental Health, 8,* 316–329.

Haley, W., Roth, D., Closton, M., Ford, G., West, C., & Collins, R. (1996). Appraising, coping, and social support as mediators of well-being in Black and White family caregivers of patients with Alzheimer's disease. *Journal of Consulting and Clinical Psychology, 64,* 121–129.

Harwood, D., Barker, W., Cantillon, M., Loewenstein, D., Ownby, R., & Duara, R. (1998). Depressive symptomatology in first-degree family caregivers of Alzheimer disease patients: A cross-ethnic comparison. *Alzheimer Disease and Associated Disorders, 12,* 340–346.

Henderson, N., & Traphagan, J. (2005). Cultural factors in dementia: Perspectives from the anthropology of aging. *Alzheimer Disease and Associated Disorders, 4,* 272–274.

Hendrie, Hall, K., & Pillay, N. (1993). Alzheimer's disease is rare in Cree. *International Psychogeriatrics, 5,* 5–14.

Hennesey, C., & John, R. (1996). American Indian family caregivers' perceptions of burden and needed support services. *Journal of Applied Gerontology, 5,* 275–293.

Hinton, L., Franz, C., Yeo, G., & Ledkoff, S. (2005). Conceptions of dementia in a multiethnic sample of family caregivers. *Journal of the American Geriatrics Society, 53,* 1405–1410.

Ho, C., Weitzman, P., Cui, X., & Leukoff, S. (2000). Stress and service use among minority caregivers to elders with dementia. *Journal of Gerontological Social Work, 33,* 67–88.

Husaini, B., Sherkat, D., Moonis, M., Levine, R., Holzer, C., & Cain, V. (2003). Racial differences in the diagnosis of dementia and its effects on the use and costs of health care services. *Psychiatric Services, 54,* 574–575.

Janevic, M., & Connell, C. (2001). Racial, ethnic and cultural differences in the dementia caregiving experience: Recent findings. *The Gerontologist, 41,* 334–347.

Jervis, L., & Manson, S. (2002). American Indians/Alaska Natives and dementia. *Alzheimer's Disease Associated Disorders, 16*(Supp. 2), S89–S95.

Jett, K. (2006). Mind loss in the African American community: Dementia as a normal part of aging. *Journal of Aging Studies, 20,* 1–10.

John, R., Hennessey, C., & Roy, L. (1996). Caring for cognitively impaired American Indian elders: Difficult situations, few options. In G. Yeo & D. Gallagher-Thompson (Eds.), *Ethnicity and the dementias* (pp. 218–231). Washington, DC: National Academy Press.

Knight, B., Silverstein, M., McCallum, T., & Fox, I. (2000). A sociocultural stress on coping model for mental health outcomes among African American caregivers in southern California. *Journal of Gerontology and Psychological Sciences, 55B,* P142–P150.

Knight, R., & McCullum, T. (1998). Heart rate reactivity and depression in African American and White dementia caregivers: Reporting bias or positive coping? *Aging and Mental Health, 3,* 212–222.

Levkoff, S., Levy, B., & Weitzman, P. (1999). The role of religion and ethnicity in the help seeking of family caregivers of elders with Alzheimer's disease and related disorders. *Journal of Cross-Cultural Gerontology, 14,* 335–356.

Li, H. (2004). Barriers to and unmet needs in supportive services: Experiences of Asian American caregivers. *Journal of Cross-Cultural Gerontology, 19,* 241–260.

Mahoney, D., Cloutterbuck, J., Neary, S., & Zhan, L. (2005). African American, Chinese, and Latino family caregivers' impressions of the onset and diagnosis of dementia: Cross-cultural similarities and differences. *The Gerontologist, 45,* 783–792.

Mausbach, B., Coon, D., Depp, C., Rabinowitz, Y., Arias, E., Kraemer, H., et al. (2004). Ethnicity and time to institutionalization of dementia patients, a comparison of Latina and Caucasian female family caregivers. *Journal of American Geriatrics Society, 52,* 1077–1084.

Miller, B., & Guo, S. (2000). Social support for spouse caregivers of persons with dementia. *Journal of Gerontology, Social Sciences, 55B,* 163–172.

Miller, B., & Mukherjee, S., (1999). Service use, caregiving mastery, and attitudes toward community services. *Journal of Applied Gerontology, 18,* 162–176.

National Alliance of Caregivers & American Association of Retired Persons. (2004). *Caregiving in the United States.* Washington, DC: Author.

National Association of Social Workers. (2001). *NASW standards for cultural competence in social work practice.* Washington, DC: Author.

Sachs-Erisson, N., & Blazer, D. (2005). Racial differences in cognitive decline in a sample of community dwelling older adults: The mediating effect of literacy and education. *American Journal of Psychiatry, 11,* 968–975.

Stevens, A., Owen, J., Roth, D., Clay, O., Bartolucci, A., & Haley, W. (2004). Predictors of nursing home placement in White and African American individuals with dementia. *Journal of Aging and Health, 16,* 375–397.

Tang, M., Cross, P., Andrews, H., Jacobs, D., Small, S., & Bell, K. (2001). Incidence of Alzheimer's disease in African Americans, Caribbean Hispanics and Caucasians in northern Manhattan. *Neurology, 56,* 49–56.

Valcour, V., Masaki, K., Curb, D., & Blanchette, P. (2000). The detection of dementia in the primary care setting. *Archives of Internal Medicine, 260,* 2964–2968.

Valle, R., & Lee, B. (2002). Research priorities in the evolving demographic landscape of Alzheimer's disease and associated dementias. *Alzheimer's Disease Associated Disorders, 16*(Supp. 2), S64–S79.

Valle, R., Yamada, A-M., & Barrio, C. (2004). Ethnic differences in social network help seeking strategies among Latino and European dementia caregivers. *Aging and Mental Health, 8,* 535–543.

Whitfield, K. (2002). Challenges in cognitive assessment of African Americans in research on Alzheimer's disease. *Alzheimer's Disease Associated Disorders, 16*(Supp. 2), S80–S81.

Yeo, G. (1996). Background. In G. Yeo & D. Gallagher-Thompson (Eds.), *Ethnicity and the dementias* (pp. 1–7). Washington, DC: Taylor & Francis.

Yeo, G., Tran, J., Hikoyeda, N., & Hinton, L. (2001). Conceptions of dementia among Vietnamese American caregivers. *Journal of Gerontological Social Work, 36,* 131–152.

Youn, G., Knight, B., Jeong, H., & Bengston, D. (1999). Differences in familism values and caregiving outcomes among Korean, Korean American and White American caregivers. *Psychology and Aging, 14,* 355–364.

CHAPTER TEN

Psychoeducational Strategies for Latino Caregivers

María P. Aranda and Carmen Morano

INTRODUCTION

This chapter highlights several salient areas to consider in adapting psychoeducational care strategies to older Latino caregivers of persons with late-life dementia. For the purpose of our discussion, *psychoeducational strategies* are defined as supportive and psychological interventions provided at the individual or family level to primarily older caregivers experiencing psychological distress in their caregiving roles. Examples of psychoeducational strategies include but are not limited to the provision of counseling services, psychotherapy, support groups, informational and educational resources, and resource linkage and navigation alone or in combination with other strategies (Crewe & Chipungu, 2006).

Although the caregiving role is challenging for all families regardless of racial or ethnic background, only a handful of studies have been published which specifically test the effectiveness of interventions designed to reduce the psychological consequences of caregiving among underserved racial and ethnic populations (Magaña, 2006). For example, a review of the published literature indicates that only two sources of intervention studies specifically addressed sociocultural adaptations to caregiver interventions for Latino caregivers in the United States (Gallagher-Thompson,

Areán, Rivera, & Thompson, 2003; Gallagher-Thompson et al., 2000; Morano & Bravo, 2002).

Commensurate with the paucity of work on caregiver interventions with racial and ethnically diverse populations is the reality that understanding the process of sociocultural adaptations in the caregiver research literature remains limited. With growing consensus that Latino caregivers have high rates of depressive symptomatology and present with different sociocultural profiles and mediators of stress and coping (Adams, Aranda, Kemp, & Takagi, 2002; Morano & King, 2005; Morano & Sanders, 2005), future studies will need to address how to tailor interventions to enhance the accessibility and acceptability of social work interventions to the Latino population.

Older Latinos (65 years and older) will make up the largest group of racial/ethnic minorities in the United States by 2028 (Administration on Aging, 2003). With recent data indicating that Latinos may be affected by dementia at an earlier age than other groups (almost 7 years earlier; Clark et al., 2005) and report low access to information and services (Aranda, Villa, Trejo, Ramirez, & Ranney, 2003), we can expect the burden of dementing illness to take a prominent toll on Latino individuals, families, and communities in the future.

We intend to follow a commonsense approach to adaptation; thus, our goal is not to "throw the baby out with the bath water" with respect to mainstream psychoeducational strategies but rather to offer specific areas for consideration in the development of psychoeducational strategies for older Latino caregivers. Toward this end, we draw from the ecological validity framework posited by Bernal and his associates (Bernal, Bonilla, & Bellido, 1995), which provides a culturally sensitive perspective to treatment outcome research with Latinos. We augment this framework by drawing from the cross-cultural practice literature (health, mental health, and social services) on Latino elderly and highlighting frequently endorsed cultural orientations that have been posited as important sociocultural considerations for practice.

ECOLOGICAL VALIDITY FRAMEWORK

Bernal and his associates (Bernal et al., 1995) present a useful framework for culturally sensitive interventions that strengthen ecological validity for treatment outcomes. Drawing from Bronfenbrenner (1977), the authors define *ecological validity* as "the degree to which there is congruence between the environment as experienced by the subject and the properties of the environment the investigator assumes it has" (p. 69). Although this framework was initially conceptualized as a heuristic tool for mental health outcome research, we posit that the concepts can be translated to social work practice with Latino caregivers of persons affected by dementia.

Table 10.1 summarizes the culturally sensitive elements and dimensions of interventions proposed by Bernal and his associates. Although a total of eight dimensions are posited by the authors, we will focus on a subset of these dimensions, namely, language, persons, metaphors, concepts, goals, and methods (Bernal et al., 1995). These dimensions represent general areas of an intervention and the corresponding culturally sensitive elements amenable to sociocultural adaptations to psychoeducational strategies. We draw from these elements not as rigid prescriptions of what to modify but to highlight possible areas to approximate a higher degree of ecological validity in social work practice with caregivers.

TABLE 10.1 Culturally Sensitive Elements and the Dimensions of Treatment for Clinical Research Interventions With Hispanics

Dimension	Culturally Sensitive Elements
Language	Culturally appropriate; culturally syntonic language
Persons	Role of ethnic/racial similarities and differences between client and therapist in shaping therapy relationship
Metaphors	Symbols and concepts shared with the population; sayings, or *dichos*, in treatment
Content	Cultural knowledge: values; customs and traditions; uniqueness of groups (social, economic, historical, political)
Concepts	Treatment concepts consonant with culture and context: dependence vs. interdependence vs. independence; emic (within culture, particular) over etic (outside culture, universal)
Goals	Transmission of positive and adaptive cultural values; support adaptive values from the culture of origin
Methods	Development and/or cultural adaptation of treatment methods. Examples: "modeling" to include culturally consonant traditions (e.g., *cuento* therapy (therapy based on folktales); "cultural reframing" of drug abuse as intergenerational cultural conflicts; use of language (formal and informal); cultural hypothesis testing; use of genograms; "cultural migration dialogue"
Context	Consideration of changing contexts in assessment during treatment or intervention: acculturative stress, phase of migration; development stage; social support and relationship to country of origin; economic and social context of intervention

Source: Bernal, Bonilla, and Bellido (1995).

Language

Language barriers are consistently cited as a major problem in conveying mental health–related information, in accessing mental health services, and in providing evidence-based psychotherapy (Lewis-Fernández, Das, César, Weissman, & Olfson, 2005). The population of persons who speak Spanish at home contains about 28% who report limited English proficiency (almost 8 million persons in 2000; U.S. Census Bureau, 2003). In particular, first-generation Latinos, which make up the majority of the Latino elderly in the United States, tend to be Spanish dominant (72%; Pew Research Center, 2005).

The issue of providing language-acceptable psychoeducational services to Latinos goes beyond the mere provision of services in the person's language of preference. Language must be familiar to the target population. Technical or medical terms may be difficult to understand—such as the term "dementia" (*demencia*), which is equated with the normal process of aging or highly stigmatized references to "craziness" or psychotic-type disorders (Mahoney, Cloutterbuck, Neary, & Zhan, 2005). Furthermore, the term "caregiver," which is still a relatively recent term in Latino households, is translated as *cuidadora* (female) or *cuidador* (male). These terms have more of a custodial and impersonal connotation that takes away the emotive and thus familial significance of the English-language term. Thus, explaining to the caregiver that this is a fairly recent term to emerge and how the term is currently utilized may increase understanding of the phenomenon. At the same time, this may raise consciousness about the unique role and experience of being a caregiver to a family member with dementia at a time when the caregiver may be trying to make sense of his or her role, expectations, and competency.

Having stated this, we follow the philosophy that it is important to introduce medical or psychiatric terms that are widely used by professional providers to the caregiver population given the problems associated with low knowledge and access to services. We suggest that technical and medical terms be followed by terms that are more familiar with the target population. This allows opportunities to increase knowledge and health literacy levels revolving around dementia, health, mental health, and the caregiving experience. For example, although the term *nervios* has been widely documented as a sociocultural expression of psychological distress in Latinos (Guarnaccia & Rodriguez, 1996; Guarnaccia & Rogler, 1999), it is still debated by some to obscure the understanding of symptom presentation because of its multiple meanings and subsequent interpretations (Givaudan, Pick, de Venguer, & Xolocotzin, 2003). Nevertheless, *nervios* is so widely utilized by Latinos that it behooves using the term in materials followed by various examples of culturally syntonic symptom presentations (decreased energy and interest in usual activities, insomnia, restlessness, and so on) by using case vignettes of Latino care-giving families (Talamantes & Aranda, 2004).

Another phrase commonly used by older Latinos is "*Me siento mal*" (I don't feel well), which speaks to the issue of a generalized, obscure sense of malaise (Aranda, 2004). Whether this phrase is the product of a paucity of language or terms to describe psychological distress or a way to open up discussion in a tentative manner regarding a potential stigma-tizing condition is not yet discerned. Thus, the social work practitioner can utilize these culturally congruent terms or phrases while augmenting them with more expansive terminology regarding the experience and treatment of dementia and caregiving.

The power differential between the social work practitioner or pro-vider and the caregiver must be taken into consideration. Aranda (1999) highlights the fact that the physician is regarded as a figure of legitimized authority and power. This legitimized power is also transferred to social workers who act in the role as agency representatives, sources of knowl-edge, and gatekeepers to needed services. Aranda (1999) also recommends that providers can attempt to minimize the power differential by watch-ing for acquiescent statements, by stating that sometimes treatments and interventions may not always work, or by introducing humor to the help-ing relationship. Such examples help "humanize" the practitioner as an ally in a way that is respectful to both parties. Another example relates to nuances of presenting information in a manner that mitigates the disparity in power between the social work practitioner or provider and the older adult consumer. For example, instead of saying, "Here is this booklet on Alzheimer's disease," it may be more culturally syntonic to say, "*Quisiera regalarle este folleto sobre la enfermedad de Alzheimer* (I'd like to offer this booklet to you on Alzheimer's disease)." *Quisiera regarlarle* is more socially graceful (thus, it tends to soften the power gap) with the word *regalar,* giving more of a semblance of "to offer a gift."

Literacy levels among Latino elderly remain low and trail signifi-cantly behind the non-Latino population: about 70% of older Latinos fail to complete high school, compared to almost 30% of the overall older adult population (Federal Interagency Forum on Aging-Related Statistics, 2004; Villa & Aranda, 2000). Most psychoeducational materi-als developed to date are targeted toward a higher level of reading lit-eracy than what is compatible with low-income, Latino older persons in general. Evidence suggests that when reading material is translated from English to Spanish, the literacy level of the Spanish version actually increases (Administration on Aging, 2003; Valle, 1998). This highlights the challenges implicated by low literacy levels in the development of consent forms, procedures, educational materials and handouts, and so on for this population (Aranda, 2001).

According to Givaudan and her associates (2003), "Written material should facilitate reading and comprehension while drawing attention and promoting identification with the contents" (p. 6). They recommend not only that materials be straightforward and clear but also that they be adapted to the lexis, grammar, and style of the targeted Latino population. Examples of successful health literacy messages and programs can be located at Hablamos Juntos (http://www.hablamosjuntos.org/default.about.asp), which includes a wealth of information on print media development and methodology for limited-English-speaking persons.

Client and Therapist Variables

Several studies in the field of mental health have addressed the cultural responsiveness/compatibility hypothesis, which purports that matching clients with mental health providers on several characteristics or attributes, namely, ethnicity and language, and/or with participation in ethnic-specific programs will be effective in increasing utilization of services. The assumption is that matching clients with providers who speak their language and are from the same ethnic group will increase the *responsiveness* and thus the acceptance of services.

Except for one study that showed no effect of ethnic matching on service use or outcomes (Ortega & Rosenheck, 2002), most studies tended to support the beneficial effects of matching client and therapist in terms of service utilization and outcomes (Gamst, Dana, Der-Karabetian, & Kramer, 2000; Gamst et al., 2002; O'Sullivan & Lasso, 1992; Snowden, Hu, & Jerrell, 1995; Takeuchi, Sue, & Yeh, 1995). Although none of these studies examined outcomes related to *older* Latinos, it is assumed that ethnic/language matching of caregivers and social work practitioners and allied providers will increase engagement, retention, successful outcomes, and overall satisfaction (Gallagher-Thompson et al., 2000; Gallagher-Thompson, Coon, et al., 2003).

While we have used the term "Latino" to describe a general group of individuals who share a common language, it is important to recognize the heterogeneity of this population (Angel & Hogan, 2004). An intervention for Cuban Americans in Miami, for example, may require modifications for Mexican Americans in rural south Texas given key differences in socioeconomic status (i.e., education, income, occupation) and sociopolitical history (immigration and migration histories, assimilation, sociopolitical policies in the country of origin) as important variables in understanding sociocultural influences on caregiver stress and well-being.

For example, in a Miami-based caregiver psychoeducational intervention, Spanish-speaking presenters were recruited to provide psychoeducational content on a variety of areas (Morano & Bravo, 2002). While both the first- and second-generation Cuban Americans requested that all the literature, presentations, and evaluations be provided in Spanish, some participants had difficulty understanding speakers because of regional Spanish-language differences. There was also some discussion about how the translated written materials were not universally understood. Other reservations arose whereby the participants believed that the Latino presenters were not as knowledgeable as their White counterparts. Similarly, participants were concerned about being negatively judged by the Latino presenters for not endorsing cultural expectations about the role of family and proscriptions against nursing home placement. Thus, although ethnic/racial matching is endorsed in the literature, we have presented some examples of the nuances and sensitivities that may arise regarding intragroup differences and perceptions of professionals and written materials even when available in Spanish.

Others have nevertheless acknowledged that adherence and satisfaction with services increase when certain person–provider relationship characteristics are in place (Paniagua, 2001). For example, it is hypothesized that the therapist's humanistic characteristics have a strong influence on whether the person adheres to provider recommendations. This in large part is due to the importance that older Latinos place on the personal or humanistic attributes (*personalismo; respeto, simpatía; cariño; orgullo*) of the helping professional (Bernal et al., 1995; Mezzich et al., 1999) and the therapeutic relationship with an authority figure (Aranda, 1999). We purport that social work practitioners evaluate the degree to which they are able to reflect these qualities in their relationship with care recipients, much like treatment fidelity strategies are used to rate interventionists' adherence to treatment protocols.

Metaphors, Images, and Sayings

Metaphors are widely used in psychotherapy with a variety of individuals and populations (Stine, 2005) and are specifically documented with Latino populations both in the United States and abroad (Altarriba & Santiago-Rivera, 1994; Aviera, 1996; Bracero, 1998). Going beyond the typical use of metaphors in common and literary speech, metaphors can take the shape of physical artifacts (symbols, images, physical environment) and communication patterns (sayings, idioms, refrains, songs) that appeal to many sensory associations rooted in daily life.

Cuentos and *dichos* have been used in psychotherapy with Latino adults (Aviera, 1996; Bracero, 1998). Reminiscent of their childhood and young adult years, metaphors such as sayings (*dichos*) and proverbs (*refranes*) are aptly suited for psychotherapy with Latinos throughout their life span insofar as these are able to communicate both simple and complex notions, concepts, and predicaments, often in lighthearted yet respectful ways. Popular sayings can succinctly capture issues that typically arise for Latino caregivers: (a) social isolation and family conflicts (*"Mas vale un vecino cercano que un hermano lejano* / A close neighbor [or friend] is better than a distant relative."), (b) feelings of being overwhelmed or unfocused (*"No dejes para mañana lo que debes hacer para hoy.* / Don't leave for tomorrow what you can do today."), (c) value of social support (*"Una mano lava la otra y las dos la cara* / One hand washes the other and both wash the face. / You scratch my back, I'll scratch yours."), and (d) problem-solving orientation and spirituality (*"Ayúdate que Dios te ayudará* / God helps those who help themselves.").

Concepts (Culturally Explanatory Models)

Culturally explanatory models (CEMs) of mental illness comprise the person's understanding of the causes, consequences, and appropriate treatment of illness (Kleinman, Eisenberg, & Good, 1978), which are influenced by the cultural background of the person and his or her community and the person's prior experience with the illness and use of services to address this illness. The degree to which there exists a consonance between the assumed tenets and mechanisms of action of the psychosocial intervention and the person's CEMs predicates in part the acceptance and thus the effectiveness of the intervention (Vera, Vila, & Alegría, 2003).

Prior work has underscored the cultural construction of dementia for a variety of racial and ethnic subgroups (see review by Henderson & Henderson, 2002). A small yet growing literature supports that low-acculturated Latino elderly are less likely to endorse biomedical models of depression (Aranda, 1999; Freidenberg & Jimenez-Velasquez, 1992; Henderson & Henderson, 2002; Valle, 1998) yet are more likely to explain depressive symptoms by the "wear and tear" hypothesis (chronic worry and suffering over life stressors, or *sufrimiento*), personal attributes (lack of will power or hope, or *sin ganas o esperanza*), interpersonal (feelings of rejection by one's intimate others), and spiritual attributions (punishment or abandonment by God) (Aranda & Ell, 2004). Social work practitioners are encouraged to include questions on caregiver beliefs and illness attributions of dementia and potential negative outcomes such as depression (Aranda, 2006) in their assessment protocols not only at the initiation of the helping relationship but throughout in order to ascertain baseline and ongoing changes in the caregiver's CEMs.

Intervention Goals (Transmission of Positive Cultural Values)

Congruence in intervention or service delivery goals and expectations is inherent in all social work practice regardless of the type of care provided or consumer population. What may be qualitatively different is how these goals are described or contextualized within the phenomenological experience of older Latinos. For example, the cultural concept of *sufrimiento* (suffering) in one's life takes on an existential meaning that needs to be clearly recognized by the therapist as an important part of the person's life. Second, the goal of treatment is to partner with the person to reduce the *sufrimiento* in ways that are culturally congruent to the person. Although this may first appear fatalistic (Choi & Gonzalez, 2005) and thus maladaptive, it really goes beyond a fatalistic posture (Aranda & Knight, 1997). This provides an opportunity to empower the person by first "publicly" (in session) acknowledging the *sufrimiento* and giving *esperanza* (hope) about the future. This accentuates the duality of life: the acknowledgment of suffering and the instillation of hope.

The role of *la familia* (family) is central to the transmission of positive and adaptive cultural values in Latino families. Lower rates of institutionalization (nursing home use) by older Latinos have been attributed to various demographic (higher fertility, larger families, multigenerational households), cultural (familism, filial obligation, low acculturation) and economic factors (low income, financial strain) (Angel, Angel, Aranda, & Miles, 2004). Included in the definition of family are nonconsanguine caregivers (personal care attendants, significant others) who act like family and are integral to the older person's psychological well-being (Aranda, 2004; Hardin & Jordan-Marsh, 2005).

It is important to include family caregivers early in the screening and assessment process to identify opportunities for family (or like-family) involvement in psychoeducational interventions. Practice models that provide the opportunity to include family in the problem-solving process are more likely to increase adherence to care regimens, and to follow with following up with assignments such as social and behavioral activation strategies (Vera et al., 2003). Moreover, older Latinos rely on family or fictive kin as "gatekeepers" to mediate such processes as informed consent, treatment adherence, coping, outcomes, and so on (Aranda, 2001; Hazuda et al., 2000).

Sometimes resistance from family may occur when caregivers attempt to use formal care services for fear that a decision will eventually be made regarding institutionalization. For this reason, reframing the reasons for service utilization can assist in the process of resource access and navigation. Morano and Bravo (2002) modified content about the use of day care services to caregivers such that services were reframed to highlight the importance of the structure and activities of day care primarily for the person with Alzheimer's disease. By contrast, the original content used in the intervention for the White caregivers focused to a larger degree on the caregiver's need for respite from the caregiving situation.

Second, the Latino participants were more likely to initiate discussion about how they made meaning of their difficult situation, how faith and prayer helped them cope with providing care and competing demands, and that the caregiving experience served as a challenge or a test of their faith. The role of religion as a mediator of caregiving strain has been documented in the literature (see Morano & King, 2005; Picot, Debanne, Namzi, & Wykle, 1997) and highlights that for many Latinos, as well as other racial/ethnic minority caregivers, religiosity and spirituality have a positive impact on well-being (Morano & King, 2005; Picot et al., 1997). Strategies such as these serve to respect cultural values such as the sociocentric goal of doing something for the common good (the family) and the spiritual goal of putting one's burdens in the realm of a Higher Power.

Methods (Procedures for Incorporating Cultural Knowledge)

An example of incorporating cultural knowledge in terms of a culturally syntonic method of service delivery is the use of *fotonovelas*. A close cousin of using *cuentos* (fictional stories) in treatment is the use of *fotonovelas* (photo novels)—stories told in pictorial formats (with typically less text). Used extensively in Latin American pop culture (Flora, 1989), *fotonovelas* have also made their way in targeting health-related messages to the U.S. Latino community for a variety of mental health conditions, such as Alzheimer's disease (Alzheimer's Association, 2005; Alzheimer's Cross Cultural Research and Development [ACCORD], 1992; Aranda, 1989; Valle, 1998) and substance abuse (http://www.hsph.harvard.edu/healthliteracy/ photonovel/drug_od.pdf), to name a few. Because *fotonovelas* rely on linguistic scaffolding—easy-to-read conversational speech in balloon captions, storyboard images that go along with the running dialogue, and text box set-asides with important health-related information—they tend to be acceptable to persons along a continuum of reading levels.

Prior work with Latino Alzheimer's disease families (ACCORD, 1992; Aranda, 1989) integrated participant involvement strategies (Rudd & Comings, 1994) in the development and production of various psychoeducational materials (*fotonovelas* and videos). Thus, real-life scenarios rooted in the lives of Latino families were highlighted, helping to destigmatize and demystify the mental health complications of Alzheimer's disease.

Another important methodological adaptation is the restructuring of schedules and group activities. For example, in order to adapt a psychoeducational intervention originally developed for primarily White European American caregivers (by the second author in previous work), Morano and Bravo (2002) conducted a structured survey to examine the appraisal and coping processes of Cuban Americans in Miami. The findings of that study, as well as from subsequent key informant interviews (providers with experience in service provision to Latinos), indicated a need to adapt some of the specific content of the sessions as well as the overall structure of the intervention.

To illustrate, from the inception of the group intervention, it was clear that the allotted time for sessions, as well as the time allowed for group processing of the presentations, would need to be adapted. Unlike the White European American caregivers who expected to start exactly at 9:00 a.m., the Latino group started closer to 9:30 to 10:00 a.m. It was not that the participants were late but that they wanted to have time to talk with each other as well as share some homemade breakfast treats. It was during this informal and unstructured time that the participants engaged with each other in intimate shared experiences that helped them put the information presented in the lectures into a more understandable and personable context.

In the evaluation of the intervention, the participants indicated that this type of flexibility was extremely useful and appreciated the time to warm-up and get to know one another better. The opportunity to reciprocate and bring something to the group was a theme that carried throughout the class sessions. This unstructured informal networking time proved to be important to the overall success of the psychoeducational group model for Cuban American Alzheimer's disease caregivers (Morano & Bravo, 2002).

CONCLUSION

Given that older Latinos will comprise the largest group of racial/ethnic minorities in the United States by 2028 and that there is ample evidence that Latinos may be affected by dementia at an earlier age, have high rates of depressive symptomology, and report low access to information and services, we can expect the burden of providing care will take a prominent toll on Latino individuals, families, and communities. Although the importance of understanding how the sociocultural profiles of Latino's might predict the caregiver's perception of and coping with providing care, there remains limited empirically supported intervention research with this vulnerable aging population.

The framework presented in this chapter offers a number of considerations and suggestions for adapting and implementing psychosocial interventions with Latino caregivers. The ecological validity framework of Bernal et al. (1995) with its focus on the use of language, metaphors, concepts, goals, and methods suggests the need to recognize and understand how these dimensions can inform the adaptation of psychoeducational interventions for Latino caregivers. The authors caution, however, that while these dimensions are informative for adapting an intervention developed for White nonethnic caregivers for Latino caregivers, social work practitioners must recognize the unique cultural and socioeconomic characteristics that come with being, for example, of Cuban, Mexican, Puerto Rican, Salvadorian, or biracial descent.

The discussion presented in this chapter recognizes the need for significantly more empirical research with culturally diverse populations. Further, the authors suggest that a collaborative approach to intervention research by providers, researchers, and, most important consumers of mental health services is required. From conception to implementation and ultimately to evaluation, culturally sensitive interventions that result from the traditional unidirectional approach, or research conceptualized in isolation by the researcher, run the risk of failing to address the real-world needs of culturally diverse caregivers.

REFERENCES

Adams, B. M., Aranda, M. P., Kemp, B. J., & Takagi, K. (2002). Ethnic and gender differences in distress among Anglo-American, African-American, Japanese-American and Mexican-American spousal caregivers of persons with dementia. *Journal of Clinical Geropsychology, 8*, 279–301.

Administration on Aging, U.S. Department of Health and Human Services. (2003). *A statistical profile of Hispanic older Americans aged 65+.* Washington, DC: U.S. Department of Health and Human Services. Retrieved July 1, 2003, from http://www.aoa. dhhs.gov/press/fact/fact.asp#Snapshots

Altarriba, J., & Santiago-Rivera, A. L. (1994). Current perspectives on using linguistic and cultural factors in counseling the Hispanic client. *Professional Psychology: Research and Practice, 25*, 388–397.

Alzheimer's Association. (2005). *What is happening to Grandpa?* Chicago: Author. Retrieved February 1, 2006, from http://www.alz.org/hispanic/downloads/fotonovela-eng.pdf (A *fotonovela* in English; Spanish-language version also available.)

Alzheimer's Cross Cultural Research and Development (ACCORD). (1992). *¿Qué le pasa al abuelito? (What happened to Grandpa?)* San Diego, CA: Author. (A *fotonovela*: Spanish and English versions; developed for the Alzheimer's Association.)

Angel, J. L., & Hogan, D. P. (2004). Population aging and diversity in a new era. In K. E. Whitfield (Ed.), *Closing the gap: Health of minority elders in the new millennium* (pp. 1–12). Washington, DC: Gerontological Society of America.

Angel, R., Angel, J., Aranda, M. P., & Miles, T. P. (2004). Risk of nursing home use among elderly Mexican Americans. *Journal of Aging and Health, 16*, 338–354.

Aranda, M. P. (1989). *Siempre Viva: An educational, illustrated booklet on a Latino family's struggle with Alzheimer's disease.* Los Angeles: Calmecac de Aztlan en Los. (A *fotonovela* in Spanish.)

Aranda, M. P. (1999). Cultural issues and Alzheimer's disease: Lessons from the Latino community. *Geriatric Case Management Journal, 9,* 13–18.

Aranda, M. P. (2001). Racial and ethnic factors in dementia caregiving research in the United States. *Aging and Mental Health, 5,* S116–S123.

Aranda, M. P. (2004, April 15). *Cultural competency in working with Latino caregivers.* Paper presented at the Joint Conference of the American Society on Aging and the National Council on Aging, San Francisco, CA.

Aranda, M. P. (2006). Social work with older Latinos: A mental health perspective. In B. Berkman (Ed.), *Handbook of social work in aging* (pp. 283–291). New York: Oxford University Press.

Aranda, M. P., & Ell, K. R. (2004, July 15). *Using in-depth interviews to understand the nature and course of depression in older adults with chronic illness.* Poster session presented at the First Annual Summer Institute, Family Research Consortium, Center on Culture and Health, University of California, Los Angeles, San Juan, Puerto Rico.

Aranda, M. P., & Knight, B. G. (1997). The influence of ethnicity and culture on the caregiver stress and coping process: A sociocultural review and analysis. *The Gerontologist, 37,* 342–354.

Aranda, M. P., Villa, V., Trejo, L., Ramirez, R., & Ranney, M. (2003). El Portal Latino Alzheimer's Disease Project: A model program for Latino caregivers of Alzheimer disease-affected persons. *Social Work, 48,* 259–271.

Aviera, A. (1996). "Dichos" therapy group: A therapeutic use of Spanish language proverbs with hospitalized Spanish-speaking psychiatric patients. *Cultural Diversity and Mental Health, 2,* 73–87.

Bernal, G., Bonilla, J., & Bellido, C. (1995). Ecological validity and cultural sensitivity for outcome research: Issues for the cultural adaptation and development of psychosocial treatments with Hispanics. *Journal of Abnormal Child Psychology, 23,* 67–82.

Bracero, W. (1998). Intimidades: Confianza, gender, and hierarchy in the construction of Latino-Latina therapeutic relationships. *Cultural Diversity and Mental Health, 4,* 264–277.

Bronfenbrenner, U. (1977). Toward an experimental ecology of human development. *American Psychologist, 32,* 513–531.

Choi, M. G., & Gonzalez, J. M. (2005). Geriatric mental health clinicians' perceptions of barriers and contributors to retention of older minorities in treatment: An exploratory study. *Clinical Gerontologist, 28,* 3–25.

Clark, C. M., DeCarli, C., Mungas, D., Chui, H. I., Higdon, R., Nunez, J., et al. (2005). Earlier onset of Alzheimer's disease symptoms in Latino individuals compared with Anglo individuals. *Archives of Neurology, 6,* 774–778.

Crewe, S. E., & Chipungu, S. S. (2006). Social work with older Latinos: A mental health perspective. In B. Berkman (Ed.), *Handbook of social work in aging* (pp. 539–549). New York: Oxford University Press.

Federal Interagency Forum on Aging-Related Statistics. (2004). *Older Americans 2004: Key indicators of well-being.* Washington, DC: U.S. Government Printing Office.

Flora, C. B. (1989). The political economy of fotonovela production in Latin America. *Studies in Latin American Popular Culture, 8,* 215–230.

Freidenberg, J., & Jimenez-Velasquez, I. Z. (1992). Assessing impairment among Hispanic elderly: Biomedical and ethnomedical perspectives. In T. L. Brink (Ed.), *Hispanic aged mental health* (pp. 131–144). New York: Haworth.

Gallagher-Thompson, D., Areán, P., Coon, D., Menendez, A., Takagi, K., Haley, W. E., et al. (2000). Development and implementation of intervention strategies for culturally diverse caregiving populations. In R. Schulz (Ed.), *Handbook on dementia caregiving: Evidence-based interventions for family caregivers* (pp. 151–185). New York: Springer.

Gallagher-Thompson, D., Areán, P., Rivera, P., & Thompson, L. (2003). A psychoeducational intervention to reduce distress in Hispanic family caregivers: Results of a pilot study. *Clinical Gerontologist, 23,* 17–32.

Gallagher-Thompson, D., Coon, D. W., Solano, N., Ambler, C., Rabinowitz, Y., & Thompson, L. (2003). Changes in indices of distress among Latino and Anglo female caregivers of elderly relatives with dementia: Site-specific results from the REACH National Collaborative Study. *The Gerontologist, 43,* 580–591.

Gamst, G., Dana, R. H., Der-Karabetian, A., Aragon, M., Arellano, L. M., & Kramer, T. (2002). Effects of Latino acculturation and ethnic identity on mental health outcomes. *Hispanic Journal of Behavioral Sciences, 24,* 479–505.

Gamst, G., Dana, R. H., Der-Karabetian, & Kramer, T. (2000). Ethnic match and client ethnicity effects on global assessment and visitation. *Journal of Community Psychology, 28,* 547–564.

Givaudan, M., Pick, S., de Venguer, M. T. T., & Xolocotzin, U. (2003). *Bridging the communication gap: Provider to patient written communication across language and cultural barriers.* Monograph prepared for Hablamos Juntos, Tomás Rivera Policy Institute, University of Southern California, School of Policy, Planning and Development and the Institute for Social and Economic Research and Policy, Columbia University.

Guarnaccia, P. J., & Rodriguez, O. (1996). Concepts of culture and their role in the development of culturally competent mental health services. *Hispanic Journal of Behavioral Sciences, 18,* 419–443.

Guarnaccia, P., & Rogler, L. H. (1999). Research on culture-bound syndromes: New directions. *American Journal of Psychiatry, 156,* 1322–1327.

Hardin, T., & Jordan-Marsh, M. (2005). Fictive kin: Friends as family supporting older adults as they age. *Journal of Gerontological Nursing, 31,* 24–31.

Hazuda, H. P., Gerety, M., Williams, J. W., Lawrence, V., Calmbach, W., & Mulrow, C. (2000). Health promotion research with Mexican American elders: Matching approaches to settings at the mediator- and micro-levels of recruitment. *Journal of Mental Health and Aging, 6,* 79–90.

Henderson, N. J., & Henderson, L. C. (2002). Cultural construction of disease: A "supernormal" construct of dementia in an American Indian tribe. *Journal of Cross-Cultural Gerontology, 17,* 197–212.

Kleinman, A., Eisenberg, L., & Good, B. (1978). Clinical lessons from anthropologic and cross-cultural research. *Annals of Internal Medicine, 88,* 51–258.

Lewis-Fernández, R., Das, A. K., César, A., Weissman, M., & Olfson, M. (2005). Depression in U.S. Hispanics: Diagnostic and management considerations in family practice. *Journal of the American Board of Family Practice, 18,* 282–296.

Magaña, S. (2006). Older Latino family caregivers. In B. Berkman (Ed.), *Handbook of social work in aging* (pp. 371–380). New York: Oxford University Press.

Mahoney, D. F., Cloutterbuck, J., Neary, S., & Zhan, L. (2005). African American, Chinese, and Latino family caregivers' impressions of the onset and diagnosis of dementia: Cross-cultural similarities and differences. *The Gerontologist, 45,* 783–792.

Mezzich, J. E., Kirmayer, L. J., Kleinman, A., Fabrega, H., Parron, D. L., Good, B. J., et al. (1999). The place of culture in DSM-IV. *Journal of Nervous and Mental Disease, 187,* 457–464.

Morano, C., & Bravo, M. (2002). A psychoeducational model for Hispanic Alzheimer's disease caregivers. *The Gerontologist, 42,* 122–126.

Morano, C., & King, D. (2005). Religiosity as a mediator of caregiver well-being: Does ethnicity make a difference? *Journal of Gerontological Social Work, 45,* 69–84.

Morano, C. L., & Sanders, S. (2005). Exploring differences in depression, role captivity and self-acceptance in Hispanic and non-Hispanic caregivers. *Journal of Ethnic and Cultural Diversity on Social Work, 14,* 27–46.

Ortega, A. N., & Rosenheck, R. (2002). Hispanic client-case manager matching: Differences in outcomes and service use in a program for homeless persons with severe mental illness. *Journal of Nervous and Mental Disease, 190,* 315–323.

O'Sullivan, M. J., & Lasso, B. (1992). Community mental health services for Hispanics: A test of the culture compatibility hypothesis. *Hispanic Journal of Behavioral Sciences, 14,* 455–468.

Paniagua, F. A. (2001). *Diagnosis in a multicultural context: A casebook for mental health professionals.* Thousand Oaks, CA: Sage.

Pew Research Center. (2005). Hispanics: A people in motion. In Pew Research Center (Ed.), *Trends 2005* (pp. 70–89). Washington, DC: Author.

Picot, S. J., Debanne, S. M., Namzi, K. H., & Wykle, M. L. (1997). Religiosity and perceived rewards of Black and White caregivers. *The Gerontologist, 37,* 89–101.

Rudd, R., & Comings, J. (1994). Learner-centered materials: An empowering product. *Health Education Quarterly, 21,* 313–327.

Snowden, L. R., Hu, T. W., & Jerrell, J. (1995). Emergency care avoidance: Ethnic matching and participation in minority-serving programs. *Community Mental Health Journal, 31,* 463–473.

Stine, J. J. (2005). The use of metaphors in the service of the therapeutic alliance. *Journal of the American Academy of Psychoanalysis and Dynamic Psychiatry, 33,* 531–545.

Takeuchi, D. T., Sue, S., & Yeh, M. (1995). Return rates and outcomes from ethnicity-specific mental health programs in Los Angeles. *American Journal of Public Health, 85,* 638–643.

Talamantes, M., & Aranda, M. P. (2004). *Cultural competency in working with family caregivers.* San Francisco: Family Caregiver Alliance. Retrieved November 29, 2004, from http://www.caregiver.org/caregiver/jsp/content_node.jsp?nodeid=1095

U.S. Census Bureau. (2003). *Language use and English-speaking ability: 2000* (Census 2000 Brief). U.S. Department of Commerce, Economics and Statistics Administration. Washington, DC: Author.

Valle, R. (1998). *Caregiving across cultures: Working with dementing illness and ethnically diverse populations.* Washington, DC: Taylor & Francis.

Vera, M., Vila, D., & Alegría, M. (2003). Cognitive-behavioral therapy: Concepts, issues, and strategies for practice with racial/ethnic minorities. In G. Bernal, J. E. Trimble, A. Kathleen Burlew, & F. T. L. Leong (Eds.), *Handbook of racial and ethnic minority psychology* (pp. 521–538). Thousand Oaks, CA: Sage.

Villa, V. M., & Aranda, M. P. (2000). The demographic, economic, and health profile of older Latinos: Implications for health and long-term care policy and the family. *Journal of Health and Human Services Administration, 23,* 161–180.

CHAPTER ELEVEN

Model Dementia Care Programs for Asian Americans

Nancy Emerson Lombardo, Bei Wu, Kun Chang,
and Jennifer K. Hohnstein

INTRODUCTION

Many members of the Chinese American community view dementia as a mental illness, which is very stigmatizing and shameful. In addition, the language barrier both causes and exacerbates this stigma. Further, the lack of services and education programs tailored to the Chinese American population leaves few options available for persons who attempt to seek help.

In this chapter, we discuss the issues and barriers that Chinese American communities face regarding dementia care. We will then introduce the Chinese Dementia Awareness and Intervention Project (CDAIP), a model we created to address the issue of dementia care among Chinese American communities in the greater Boston area.

DEMOGRAPHIC TRENDS

Asian Americans are one of the fastest-growing ethnic minority groups; there are currently nearly 12 million Asian Americans in the United States, and that number is expected to reach 22 million by 2025 (U.S. Census Bureau, 1996). A large percentage (23.8%) of Asian Americans are Chinese Americans. Among the Asian population, 8% are elders aged 65 and older (Reeves & Bennett, 2004).

In the city of Boston, where the CDAIP was located, the Asian American population grew 46.7% from 1990 to 2000. In the Greater Boston area, in a 1990 census of three counties, there were about 6,750 Asian and Pacific Islanders over the age of 60, of which most are Chinese. Based on some recent prevalence studies, the prevalence of dementia among those age 65 and older will be more than 10% (Manton, Gu, & Ukraintseva, 2005), and that number is expected to more than triple by 2025 (Evans et al., 1989).[1]

Despite the growing need, dementia services and educational resources within the Chinese American community were seriously deficient. In the late 1990s, there were no existing bilingual programs for Chinese Americans in all of New England. Even today, in the Boston area, there is insufficient housing, no available assisted living program, and only one nursing home with Cantonese/Mandarin-speaking staff for Chinese American elders.

BARRIERS TO SEEKING HELP

Barriers experienced by Chinese American families exemplify the knowledge, access, and intent barriers described for other elderly populations (Silverstein, 1984; Yeatts, Crow, and Folts, 1992). Research shows that Chinese families providing care to an elder with dementia tend to use fewer support services than families from other ethnic groups (Ho, Weitzman, Cui, & Levkoff, 2000; Wu, 2000). Explanations for the low use of services by Chinese include the view that dementia symptoms are part of normal aging, a stigma toward Alzheimer's disease, the Confucian value of piety (the importance of children taking care of elders), and a lack of culturally competent service and educational information (Chow, Ross, Fox, Cummings, & Lin, 2000; Delgado, 2000; Elliott, Minno, Lam, & Tu, 1996; Guo, Levy, Hinton, Weitzman, & Levkoff, 2000; Levkoff, Levy, &, Weitzman, 2000; Ren & Chang, 1998; Tabora & Flaskerud, 1997).

One of the most common responses to dementia (among Chinese Americans as well as many other groups) is viewing the symptoms as a normal consequence of aging. Since many Chinese American families do not perceive dementia as an illness, they do not seek services at all or may only seek services late in the disease process. An ethnically Chinese Western-trained primary care physician may even share and reinforce this perception of aging.

Alternatively, some Chinese Americans interpret the signs and symptoms of dementia as indicative of mental disorder. When translated to

Chinese, the word *dementia* uses two characters, one meaning "crazy" and the other meaning "catatonic." This perception of dementia as a shameful mental illness triggers a strong negative response among Chinese families and often inhibits their seeking diagnosis and assistance (Elliott et al., 1996; Guo et al., 2000).

The stigma and shame associated with mental illness not only adheres to the individual with dementia but may also reflect on the entire family and is sometimes feared to detract from, for instance, the attractiveness of a granddaughter for marriage or any adult for membership in important groups. Therefore, elderly Chinese and their families have a strong tendency not to seek help (especially formal services) because of the fear of exposing family disgrace (Ren & Chang, 1998; Tabora & Flaskerud, 1997).

This complex situation places a difficult burden on the individual with dementia and the caregiver since dementia stigmatizes not only the individual but also the entire family. The family and the caregiver find themselves facing a traditional culture that regards dementia not as an illness or disease but as the punishment for past moral transgressions or other failings.

Knowing that a label of dementia can bring shame to the entire family, Chinese doctors may not voice their suspicions about Alzheimer's disease or dementia if the family has adapted to the changing needs of the elder with dementia. Even mainstream primary care physicians are often reluctant to make the diagnosis or share with the family because of concerns over lack of treatment options (Emerson Lombardo, 1997; U.S. Department of Health and Human Services, 1996). Thus, only when the situation seems to have deteriorated to the point that the family can no longer handle things on their own is a diagnosis sought or offered by a Chinese health care provider. By the time families seek help, the situation is usually desperate, and there is immediate need for assistive services or nursing home placement.

Additionally, a large percentage of Asian caregivers are immigrants with limited English proficiency, which is another barrier to obtaining services. Immigrants face many stressors, including those created by the acculturation process, stressful life events, employment, and economic hardships. They may have higher levels of stress than the general White population (Kuo, 1984; Kuo & Tsai, 1986). As Liu (1986) points out, most new immigrants are either unreachable or neglected by health and home care organizations.

Asian American's lack of knowledge regarding the availability of services and means of assistance is another key reason why Asian Americans have not sought social services as often as others (Calsyn & Roades, 1993; Die & Seelbach, 1988; Krout, 1983; Lee, 1992; Nah, 1993; National Alliance for Caregiving & American Association of Retired Persons,

1996; Uba & Sue, 1991). English-speaking Asian caregiving responding to a national telephone survey also were less likely to provide assisted day living care for the elder, and 50% said they did not know what kind of help they needed (compared to only 34% to 38% for other ethnic groups) (National Alliance for Caregiving & American Association of Retired Persons, 1996).

The reluctance of Chinese Americans to seek social services may cause the underdocumentation of dementia prevalence rates in this population. For example, while many Chinese studies provide lower rates of dementia than in the United States, people with dementia often are diagnosed at much later stages in China and have more severe symptoms than their U.S. counterparts (Yu et al., 1989; Zhang et al., 1990). Dementia does not seem to be as well recognized in China as in the United States. Wu's (2000) study, using a nationally representative telephone survey with English-speaking caregivers, showed that a much lower percentage of Asian care-givers (13%) compared to Hispanic (20%) and White (21%) caregivers reported that they were caring for persons with dementia. However, the low percentage of the dementia patients reported by Asian American care-givers may not reflect the actual prevalence of dementia in the population because of the stigma and denial issues just described.

THE CDAIP

To address problems surrounding dementia care in the Chinese communities of the greater Boston area, the Chinese Dementia Aware-ness and Intervention Project (CDAIP) was launched in 1998. The CDAIP was spearheaded by the primary author of this chapter, along with the Greater Boston Chinese Golden Age Center (GBCGAC), the Wellesley Center for Research on Women, Midtown Health Care, Inc., and the Massachusetts Chapter of the Alzheimer's Association.

Funded by the Boston Foundation and subsequently by the EHA Foundation, this community-based collaborative project accomplished the following tasks:

1. Reaching out to the Boston Chinese community and raising awareness about dementia
2. Increasing institutional awareness and commitment to caregiving for Chinese elders with dementia
3. Enhancing the knowledge of dementia and skills among Chinese pro-fessional caregivers and family caregivers of persons with dementia
4. Increasing the availability of educational and assessment materials concerning culturally appropriate services related to coping with the pressures of caregiving

5. Increasing access to existing services for Chinese elders with dementia and their family members
6. Creating new services for family caregivers: a help line and an individualized family caregiver intervention
7. Ensuring the sustainability of new services for Chinese elders with dementia by obtaining continuous funding

Through this project, we were able to identify and successfully serve a group of caregivers and persons with dementia who probably would not have been identified and served by the mainstream service system. In 2 years, our team created an outreach/public education effort, a train-the-trainer program (called the Chinese Dementia Specialist Education Program), a phone help line, a bilingual brochure, public access bilingual educational materials, and an individualized caregiver counseling and support program. Each of these efforts is discussed in turn later in the chapter.

Collaboration Efforts

The model we created was a three-way collaboration of an academic institution (Wellesley Centers for Women), Chinese American community-based agencies, and a mainstream agency (the Massachusetts chapter of the Alzheimer's Association), with each of the organizations learning from and empowering the others.

The Greater Boston Chinese Golden Age Center (GBCGAC) was an important community-based agency collaborator. The GBCGAC is the largest organization to serve Chinese Americans in the greater Boston area. Currently, the GBCGAC services about 1,000 Chinese elderly clients each year, together with more than 1,000 family members. It provides many services, such as adult day health/transportation programs, independent living residences, an extensive nutrition program, a Lifeline medical emergency program, drop-in social service programs, and a variety of health promotion programs to help people navigate the health, insurance, and social service systems. A key to the project's success was the mutuality of exchanges of information, empowerment, and resources between all participating organizations, a finding consistent with the Relational-Cultural Theory of Human Development (Jordan, Miller, & Walker, 2000).

As Figure 11.1 depicts, the community agency staff offered concrete experiences and authentic perspectives from persons who work with Chinese Americans. The Alzheimer's Association learned how to better serve the Chinese American community while in turn offering their expertise about the disease and providing help-line training, speakers,

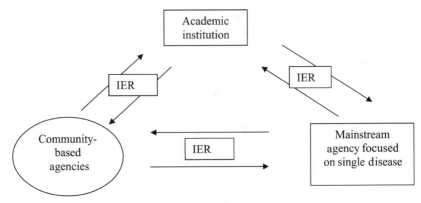

IER-information, empowerment, and resources

FIGURE 11.1   Model of collaborative efforts to raise awareness about a specific disease.

and materials for the CDSEP. The researchers provided funding (through foundation grants), information and an infusion of additional time, effort, and expertise to organize and facilitate intensive sustained education and service development efforts. This program shows a model for a successful effort to build enduring capacity to serve Chinese Americans dealing with dementia that could be replicated in other multilingual communities.

Process-wise, our project began with team meetings composed of representatives from the three groups (some of whom were social workers), then focused on the staff training program to build staff awareness and focus groups to solicit staff suggestions and buy-in for services development.

Issues in Community Outreach

Outreach efforts in minority communities require a clear understanding of the target populations, intracommunity linkages, service accessibility (e.g., location and cost), sensitivity to the cultural and ethnic characteristics of the clients to be served, and knowledge of existing barriers (Alzheimer's Association, Columbus Chapter, 1989; Ballard, 1990, 1993; Belleville-Taylor et al., 1993; Cox, 1999; Emerson Lombardo, Dresser, Belleville-Taylor, Wu, & Ooi, 2000; Emerson Lombardo, Dresser et al. 2001; Emerson Lombardo & Ooi, 1998; Sinclair et al., 2000; Valle, 1988–1989, 1989, 1990, 1990, June; Wykle, 1993; Wykle & Segal, 1991).

The most effective outreach efforts occur when the staff remains flexible in their approach and open to modifications as they learn to interact with the community. An awareness of community needs and experiences is central to success, while rigid preconceptions appear to result in failed efforts (Valle, 1988–1989). Sensitive approaches begin with cultural knowledge, awareness of the use of language, and ultimately the translation of this information into targeted staffing and programmatic decisions. Success requires a focus on community linkages among agencies and a willingness to work with and through existing support networks (Ballard, 1990, 1993; Valle, 1989).

Minorities have been treated as an underclass in our society. Thus, their faith in mainstream institutions is not high, as promises have often been broken and services to the minority community limited. Many minority elders are discouraged, worn down by historic prejudices and exclusionary service practices (Valle, 1988–1989, 1990, 1990, June). We focused on these important issues in our Boston needs assessment.

Our effort had to emphasize service as its priority rather than research data collection. In addition, we encountered communication barriers between the underserved populations and the research community. To best meet the needs of Chinese Americans with dementia and their caregivers, researchers and outreach workers need to develop collaborative and cooperative relationships between informal and formal support systems. The formal system, as such, should be recognized as parallel and complementary to the informal system (Mindel, Wright, & Starrett, 1986). Knowledge gained by researchers concerned with recruitment for their studies also helped guide our efforts (Belleville-Taylor et al., 1993; Gurland et al., 1995; Guthrie & Pegelow, 1993; Valle, 1990; Wykle, 1993; Wykle & Segal, 1991). Helpful strategies for outreach and recruitment to minority populations include collaborating with relevant "gatekeepers" and using focus groups to shape recruitment materials and approaches (Sinclair et al., 2000). A key ingredient for success is having outreach carried out by a bicultural person who either lives in the target community or has a familiarity with it. Personal ties can add further legitimacy to an effort.

Our survey at the time of other outreach efforts confirmed that a primary barrier to utilization arises from the lack of knowledge concerning the disease, services, procedures, and needs. We found that networking with preexisting minority community organizations, especially religious groups, facilitates minority outreach efforts. In addition, existing services and informational materials need to be modified to meet the cultural and language needs of the minority group. Our previous African American outreach/education and caregiver intervention project staff formed partnerships with and worked through community organizations and institutions to this end (Belleville-Taylor, 1993; Emerson Lombardo, Dresser, et al., 2001; Emerson Lombardo & Ooi, 1998). We knew that success depended on the effort becoming "owned" or at least partnered by the community to which it was directed. White middle-class suburban faces and ownership could have invited failure. Our long-term commitments to minority outreach efforts necessitated a sustained investment of time and effort and helped us achieve sufficient penetration into ethnic communities.

Henderson, Gutierrez-Mayaka, Garcia, and Boyd (1993) also developed a successful outreach program of support groups for African American dementia caregivers. They emphasize the importance of "ethnic competence," the knowledge of the salient social and cultural aspects of ethnic communities to maximize program effectiveness. They also underline the importance of repeated and frequent personal contacts with minority caregivers and flexibility of project design to tailor interventions to the needs of an individual family. Henderson et al. (1993) also emphasized the importance of indigenous support leaders. Their conclusions point to the critical role of information, cultural familiarity, perception, and problem definition in determining use of existing resources.

How best to focus resources depends on the cultural history, geographic distribution, and social network patterns of ethnic minorities within a particular city. Various reports on sources of referrals for Alzheimer's Disease and Related Dementias (ADRD) case finding, programs, or services indicate that, to some extent, the most successful recruiting/publicity strategies varies by geographic area or city as well as by ethnic or cultural groups (Gurland et al, 1995; Guthrie & Pegelow, 1993). Where care partners are better informed, service use improves (Barresi, 1992; Valle, 1988–1989, 1990; Wykle, 1993). We believe open discussion, analysis and negotiation of differences that create barriers to recruitment can lead to a successful effort by evolving a better match between ethnic minority groups and researchers at the macro, mediator, and individual levels (Levkoff, Levy, & Weitzman, 2000).

THE CHINESE DEMENTIA SPECIALIST EDUCATION PROGRAM

In order to reach successfully both recent immigrants and later generations of Chinese Americans and to provide culturally appropriate services, special training programs are needed in their communities. Staff at ethnic community service agencies have the potential to successfully provide dementia-related services and outreach to their clients because they speak the same language as their clients, are familiar with their culture, and are not viewed as outsiders. On the basis of our previous work with African Americans, we believed that training ethnic minority providers about dementia and service availability and, in turn, asking them to reach persons with dementia and their caregivers is an effective way to provide outreach and perform caregiver interventions (Belleville-Taylor et al., 1993; Emerson Lombardo, Dresser, et al., 2001; Emerson Lombardo & Ooi, 1998).

Our train-the-trainer program, called the Chinese Dementia Specialist Education Program (CDSEP), reflected both the literature and the team members' experience and belief in the importance of capacity building for existing staff as opposed to continually bringing in outside experts for in-service training. Its design was based on previous informal need assessments by our own team and another one at Harvard Medical School.

The CDSEP was launched in 1998 and had three goals:

1. To train Chinese American bilingual professionals as dementia specialists so they could improve services to the elderly
2. To encourage the dementia specialists to spread their knowledge throughout their agencies and to others within the Chinese American communities
3. To engage CDSEP participants to shape and support a new dementia outreach and service development effort

Methods

The CDSEP was a collaborative effort among academic researchers, executives from three community-based agencies serving Chinese American elders, the local Alzheimer's Association chapter, and three consultants from mainstream agencies. The course was 17 hours in total. Classes were conducted in English at the request of the community-based agencies that wished to encourage participants to improve their English proficiency (Emerson Lombardo, Wu, & Hohnstein, 2001; Emerson Lombardo, Wu, Hohnstein, & Chang, 2001).

As incentives for participant retention, top agency executives attended all of the classes themselves and dementia specialist certificates were awarded to all CDSEP participants who graduated with perfect attendance and completed evaluation forms for each class. We also offered continuing education units for nurses and social workers and created videotapes that attendees could watch to make up missed classes.

The CDSEP featured 11 lecture topics, presented by various faculty experts and chosen for their relevance to the prospective participants. Topics included the signs and symptoms of dementia, the differences between dementia and normal aging, the latest research and medical treatment, drug reactions, cultural issues, communication issues, behavioral issues, services offered by the Alzheimer's Association, therapeutic activities, Chinese medicine, acupuncture, and more.

Cultural issues related to dementia services were introduced in the first two classes and then integrated into each later session. Participants were encouraged to share their experiences with Chinese elders and families. As part of the cultural appropriateness efforts, most speakers were knowledgeable about both Chinese American culture and dementia including four Chinese American physicians and clinicians.

The final two classes focused on small-group discussions designed (successfully) to encourage staff to take ownership of emerging outreach and dementia service efforts. Participants also discussed the resources they believed were needed to carry out their own roles more effectively.

The CDSEP participants received more than 300 pages of written materials in both English and Chinese on designated curriculum topics, including a Chinese language "activity guidebook" (Hong Kong Alzheimer's Disease and Brain Failure Association, 1997). We purposely distributed a considerable amount of materials so that each dementia specialist would have them readily available both for personal reference and to share with others and to use for subsequent training of other people.

To gain a better understanding of how effective the course was, CDSEP participants took baseline and posttests about Alzheimer's disease and caregiving. Finally, 10 months after the completion of the course, we sent participants a monitoring tool. This instrument asked participants to enumerate the number of services and lectures they had given and about the perceived usefulness of the course in both their personal and their professional lives.

Results and Discussion

The CDSEP trained 22 people from various agencies, of which 16 were certified as bilingual dementia specialists. The CDSEP graduates helped more than 70 families within 10 months of completing the training program. In addition, they held 76 workshops and discussions that we estimate reached approximately 300 to 400 people. Furthermore, one CDSEP graduate served as a panelist on a television show on Alzheimer's disease and another spoke about Alzheimer's on a local Cantonese radio station.

Since the course, evaluation materials, and many of the handouts were in English, people with limited English proficiency experienced difficulties that appeared to affect their test scores, attendance, and participation in the follow-up surveys. They were also less likely to receive certification as dementia specialists. For future classes that target multilingual communities, it is recommended that participants first be surveyed to determine their language/dialect preference and whether translators are needed for key sessions. Furthermore, both the audio and the visual course materials should reflect the participants' primary language preference in addition to English.

We also recommend creating continuing education and peer support services. Continuing education would involve periodically updating dementia knowledge after the completion of the initial formal training. Peer support activities could provide on-the-job troubleshooting and emotional support. These services would aid the solidification of new knowledge, ensure appropriate handling of client cases, and encourage frontline workers to take on more dementia clients and caregivers.

Feedback from participants on improving the course included having information about new research, including alternative treatments for Alzheimer's disease; using more case studies; adding more tests and quizzes to reinforce learning; and adding additional information on patient advocacy and how to help caregivers address behavior issues. Also suggested was training participants on how to administer simple cognitive screens in Chinese and English to help staff recognize persons with dementia. This request highlights the need for culturally sensitive cognitive screening tools that are also short and easy to administer.

The success of the CDSEP demonstrates that the train-the-trainer model is an effective approach for building dementia care capacity in community-based agencies, increasing outreach to people with dementia and their families, and raising dementia awareness in bilingual and minority communities. In addition, once staff are trained, they can be effectively involved in choosing priorities and shaping programs to meet the needs of clients about whom they have become more knowledgeable.

BILINGUAL HELP LINE

An important component of the CDAIP was the creation of a Chinese-language dementia help line. The help line offered an immediate solution to people who needed information about the process, treatments, and services associated with dementia.

To disseminate information about the helpline, we stepped up outreach efforts (radio, presentations, newspapers, etc.) and created and distributed the world's first bilingual Chinese/English Alzheimer's brochure, which included help-line contact information. Bilingual brochures are necessary to reach simultaneously elders, who mostly read only Chinese, and younger family members and mainstream professionals, who mostly read only English; each party wants to know what the others are reading. For example, English-speaking referral sources could read the English portion and feel comfortable referring their Chinese American clients to these new services.

Next, the teams choose people who would actually run the help line. The skills needed for this job included a fluent knowledge of Alzheimer's disease and dementia; an ability to locate key services needed by clients, proficiency in Cantonese, English, and Mandarin; and an established reputation within the Chinese community. The team chose two social work staffers on the basis of these criteria.

The Alzheimer's' Association of Eastern Massachusetts provided the initial help-line training, follow-up training, peer support, and backup for questions and concerns. The two help-line staffers were also trained through the CSDEP program. We also collected Chinese-language materials on dementia and aging from around the world; when Chinese-language materials simply did not exist, the team translated materials from English. We created three libraries on Chinese dementia in the GBCGAC branch offices, from which the help-line workers could retrieve, copy, and distribute relevant information. In addition to running the help line, they also offered longer-term services, including consultation and counseling.

Summary of Help-Line Results and Discussion

The help line quickly became a key aspect of our efforts, proved itself to be a great asset to the Chinese-speaking communities, and helped approximately 40 to 50 families per year who found it a convenient and culturally appropriate service. The topics counseled on included home safety, available services, transportation, dementia symptoms, care methods, home-based activities for the person with dementia, and emotional and behavior issues. Encounters included emotional support for the client and families.

Statistics gathered for 11 client dyads during a 6-month period in 1999–2000 by one of the two help-line counselors showed that the average age of the elders was 76; 65% were female, 57% lived alone, and 78% lived in Boston, and none of the dementia patients spoke English. Of 91 telephone interactions that were tracked, 26% were information requests, 4% were referrals, 42% were assistance to caregivers in acquiring services, and 27% were follow-up calls. Topics discussed, tracked for 33 clients, included 30% about adult day health, 12% home safety, 24% elders at risk concerns, 21% behavioral problems, and 2% assorted other topics.

Among both the help-line and the caregiver advocacy families, almost none of the Chinese elders with probable dementia spoke English, and less than half of their family caregivers did. Most of the caregivers who did speak English were not fluent enough to deal with complicated issues involved in gaining service in the long-term care system. Since our help-line staffers spoke English, Mandarin, Cantonese, Taishanese, and various dialects, they were equipped to overcome the language barrier within this community and to help introduce and even escort families to appropriate services. Thus, this bilingual, bicultural service was essential; no other providers exist in the greater Boston area.

The pictures we present about these model services can provide valuable information for policymakers that may be missing from mainstream studies. Unfortunately, for the Chinese community, policymakers usually base programs on national databases, such as the census and the National Caregiver Alliance Survey. These databases usually exclude non-English-speaking persons.

For example, the National Caregiver Alliance Survey was the only nationally representative survey that included Asian caregivers. However, even their sample was skewed and biased because it excluded all non-English-speaking persons and excluded all those without telephones. The result was that many Asian caregivers in their survey had higher incomes and education than those in census data. The census may also undercount those Chinese-speaking persons who, because of age or lack of English, are missed by the census forms, which are in English.

INDIVIDUALIZED CAREGIVER COUNSELING AND SUPPORT INTERVENTION

In the past few decades, caregiver research has burgeoned to being one of the most frequently studied issues in gerontology (Emerson Lombardo & Eisdorfer, 1993; Zarit, 1990, 1991). Family caregivers of persons with Alzheimer's disease provide the majority of informal care (that provided by nonprofessionals) and have a critical role in initiating and directing the formal care for community-dwelling Alzheimer's victims (Emerson Lombardo & Eisdorfer, 1993; Schultz & O'Brien, 1994).

However, at the time the CDAIP was launched, there was still a pressing need for documentation to reveal and clarify caregiving experiences in the minority communities so that agencies can provide culturally appropriate and informed services (Advisory Panel on Alzheimer's Disease, 1991; Ballard, 1993; Emerson Lombardo & Aronson, 1995; Gallagher-Thompson, 1994; Gallagher-Thompson et al., 2003; Gelfand, 1994; Henderson et al., 1993; Shultz & O'Brien, 1994; Valle, 1990). Thus, the Chinese Caregiver Intervention was created. It was an adaptation of a National Institute on Aging (NIA) grant titled the Multicultural Memory Loss Awareness Project (MMLAP) (Emerson Lombardo, Dresser, et al., 2001; Emerson Lombardo & Ooi, 1998) and with some similarities with interventions being developed elsewhere (Brodaty, 1994; Brodaty, Peters, 1991; Brodaty, Mittelman, & Burns, 2003; Emerson Lombardo, Wu, & Harden, 2000; Emerson Lombardo, Wu, Malivert, et al., 2002; Mittelman, 2003; Mittelman, Ferris, Steinberg, et al., 1993; Mittelman, Ferris, Shulman, Steinberg, & Levin, 1996).

Participants

The primary subjects in this study were caregivers of persons with dementia. For eligibility purposes, all elders with dementia in the caregiver/elder dyads (n = 11) had symptoms of memory loss and were not expected to die, move, or enter a nursing home throughout the 6-month intervention. Recruitment occurred via hospitals, home care agencies, clinics, and day care services. In addition, advertisements were placed in Chinese newspapers and on radio programs.

The interventionist received training and certification through the CDSEP. Then the interventionist was trained for an additional 4 weeks on (a) becoming a caregiver advocate, (b) assessing caregiver needs, (c) using the assessment instrument, and (d) conducting in-home skill training intervention consisting of education, counseling, and service acquisition.

Beginning in May 1999, this specialist made home visits to families, teaching them skills for caring for their elders with dementia and offering them information about caregiving options and assistance in securing supportive services and community support. She offered counseling and emotional support as needed and guided them in relieving their own stress.

Bilingual Assessment Instrument

This program included piloting of a complete assessment of patient and caregiver status and issues adapted from a previous caregiver intervention assessment developed under the NIA-funded MMLAP effort and translated into Chinese. The assessment instrument was designed to be completed over several meetings and be part of the therapeutic intervention. Domains covered by the instrument included caregiver status; caregiver moods and sense of burden/stress; history of client memory and cognitive issues; client physical, cognitive, and emotional condition; behavioral symptoms; and client and family financial and legal status. In addition, the MMSE (in Chinese) was used to give a direct assessment of cognitive status. The assessment guided the interventionist and family in setting priorities and making decisions.

The assessment, education, and training occurred in the caregiver's home to allow firsthand observation of the caregiving situation to accommodate caregivers with limited free time. All documentation was made in English so that the answers, orally given in Chinese, did not require translation. Evaluations were also based on the interventionist's case notes.

Results

Approximately 15 families were helped during the 18-month intervention demonstration and others after the demonstration period. Caregivers were very satisfied with this individualized, personalized program. We gathered statistics on 10 caregiver/patient dyads. Of these caregivers, 50% were women, and 50% were men. The majority of caregivers (60%) resided with the person with dementia. The caregivers' ages ranged from 42 to 80 (mean 59 years);[2] 70% lived in Boston. Only four (40%) caregivers spoke English, seven spoke Cantonese (70%), two spoke Mandarin (20%), and two spoke Taishanese (20%).

The elders with dementia ages ranged from 68 to 93 years (average age was 83)[3] and were mainly women (90%); 40% of elders lived alone and 60% with their caregivers. None of the elders spoke English but instead spoke Cantonese (50%), Taishanese (30%), and Mandarin (20%).

Types of counseling/consultation services used included needs assessments (29%), counseling (33%), service acquisition (13%), follow-up (17%), and referral (8%). Service-related topics discussed during sessions with caregivers included adult day health (50%), Medicaid (21%), "general questions" (13%), nursing homes (13%), and home safety (4%). Other issues addressed most frequently included embarrassing behaviors, verbal abuse, isolation, learning how to make positive financial arrangements, and handling challenging behaviors as well as emotional support for the caregiver.

Because of the stigma associated with dementia, some families meet the interventionist with great reluctance and wanted a shorter intervention length. Thus, the length of visits varied greatly, with some families wanting between one and four visits and others wanting more than 10. The planned 24 hours of the intervention was divided among approximately 10 to 14 home visits at mutual convenience and visits to the caregiver's home as well as caregivers coming into the office to see the social worker.

Barriers to Services

The lack of knowledge and training for social services workers serving the Chinese communities, especially the direct social services providers, caused delays in caregivers and persons with dementia receiving needed services and support. For instance, one case manager working in a local agency serving the Chinese communities stated that he did not know what Alzheimer's disease was and how to differentiate Alzheimer's from normal aging. He could identify the signs of dementia only with great difficulty. He also was unfamiliar with community services available for persons with dementia and their families. As a result, he could not develop comprehensive long-term care plans needed to serve the persons with dementia.

As mentioned earlier in the chapter, many caregivers neglect the signs of dementia at the early and middle stage of the disease because they often confuse the symptoms of dementia as the normal signs of aging. This belief builds up barriers for social services workers to aid those who need help and information.

This lack of knowledge caused many Chinese family caregivers to exhaust their own resources before seeking help. For example, a daughter sought day care services for her mother with dementia; the mother had had Pick's disease for years. The screening and assessment revealed the mother to be in a late stage of Pick's disease; she required one-on-one individual supervision with intensive care. During the intervention, the daughter was surprised to discover the existing social and community services that, for years, could have better supported her to perform the tasks of caring for her mother.

As mentioned earlier, language problems limit the service choices for Chinese-speaking persons with dementia and their caregivers. One caregiver/elder dyad in the intervention had become housebound and felt socially isolated despite trying to seek help by putting themselves on a nursing home waiting list. While the couple was assisted in obtaining other services during the wait, a year after the intervention they still had not entered the nursing home. Chinese-speaking elders also have difficulties using transportation services.

The lack of culturally appropriate hospitals and nursing homes cause many family caregivers to spend long periods of time daily in institutions caring for the elder; they aid the English-speaking staff to deliver services to the patient. Even once the elder is in the hospital or care facility, non-Chinese-speaking primary physicians, because of language barriers, have difficulty identifying dementia and suggesting appropriate treatments. Compounding this problem, many family caregivers are unaware of the signs of memory and/or cognitive problems in the early stage, so they cannot bring them to attention of the physician.

Another complication arising from language barriers occurs within the Chinese-speaking community itself because of the multiple languages/dialects spoken. In one family, the person with dementia spoke Taishanese; her daughter/caregiver spoke Cantonese, Taishanese, and limited English; and her granddaughter-in-law spoke English and limited Cantonese. This intervention focused on mediation between the different family members to bridge the generational and cultural gaps. Thus, the language barrier not only separates the Chinese-speaking community from many English-speaking people and services but also internally fragments the Chinese-speaking community.

Many Chinese-speaking primary physicians do not aggressively advocate for Chinese persons with dementia and their families, even if they suspect memory problems in their patients, because of the stigma surrounding deterioration of mental health and the lack of physician education. Concurrently, many providers follow the popular use of Aricept and/or vitamin E to treat memory problems of patients but do not ask them to have a neurological assessment. This may cause the underdiagnosis or misdiagnosis of Alzheimer's and related diseases. This lack of diagnosis causes skewed statistics about the actual demands and needs of Chinese patients with dementia. This in turn results in uncertainty among legislative members and community leaders concerning development of linguistically and culturally appropriate services or programs.

Suggestions for Future Caregiver Intervention Programs

On the basis of her experiences with Chinese community caregivers, the interventionist created the following recommendations for caregiver interventions:

1. Provide informal peer support sessions that could be facilitated by Alzheimer's and dementia experts and a social worker on a regular basis
2. Encourage community-based agencies to network and publicize each other's services
3. Make more time available for home visits to meet caregiver schedules
4. Form support groups for caregivers
5. Train students or other responsible people as "relief" caregivers to allow primary caregivers some time off
6. Initiate a 3- to 6-month follow-up to assess whether new needs have arisen with the client and the family

Discussion

This 1-year caregiver intervention successfully identified and served a group of caregivers and persons with dementia who were overlooked by the mainstream service system. During this intervention, barriers that inhibit Chinese-speaking Americans from obtaining proper services were uncovered including: lack of trained health care professionals, lack of knowledge among Chinese-speaking caregivers, language barriers, and the lack of advocacy, diagnosis, and statistics.

LESSONS LEARNED FROM THE CDAIP

The Chinese Dementia Awareness and Intervention Project (CDAIP) demonstrated that, contrary to much popular wisdom, Chinese American elders and families responded as positively to caregiver support programs as any other ethnic group once they were created and offered them in a bilingual format with culturally attuned staff delivering the services in familiar settings and organizations.

A key to the success of this project was that the community-based agency took the lead, with the academic institution and the mainstream agency playing the facilitative and supportive roles and each of the three organizations learning from and empowering the other two. Another important aspect to our strategy was to create "experts" within the Chinese community who were likely to stay in place to continue delivering needed services and lead efforts to disseminate knowledge.

Agency executives modeled the priority they gave this effort through their own active participation and empowered and encouraged staff to help shape the new programs and volunteer to staff them. Thus, another important component of the CDAIP's success was making sure that agency staff knew they were expected to pass on their knowledge to other staff members as well as to clients and the general public with whom they had contact. Some conducted additional outreach efforts, gave talks or trainings on dementia and care, or helped implement or refer clients to the new programs.

Furthermore, this program demonstrated that staff initiative in taking on a new challenging program was rewarded by their employer. One employee was promoted after these programs and has since become a leader in the Chinese American aging services community.

In the Boston area, the pilot programs originally launched through the CDAIP have become an ongoing program of the GBCGAC through funding from the federal Family Caregiver Support program via the state, and the city of Boston. In addition, the CBCGAC has since become involved in other collaborative dementia research projects. However, additional funds are needed to revitalize and expand these programs supporting Chinese family caregivers of persons with dementia.

CONCLUSION

The CDAIP had three key factors behind its success:

1. Educating all staff members, from top executives to direct services workers, about dementia and engaging them in developing the new dementia care services ensured that each organization, its branch offices, and specialties could more successfully identify and serve persons with dementia and their families.
2. The train-the-trainer (CDSEP) program ensured that information was spread throughout the entire staff and communities.

3. The codevelopment of the outreach, help-line, and caregiver intervention programs and the increased capacity of all three types of partners would not have been possible without mutual exchanges of information, empowerment, and resources between the researchers, community-based agencies, and the mainstream agency.

While these were the elements that made the program successful, foundation funding was a prerequisite for the program's existence and development of the services. Government funding may be essential for their continuance. In addition, this project was greatly aided by a top-down commitment from community agencies' leadership who continually generated support and enthusiasm for this project.

Our explorations and findings in the Chinese American community provide valuable information for researchers who have traditionally had access only to mainstream findings in this area. This program shows a model for a successful service that could be replicated in other multilingual communities.

From this project, we developed some recommendations for future efforts. While these are addressed to Chinese American communities in Massachusetts, they can be applied to any Asian community, and they have been so applied in several regions of the United States thanks to the leadership of several other chapters of the Alzheimer's Association, other Asian-led community organizations, and funding through the federal State Alzheimer's Demonstration Program. The recommendations are the following:

1. Create, maintain, and expand existing Chinese-language help-line and individualized counseling and skills training and support system-building services for Chinese American family caregivers of persons with dementia.
2. Increase caregiving information available in the Chinese language about dementia and dementia-related services.
3. Adequately fund the creation of a complete continuum of care for Chinese American persons with dementia and fill any gaps. Quality services include adequate training of staff about dementia care.
4. Raise public awareness through ongoing publications, media outlets, and workshops in senior housing and centers. In addition, creating Web sites for patients and Chinese caregivers can be an effective way to raise awareness and reach out to our targeted population.
5. Raise health care and social service providers' awareness through training or education courses, information dissemination, and requests for culturally and linguistically appropriate services.

Acknowledgments

We thank Ruth Moy, executive director of the Greater Boston Chinese Golden Age Center (GBCGAC), and Nelson Wong, M.S.W., originally at the GBCGAC and later program director of the Asian Mental Health Program at the New England Medical Center, for their leadership and Jennifer K. Hohnstein, B.A., J.D., then the project coordinator in the latter years of the project when an undergraduate student at Wellesley College, coauthor of several papers, and now a graduate of University of Colorado, Boulder, School of Law and a practicing lawyer in Colorado; Pauline Belleville Taylor, R.N., C.N.S., of the Hebrew Rehabilitation Center for Aged, who helped design and lead the CDSEP effort; Wee Lock Ooi, Dr. P.H., of the Massachusetts Department of Public Health; and Zibin Guo, Ph.D., of the University of Tennessee for their contributions to this project. We would also like to thank Katherine Schleyer, then administrative assistant at the Wellesley College Center for Research on Women, for her assistance and other Wellesley undergraduate students who served as research assistants: Jennifer Choe, Wendy Fong, and Sharon Ng. The project team is grateful for funding by the Boston Foundation and the EHA Foundation and in-kind support from the Wellesley College Center for Research on Women and the GBCGAC that made this project possible.

NOTES

1. This number is based on calculations estimating that 5% of the 65+ Americans have Alzheimer's disease.
2. Only six caregivers gave their age, and the caseworker estimated three caregivers' ages.
3. The caseworker estimated two elders' ages.

REFERENCES

Advisory Panel on Alzheimer's Disease. (1991). *Second report of the advisory panel on Alzheimer's disease, 1990.* DHHS Pub. No. (ADM) 91-1791, Washington, DC: Superintendent of Documents, U.S. Government Printing Office.

Alzheimer's Association, Columbus Chapter. (1989). *Black Church Network Program.* Columbus, OH: Author.

Ballard, E. L. (1990). Minority recruitment in CERAD: Reaching ethnic populations and those with low education. *The Caregiver,* 9: 16–17.

Ballard, E. L. (1993). Recruitment of black elderly for clinical research studies of dementia: The CERAD experience. *Gerontologist, 33*(4), 561–565.

Barresi, C. M. (1992, March). *The impact of ethnicity on aging: A review of theory, research and issues.* Symposium presented at the 38th annual meeting of the American Society of Aging, San Diego, CA.

Belleville-Taylor, P., Rosenberg, R., Ooi, W. L., Gornstein, E., Emerson Lombardo, N. B., Wykle, M., et al. (November, 1993). *Building bridges for Alzheimer's: Developing an effective strategy to overcome cultural and economic challenges in the urban setting.* Symposium presented at the 46th annual scientific meeting of the Gerontological Society of America, New Orleans, LA.

Brodaty, H. (1994). Quasi-experimental evaluation of an educational model for dementia caregivers. *International Journal of Geriatric Psychiatry, 9,* 195–205.

Brodaty, H., & Peters, K. (1991). Cost effectiveness of a training program for dementia caregivers. *International Psychogeriatrics, 3,* 11–22.

Brodaty, H., Mittelman, M., & Burns, A. (2003, October 16-18). *3-country study: Added benefit of caregiver intervention to treatment of Alzheimer's disease with Aricept,* 19th international conference of Alzheimer's Disease International, Santo Domingo, Dominican Republic.

Calsyn, R. J., & Roades, L. A. (1993). Predicting perceived service need, service awareness, and service utilization. *Journal of Gerontological Social Work, 21,* 59–76.

Chow, T. W., Ross, L., Fox, P., Cummings, J. L., & Lin, K. M. (2000). Utilization of Alzheimer's disease community resources by Asian-Americans in California. *International Journal of Geriatric Psychiatry, 15*(9), 838–847.

Cox, C. (1999). Race and caregiving: Patterns of service use by African American and White caregivers of persons with Alzheimer's disease. *Journal of Gerontological Social Work, 32*(2), 5–19.

Delgado, M. (2000). *Chinese elders and the 21st century: Issues and challenges for culturally competent research and practice.* Binghamton, NY: Haworth.

Die, A. H., & Seelbach, W. C. (1988). Problems, sources of assistance, and knowledge of services among elderly Vietnamese immigrants. *The Gerontologist, 28,* 448–452.

Elliott, K. S., Minno, M. D., Lam, D., & Tu, A. M. (1996). Working with the Chinese family in the context of dementia. In G. Yeo & D. Gallagher-Thompson (Eds.), *Ethnicity and the dementias* (pp. 89–108). Washington, DC: Taylor & Francis.

Emerson Lombardo, N. B. (1997). Recognition and initial assessment of Alzheimer's disease, commentary 2, from the guideline developer's perspective. *Abstracts of Clinical Care Guidelines, 9,* 6–7.

Emerson Lombardo, N. B., & Aronson, M. K. (1995). Caregiving research: An overview. In K. Iqbal, J. Mortimer, B. Winblad, & H. Wisniewski (Eds.), *Research advances in Alzheimer's disease and related disorders* (pp. 337–348). Sussex: Wiley.

Emerson Lombardo, N. B., Dresser, M., Belleville-Taylor, P., Wu, B., Boi, W. L., et al. (2001). *Boston minority dementia outreach and educational program.* Unpublished final report to the National Institute on Aging. Wellesley: Wellesley Centers for Women.

Emerson Lombardo, N. B., & Eisdorfer, C. (1993). The role of the family in the provision of care for people with Alzheimer's disease. In B. Corain, K. Iqbal, M. Nicolini, B. Winblad, & H. M. Wisniewski (Eds.) *Alzheimer's disease: Advances in clinical and basic research* (pp. 613–615). Sussex: Wiley.

Emerson Lombardo, N. B., & Ooi, W. L. (1998). A multicultural in-home skills training/ support systems building program for family and informal caregivers of persons with dementia. *Neurobiology of Aging, 19,* 892.

Emerson Lombardo, N. B., Wu, B., & Harden, T. (2000). Individualized interventions for dementia family caregivers: Results of a national policy study. *Neurobiology of Aging, 21*(1S), S366.

Emerson Lombardo, N., Wu, B., & Hohnstein, J. (2001). The Chinese Dementia Awareness and Intervention Project: Raising awareness in the Chinese community. *Asian Pacific Affairs, 8–9,* 14.

Emerson Lombardo, N., Wu, B., Hohnstein, J., Chang, K. (2001). Training community providers as dementia care specialists for Chinese-speaking elders. *Dimensions, 8,* 3.

Emerson Lombardo, N. B., Wu, B., Hohnstein, J. K., & Chang, K. (2002). Chinese Dementia Specialist Education Program: Training Chinese American health care professionals as dementia experts. *Home Health Care Services Quarterly, 21,* 67–86.

Emerson Lombardo, N. B., Wu, B., Malivert, M., Dresser, M. V. B., Washko, M., & Stott, C. (2002). Individualized interventions for dementia family caregivers: Findings from a USA national policy study. *Neurobiology of Aging, 23,* S1994.

Evans, D. A., Funkenstein, H. H., Albert, M. S., Scherr, P. A., Cook, N. R., Chown, M. J., et al. (1989). Prevalence of Alzheimer's disease in a community population of older persons. Higher than previously reported. *Journal of the American Medical Association, 262,* 2551–2556.

Gallagher-Thompson, D. (1994). Direct services and interventions for caregivers. In M. H. Cantor (Ed.), *Family caregiving: Agenda for the future* (pp. 102–122). San Francisco: American Society on Aging.

Gallagher-Thompson, D., Haley, W., Guy, D., Rupert, M., Arguelles, T., Zeiss, L. M., et al. (2003). Tailoring psychological interventions for ethnically diverse dementia caregivers. *Clinical Psychology, 10*(4), 423–438.

Gelfand, D. (1994). *Aging and ethnicity: Knowledge and services.* New York: Springer.

Guo, Z., Levy, B., Hinton, L., Weitzman, P., & Levkoff, S. (2000). The power of labels: Recruiting dementia-affected Chinese American elders and their caregivers. *Journal of Mental Health and Aging, 6,* 103–111.

Gurland, B., Wilder, D., Cross, P., Lantigua, R., Teresi, J., Barrett, V., et al. (1995). Relative rates of dementia by multiple case definitions: Over two prevalence periods, in three socio-cultural groups. *American Journal of Geriatric Psychiatry, 3*(1), 6–20.

Guthrie, M., & Pegelow, B. (1993, November). *Outreaching minority populations: Experiences from Medicare Alzheimer's Project (MAP).* Presented at a symposium at the 46th annual scientific meeting of the Gerontological Society of America, New Orleans, LA.

Henderson, N., Gutierrez-Mayaka, M., Garcia, J., & Boyd, S. (1993). A model for Alzheimer's disease support group development in African-American and Hispanic populations. *The Gerontologist, 33,* 409–414.

Ho, C. J., Weitzman, P. F., Cui, X., & Levkoff, S. E. (2000). Stress and service use among minority caregivers to elders with dementia. *Journal of Gerontological Social Work, 33*(1), 67–88.

Hong Kong Alzheimer's Disease and Brain Failure Association. (1997). *Activity guidebook on care of dementia.* Hong Kong: Author.

Jordan, J. V., Miller, J. B., & Walker, M. (2000). *An introduction to relational-cultural theory: Excerpts from training institutes.* Wellesley: Wellesley Centers for Women and Jean Baker Miller Training Institute.

Krout, J. A. (1983). Knowledge and use of services by the elderly: A critical review of the literature. *International Journal of Aging and Human Development, 17,* 153–167.

Kuo, W. H. (1984). Prevalence of depression among Asian-Americans. *Journal of Nervous and Mental Disease, 172,* 449–457.

Kuo, W. H., & Tsai, Y. (1986). Social networking hardiness and immigrants' mental health. *Journal of Health and Social Behavior, 27,* 133–149.

Lee, J. J. (1992). *Development, delivery, and utilization of services under the Older American Act: A perspective of Asian American elderly.* New York: Garland.

Levkoff, S. E., Levy, B. R., & Weitzman, P. F. (2000). The matching model of recruitment. *Journal of Mental Health and Aging, 6*(1), 29–38.

Liu, W. T. (1986). Health services for Asian elderly. *Research on Aging, 8,* 156–175.

Manton, K. C., Gu, X. L., & Ukraintseva, S. V. (2005). Declining prevalence of dementia in the U.S. elderly population. *Advances in Gerontology, 16,* 30–37.

Mindel, C., Wright, R., & Starrett, R. (1986). Informal and formal health and social support systems of Black and White elderly: A comparative cost approach. *The Gerontologist, 26,* 279–285.

Mittelman, M. (2003). The role of counseling and support for family caregivers in the management of Alzheimer's disease: Evidence from the Three Country Study. *International Psychogeriatrics.*

Mittelman, M. S., Ferris, S. H., Steinberg, G., Shulman, E., Mackell, J. A., Ambinder, A., et al. (1993). An intervention that delays institutionalization of Alzheimer's disease patients: Treatment of spouse-caregivers. *The Gerontologist, 33,* 730–740.

Mittelman, M. S., Ferris, S. H., Shulman, E., Steinberg, G., & Levin, B. (1996). A family intervention to delay nursing home placement of patients with Alzheimer disease. A randomized controlled trial. *JAMA, 276,* 1725–1731.

Nah, K. H. (1993). Perceived problems and service delivery for Korean immigrants. *Social Work, 38,* 289–296.

National Alliance for Caregiving & American Association of Retired Persons. (1996). *National caregivers survey.* Washington, DC: Author.

Reeves, T. J., & Bennett, C. E. (2004). *We the People: Asians in the United States.* Census 2000 Special Reports. Washington, DC: U.S. Census Bureau.

Ren, X. S., & Chang, K. (1998). Evaluating health status of elderly Chinese in Boston. *Journal of Clinical Epidemiology, 51,* 429–435.

Schultz, R., & O'Brien, A. T. (1994, July 30). Alzheimer's disease caregiving: Prevalence and health effects. Presented at the 4th ICADRD-MN'94. *Neurobiology of Aging, 15*(S1), S1.

Silverstein, N. M. (1984). Informing the elderly about public services: The relationship between sources of knowledge and service utilization. *The Gerontologist, 24,* 37–40.

Sinclair, S., Hayes-Reams, P., Myers, H. F., Allen, W., Hawes-Dawson, J., & Kington, R. (2000). Recruiting African Americans for health studies: Lessons from the Drew-RAND Center on Health and Aging. *Journal of Mental Health and Aging, 6,* 53–66.

Tabora, B. L., & Flaskerud, J. H. (1997). Mental health beliefs, practices, and knowledge of Chinese immigrant women. *Issues in Mental Health Nursing, 18*(3), 173–189.

Uba, L., & Sue, S. (1991). Nature and scope of services for Asian and Pacific Islander Americans. In N. Kokuau (Ed.), *Handbook of social services for Asian and Pacific Islanders* (pp. 21–35). New York: Greenwood.

U.S. Census Bureau. (1996). *Population projections of the United States by age, sex, race, and Hispanic origin: 1995 to 2050, Current population reports.* Washington, DC: U.S. Census Bureau.

U.S. Department of Health and Human Services. (1996). *Recognition and initial assessment of Alzheimer's disease and related dementias* (Report No. 97–0702). Rockville, MD: Agency for Health Care Policy and Research.

Valle, R. (1990). Cultural and ethnic issues in AD family research In E. Light & B. Lebowitz (Eds.), *Alzheimer's disease treatment and family stress: Directions for research.* (pp. 122–154). New York: Taylor & Francis.

Valle, R. (1988–1989). Outreach to ethnic minorities with AD: The challenge to the community. *Health Matrix, 6,* 13–27.

Valle, R. (1989). US ethnic minority group access to long-term care. In T. Scwab (Ed.), *Caring for an aging world: International models for long-term care, financing, and delivery* (pp. 339–365). New York: McGraw-Hill.

Valle, R. (1990, June). *A multi-cultural outreach strategy for ethnically diverse Alzheimer's disease and dementia-affected patients and their caregivers.* Paper presented at the

2nd Annual Multicultural Symposium at the 10th annual meeting of the Alzheimer's Association, Chicago, IL.

Wu, B. (2000). Supplementing informal care of frail elders with formal services: A comparison of White, Hispanic, and Asian non-spouse caregivers (Doctoral dissertation, University of Massachusetts, Boston).

Wykle, M. (1993). *FOCUSSED: Communicating with the AD Residents*. Presentation.

Wykle, M., & Segal, M. (1991). A comparison of Black and White family caregiver experiences with dementia. *Journal of National Black Nurses' Association, 5*, 29–41.

Yeatts, D. E., Crow, T., & Folts, E. (1992). Service use among low-income minority elderly: Strategies for overcoming barriers. *The Gerontologist, 32*, 24–32.

Yu, E. S. H., Liu, W. T., Levy, P., Zhang, M. Y., Katzman, R., Lung, C. T., et al. (1989). Cognitive impairment among elderly adults in Shanghai, China. *Journal of Gerontology: Social Science, 44*, S97–S106.

Zarit, S. (1990, June). *Concepts and measures in family caregiving research*. Paper presented at the Conference on Conceptual and Methodological Issues in Family Caregiving Research, University of Toronto, Toronto, Ontario, Canada.

Zarit, S. H. (1991). Intervention with frail elders and their families: Are they effective and why? In M. A. P. Stephens, J. H. Crowther, S. E. Hobfoll, & D. L. Tennebaum (Eds.), *Stress and coping in later life families* (pp. 241–266). Washington, DC: Hemisphere.

Zhang, M. Y., Katzman, R., Salmon, D., Jin, H., Cai, G. J., Wang, Z. Y., et al. (1990). The prevalence of dementia and Alzheimer's disease in Shanghai, China: Impact of age, gender, and education. *Annals of Neurology, 27*, 428–437.

CHAPTER TWELVE

Models From Other Countries: Social Work With People With Dementia and Their Caregivers

Jill Manthorpe and Jo Moriarty

INTRODUCTION

Every 7 seconds, another person in the world develops dementia (Ferri et al., 2005). Although dementia remains a comparatively rare disability in terms of the overall numbers of people affected, its impact is profound because of the effects on individuals, their families, and the health and care systems set up to support them.

We begin the chapter by highlighting some principles of social work with people with dementia that would seem to have relevance across different cultures and care systems. We then set the context in which social work with dementia takes place in different countries by giving an overview of the numbers of people affected by dementia in the developing world (Europe and Japan) and the systems for care within these regions. This is followed by examples of the different ways that social workers have been involved in practice in different parts of the world.

However, before going any further, an important caveat should be made. Outside the United States, social work with people with dementia remains a neglected subject in both academic and practice circles. For example, with the exceptions of Chapman and Marshall (1993), Tibbs (2001), and Marshall and Tibbs (2006) very few textbooks devoted solely to social work and dementia have been published in the United Kingdom.

This means that the social work evidence base remains very limited and often draws widely on the wider gerontological literature or that of other health professionals.

DEMENTIA: A GLOBAL PHENOMENON

There are two key reasons why it is important for today's social workers to have an understanding of the various ways that different countries are approaching the challenge of dementia.

First, the impact of globalization is such that social workers are working with an increasingly diverse group of people and their families. Social workers need to be culturally competent so that, for example, they have an understanding of any expectations that individuals may hold that are based on their cultural or ethnic identities or their experiences in their countries of origin.

Second, no single country has a monopoly on good-quality care. As we will show, developments in one country have gone on to be adopted in others, often becoming integrated into mainstream provision in the process.

In this context, the social work response to people with dementia is threefold and aims to do the following:

- Look at ways of minimizing the difficulties that people with dementia face—not just as a result from living with dementia but because of the way that we organize society so that we can improve or maintain their quality of life. This is an idea that has its origins largely in the concept of the social model of disability expounded by the British disability movement (Campbell & Oliver, 1996).
- Ensure that access to timely and tailor-made support is available.
- Work collaboratively with others in difficult times, crises, or transitions.

These aims reflect the *Statement of Principles About Ethics in Social Work* made by the International Federation of Social Workers and International Association of Schools of Social Work (2004), which point out social workers' responsibility to respect the right to self-determination, to promote participation, to treat each person as a whole, and to identify and develop strengths. For people with dementia, the principle of social justice is especially important because, as we describe in this chapter, dementia is often viewed negatively and the quality of care for individuals may be poor. The *Statement of Principles* also expects social workers to challenge negative discrimination, to recognize diversity, to distribute resources equitably, and to challenge unjust polices and practices and to work toward an inclusive society.

In saying this, we recognize that there is much debate about the existence of universal values in social work (Gray, 2005). In discussing social work practice with people with dementia in different countries, we are not seeking to imply that we are necessarily in favor of the idea of universal values. Rather, we are trying to show how providing support that is tailored to the needs and preferences of the person with dementia is central to social work practice.

Neither can a short chapter such as this provide an in-depth picture of dementia across the globe. Our aim, therefore, is to make connections among the tasks and roles of social workers. We argue that wherever you practice as a social worker, if you work with people with dementia, then you will have much in common with colleagues in similar contexts. While local circumstances affect our roles, the systems in which we work, and their rules, we believe that social work with people with dementia has at its essence the task to listen to individuals, empower them, and enhance their quality of life.

CORE PRINCIPLES OF SOCIAL WORK WITH DEMENTIA

Alzheimer's Disease International is the umbrella organization of Alzheimer's associations around the world. In 1999, it issued a *Charter of Principles for the Care of People With Dementia and Their Carers,* which was updated in 2002 (Alzheimer's Disease International, 2002). It suggests the variety of roles open to professionals such as social workers supporting people with dementia and their caregivers (see Figure 12.1). We set it beside summarized sections (in italics) from the *Statement of Principles About Ethics in Social Work* referred to earlier to make the links evident.

NUMBERS OF PEOPLE AFFECTED BY DEMENTIA IN THE WORLD

There are currently 24.3 million people in the world living with dementia, with 4.6 million new cases occurring every year (Ferri et al., 2005). Over the next 20 years, their numbers are set to almost double, reaching 42.3 million in 2020 and doubling again to 81.1 million in 2040. However, not all countries will be similarly affected. At the moment, it

1. Alzheimer's disease has a profound impact on individuals and families —*Social workers are responsible for promoting social justice and challenging unjust polices and practices (section 4.2.4)*

2. A person with dementia continues to have worth and deserves respect —*Social work is based on respect for the inherent worth of individuals and should uphold and defend their integrity and wellbeing (section 4.1)*

3. People with dementia should be protected from exploitation and abuse —*Social workers should challenge negative discrimination (section 4.2.1)*

4. People with dementia need information and access to ongoing, coordinated services — *Social workers should respect the right to self-determination (section 4.1.1) and distribute resources equitably (section 4.2.3)*

5. People should participate in their care and plans for their future— *Social workers should promote the right to participation and involvement (section 4.1.2)*

6. Family caregivers should have their own needs assessed and met— *Social workers should identify and develop strengths (section 4.1.4)*

7. Adequate resources should be available to support people with dementia and their caregivers—*Social workers should ensure resources are distributed equitably (section 4.2.3), challenge unjust polices and practices (section 4.2.4) and work in solidarity to challenge social exclusion and stigma (section 4.2.5)*

8. Information, education and training must be available to everyone supporting a person with dementia—*Social workers are expected to have the skills necessary for their job (section 5.1) and recognize diversity and difference (section 4.2.2)*

FIGURE 12.1 Alzheimer's Disease International *Charter of Principles* summarized and linked to social work.

is estimated that 46% of those affected by dementia across the world live in Asia, 30% in Europe, and 12% in the North America (Wimo, Winblad, Aguero-Torres, & von Strauss, 2003). With the so-called graying of the population in the developing regions due to increased life expectancy, the largest increases in the numbers of people with dementia will take place not in North America or Europe but in China, India, and Latin America (Ferri et al., 2005).

This is one of the major demographic challenges of our time, yet social work has not always reflected this immense change in the disability of populations and the impact it will have on the lives of individuals and their families or even care services. A recent book on international social work, for example (Cox & Pawar, 2005), did not mention this subject despite the fact that the countries facing the largest growth in the numbers of people with dementia are those with the least developed health and social welfare infrastructures needed to support them.

The Developing World

There is a symbolic importance in beginning by discussing the numbers of people with dementia in the developing world. Although 60% of people with dementia live in the developing world, less than one-tenth of population-based research into dementia has been directed there (10/66 Dementia Research Group, 2000). As a result, comparatively little is known about what it is like to be a person living with dementia in a developing country.

What is clear is that the majority of people with dementia rely on their families for care and support. In many ways, their caregivers share similarities with their counterparts in the developed world in that the majority of them are wives caring for husbands or adult daughters and daughters-in-law caring for parents. Many caregivers experience considerable levels of stress, although there is some evidence that the greater prevalence of three-generational households slightly reduces both the risk of psychological distress among caregivers and the amount of time that they have to spend caregiving (10/66 Dementia Research Group, 2004).

However, too much emphasis should not be placed on the advantages deriving from the presence of other household members. A small study of 17 caregivers who were mostly young daughters-in-law in south India found that other family members did not always support them; indeed, some were hostile, and there was little back up from local health services. The authors pointed out that aspects of physical care, such as dealing with incontinence, were especially difficult in houses without bathrooms. They also suggested that people with dementia and their carers could be helped by the development of more *multipurpose health workers,* a model used in many developing countries that is based on training workers in simple medical tasks who can then undertake outreach work with families living in their locality (Shaji, Smitha, Praveen Lal, & Prince, 2003).

A further difficulty stems from the lower levels of public awareness of dementia in the developing world, meaning that its symptoms are often mistaken for normal aging. This, in combination with less well developed health and welfare systems, means that

> many families burdened with caregiving suffer from lack of information about the illness, lack of information about management issues, lack of support systems, and lack of respite services. Since deeply entrenched traditional values make parent care obligatory, many families suffer from stress and guilt due to their inability to provide quality care. (Prakash, 2003, p. 95)

However, some improvements have begun. For example, dementia diagnosis in developing countries has recently been made easier by the development of a one-stage, culturally and educationally sensitive diagnostic instrument that has been tested in India, China, Nigeria, South America, and the Caribbean (Prince, Acosta, Chiu, Scazufca, & Varghese, 2003). This will help social workers in supporting families and care workers because they will be able to explain that any problems experienced by the person with dementia are not an inevitable part of aging, nor a sign that he or she is deliberately behaving in a particular way.

Nevertheless, we are still at the beginning of learning about cultural responses to dementia and how societies with limited health and welfare networks can support growing numbers of older people with dementia. Many such societies have few social work services, and, should they exist, it is arguable that their role should consist mainly of educational and organizational activities, such as supporting community development and self-help networks.

There is also an issue about social work education, with some concerns being expressed that Western models of social work education have been too influential in developing countries and may not be suited to the systems of care that are available (Cox, Gamlath, & Pawar, 1997; Desai & Narayan, 1998). This is why some commentators favor a process of indigenization whereby social work is adapted to fit the ideologies and epistemologies of each country in which it is practiced (Chung Yan & Ka Tat Tsang, 2005; Kat Tat Tsang & Yan, 2001).

Europe

Dementia affects more than 5 million Europeans (Ferri et al., 2005), and the costs of care exceed those for people with cancer, heart disease, and stroke combined (Wilkinson, 2005). Across Europe, there is policy convergence about the best way to address the continued growth in the numbers of people with dementia and to improve the quality of their care. Longley and Warner (2002) summarize a set of five principles that are espoused by all the (then) European Union member states:

- People with dementia should remain at home as long as possible.
- Caregivers need support.
- People should have as much control over their support as possible.
- Support should be locally coordinated.
- Institutional care should be as "homely" as possible.

As they point out, barriers to implementation of these policies also exist and consist of resource inadequacies, the low status of dementia care, professional power, and the complexities of balancing between the needs of people with dementia and those of their caregivers.

Officially, there is much emphasis on the primacy of community-based support, and Longley and Warner (2002) note that in most European Union countries

> social workers or their equivalents play a crucial role for individual sufferers and their carers in identifying their potential entitlements and advising on inappropriate ways of accessing them. (p. 23)

However, there are reasons why people with dementia and their families do not always receive this type of help. The *Facing Dementia* survey was undertaken to assess the awareness of dementia in six European countries (France, Germany, Italy, Poland, Spain, and the United Kingdom). More than 2,500 people participated, including caregivers, members of the general public, physicians, people with dementia, and policymakers. Four key messages emerged from the results.

First, on a positive note, a substantial majority of caregivers, physicians, and the general population acknowledged the wide-ranging impact that dementia can have on the quality of life of both the people who are affected by it and their caregivers. Second, and less positively, the survey found that dementia often remains undiagnosed until the symptoms become moderate or severe. These delays may stem from the difficulties in recognizing the symptoms of early dementia and the attribution of symptoms to so-called normal aging, the fear of dementia common among older people, inadequate screening tools for use by physicians, and/or delays in the confirmation of the diagnosis once suspicion is raised. Third, it emerged that most caregivers and members of the general public do not have sufficient information about the benefits of treatment and care. Finally, a majority of respondents perceive their governments as indifferent to the economic, social, and treatment burdens associated with dementia (Bond et al., 2005). For example, around 80% of caregivers consider that their government gives inadequate support to people with dementia and their families (Rimmer, Wojciechowska, Stave, Sganga, & O'Connell, 2005).

These findings help explain why for many social workers, people are often referred to their services only when their disabilities are getting worse and when informal support from social networks has begun to be under stress. Help, if it does arrive, is sometimes very late in the day, and social work interventions are often based on responding to breakdowns in caregiving relationships rather then being able to support people in the initial stages of their dementia.

Throughout Europe, in common with research undertaken in the United States, caregivers of people with dementia, especially spouses and partners, often show high levels of psychological distress or burden. The EUROCARE study (Schneider, Murray, Banerjee, & Mann, 1999) found that although there were differences between caregivers living in different countries, the results suggested that it would be possible to develop four cross-national preventive strategies for supporting caregivers:

- Developing interventions aimed at helping carers deal with aspects of dementia such as behavioral problems or elements of cognitive impairment such as disorientation
- Improving public education so that caregivers and people with dementia are less likely to experience negative social reactions, such as laughter or ridicule
- Providing better financial support to cover the extra expenses incurred as a result of dementia
- Identifying caregivers likely to be at greater risk of experiencing distress, such as younger caregivers

We think that these conclusions are particularly relevant to social work activity, namely, their ability to recognize the stressors affecting caregivers and to help marshal social support and behavioral or cognitive coping strategies. This means developing local knowledge of groups for caregivers, notably but not exclusively through Alzheimer's Associations, supporting their development if necessary; ensuring that caregivers receive financial entitlements; helping to put caregivers in touch with other practitioners to help address behavioral problems and not to see these as inevitable or impossible to modify; and contributing to wider public education about dementia and so alleviating stigma and enhancing social recognition of the caregivers' tasks and stress.

While these points suggest that within Europe social work with people with dementia and their caregivers is likely to be similar, there are, of course, differences between countries. These depend on policy and service traditions related to care of older people but also of people with mental health problems. Warner and Furnish (2002) recommend setting targets to increase the quality of assessment and diagnosis of early dementia, and while this may sound like a medical activity, we know that such policy moves have important implications for social workers who are likely as a result to receive earlier calls for support and information (Manthorpe & Iliffe, 2005).

Of course, the benefits to individuals and their families of identifying dementia are limited if no supportive services are available. For example, in Lithuania, although medical services are in place, comprehensive care for people with dementia has been hindered by the lack of social services and social work services (Macijauskiene & Engedal, 2005). The increase in the numbers of admissions to long-term care caused by a lack of supportive services in Italy (Bianchetti et al., 1995) has been recognized by providing new forms of home support that have benefited both people with dementia and their caregivers (Di Gioacchino et al., 2004; Ponzetto et al., 2004).

These different structural and cultural elements across different countries can, in turn, lead to important differences in services. The comparison of approaches to dementia care in the Netherlands and in England shows how different traditions lead to divergence in emphasis between countries that are otherwise quite similar in terms of the population age structure and the length of time over which services for people with dementia have been developed.

Kümpers, Mur, Maarse, and van Raak (2005) reviewed the literature and interviewed experts in dementia care in the two countries. They found that in England there was a strong focus on independence for vulnerable people, including people with dementia, that helped explain the priority of community support over long-term care and the widespread negative attitudes toward institutional provision. In the Netherlands, the historically high level of institutional care, based on societal views about old age and the welfare state, and the significant influence of nursing home professionals' perspectives had molded dementia care pathways in which institutional provision was more common. However, the higher rate of care home provision in the Netherlands could be viewed as placing less pressure on community care services. They concluded that services in England could learn from the Netherlands about achieving higher societally accepted rates of care home support and improving specialist dementia care provision. These helped avoid bottlenecks in other services. In turn, the authors recommended that dementia care practitioners in the Netherlands should rethink their attitudes toward the person with dementia, moving toward services that are better at involving and empowering people with dementia and placing greater emphasis on caring *with* the person with dementia rather than caring *for* him or her.

Japan

There are 1.1 million people with dementia in Japan (Ferri et al., 2005). This has been an important issue for Japanese health and welfare services policymakers for some time because, with a life expectancy at birth of 84.6 years for woman and 77.7 years for men in 2000, Japanese people have the highest rates of life expectancy in the world (Yoshinaga & Une, 2005). There are still considerable cultural pressures on Japanese families to care without seeking support from services, especially in rural areas (Arai, Sugiura, Miura, Washio, & Kudo, 2000), and, in common with every country that has undertaken studies looking at what it is like to care for someone with dementia, many caregivers experience high levels of stress and strain (Takahashi, Tanaka, & Miyaoka, 2005). Along with spouses, daughters-in-law make up a higher proportion of caregivers than in Western countries because of the Confucian tradition of filial piety (Arai, Zarit, Suguira, & Washio, 2002). Interestingly, there has been an expansion in the number of care homes in Japan, and it is expected that, in the future, more Japanese people will choose to live in these rather than be cared for by their families (Hirakawa et al., 2006).

Concern about the numbers of older people needing support in Japan led to the introduction of a long-term care insurance (LTCI) scheme in 2000. This is a compulsory, universal scheme, and, in return, those who are deemed eligible receive both long-term and community care services (Ito, Tachimori, Miyamoto, & Morimura, 2001).

Social work in Japan has a comparatively short history (Inaba, 2002; Ito, 1995), and the LTCI system is administered mainly by care managers who are mostly local government employees who have received some training. There is a high reliance on computer programs to assess a person's eligibility for LCTI (Tsutsui & Muramatsu, 2005). This may be significant because, although generally well received, the LCTI has been criticized for failing to take account of the needs of people with dementia (Arai, Zarit, Kumamoto, & Takeda, 2003; Ito et al., 2001) and for poor levels of knowledge of dementia among care managers and their failure to recognize the needs of family caregivers (Homma, 2005). This has led to the suggestion that social work should play a greater role within the LTCI system (Inaba, 2002).

PRACTICE PERSPECTIVES

Discussions on international policy developments can sometimes seem very remote from the individual experiences of dementia. This last section looks at some developments in dementia care internationally that may be of interest to a U.S. audience.

Person-Centered Care

Social workers can play a part in remembering that each individual with dementia is unique. One key influence in developing ideas about the importance of the social model in dementia care was the English writer Tom Kitwood, whose ideas have been influential in the United Kingdom and more widely in Europe. Books such as *Dementia Reconsidered* (Kitwood, 1997) have been inspirational to both social workers (Tibbs, 2001) and nurses (Adams, 1996), giving them a strong value base about the behaviors and practices that promote person-centered dementia care. From this have come two particular practice changes: the use of *Dementia Care Mapping* and the wide acceptance of person-centered approaches as the hallmark of good quality care.

Dementia Care Mapping is an observational tool that links measures of quality of life and quality of dementia care by looking at the perspective of care as if from the person with dementia. Each "mapper" observes a small group of people over a period of time, such as a few hours a day, in a care home or a day care center. Behavior is linked to categories that group together behavior that promotes well-being or, what Kitwood termed its opposite, ill-being. Signs that suggest that interpersonal communication by a person with dementia is being devalued, albeit unintentionally, such as ignoring what they say (what Kitwood described as malignant social psychology), are also recorded. Staff are encouraged to look at the results of the observations and to consider possible changes in care plans and activities (Brooker, 2003a).

In the United Kingdom, mapping is a common quality assurance method, and social workers will often be aware of its potential to improve residential care practice. Its applications across cultures are also promising and have been studied in Germany, Hong Kong, and Australia (Innes, 2003). Social workers may also seek to influence the practice of dementia care by acting as a resource for care staff, helping them see the links between theory and practice and become more reflective about how they care for people with dementia (Emilsson, 2005).

In recent years, references to person-centered approaches have become increasingly widespread. Some use it to refer to individualized support, others use it to describe a value base, and the more cynical have adopted it as rhetoric (Brooker, 2003b). However, despite this lack of clarity, person-centered approaches can be seen as encompassing four main elements:

- Valuing people with dementia and those who care for them
- Treating people as individuals
- Looking at the world from the perspective of the person with dementia
- [Creating] a positive social environment in which the person living with dementia can experience relative wellbeing (Brooker, 2003b, p. 215)

Like many developments, the concept has roots in other contexts, especially in the work of Carl Rogers (1961), but a person-centered approach has a long history relevant to social work. For example, awareness of a person with dementia's biography may help a social worker understand their preferences and possible concurrent disabilities such as deafness and the impact of these on an assessment.

Person-centered approaches have also led to greater appreciation of the perspectives of the person with dementia. Phillips, Ray, and Marshall (2006) ask,

> How does it feel to us to be with someone who has a disrupted short-term memory and serious difficulties communicating with the spoken word? How easy is it for us to change our practice to adopt other strategies that rely less on spoken word and more on emotion, observation, non-verbal cues and other means of aiding communication such as visual materials? (p. 116)

The voices of people with dementia are providing us with some answers to this question. The inclusion of people with dementia in service planning and training for professionals such as social workers is slow but is developing in many countries. In Scotland, for example, there have been examples such as leaflets written *by* people with dementia *for* people with newly diagnosed dementia (Alzheimer Scotland—Action on Dementia, 2003). Many research projects have also begun to engage with people with dementia not as passive respondents but as active participants in the research process (Wilkinson, 2002). These methods have much in common with good assessment practice.

Crisis Theory

However, lessons from social work practice around the globe reveal that while there are islands of good practice, in many cases social work with people with dementia is undertaken at a time of crisis. Crisis theory tells us that social workers can use this opportunity to effect change and can make a positive difference; however, the crisis might have been averted if social work support could have been available earlier.

The difficulties of caregivers struggling on unsupported until they become ill themselves might be alleviated by earlier support and advice from social workers. For example, a study from Australia asks why caregivers of people with dementia and memory loss make infrequent use of services (Brodaty, Thompson, Thompson, & Fine, 2005). The main reasons why a third of the caregivers interviewed said they used none and a fifth only used one service were that they did not think they needed them; also, people with dementia were reluctant to use them. Many did not know about services, although some said they were in the process of applying. Having a social worker was associated with service use, suggesting the importance of the social work role in helping people make decisions about the help that they would like.

Assistive Technology

Many European governments are investing in supporting people with dementia through assistive technology. While some developments such as "smart houses" (Gann, Barlow, & Venables, 1999) require considerable investments, others do not (Gilliard & Hagen, 2004). For example, an older person living alone in fear of having to leave a much-loved house may benefit from being told about ways in which he or she can make the most of assistive technology in his or her own home, for instance, by providing a telephone with photos of familiar contacts in place of numbers on the pad.

Cash or Care?

An increasing challenge for social workers in many parts of the world is that they will work in systems whereby governments are moving to offer people the choice of services or cash (Glendinning, Davies, Pickard, & Comas-Herrera, 2004; Glendinning, Halliwell, Jacobs, Rummery, & Tyrer, 2000; Ungerson, 1997). This means that social workers may still be involved in assessment but that individuals with dementia or their caregivers may have greater say in how they wish their support to be organized. For example, people may prefer to employ a support worker to help them go for a walk in the park rather than attend a day care facility.

Social workers who are the gatekeepers to such schemes will have key roles in making sure as far as possible that people are not being abused, neglected, or exploited. The work of social workers in preventing elder abuse among older people with dementia is a part of their work that is increasingly acknowledged, shown by the development of organizations such as the *International Network for the Prevention of Elder Abuse* (http://www.inpea.net/).

Balancing Resources

Financial pressures have led to the growth of systems whereby the social work role is seen as allocating and controlling resources. This can lead to conflicts. For example, although there have been experiments in the United Kingdom to adapt "classic" care management approaches based on assigning specialist and more intensive support to people with dementia (Challis, von Abendorff, Brown, Chesterman, & Hughes, 2002), the way that care management has been interpreted in the United Kingdom has led to systems that have more in common with managed care and where there are considerable pressures to limit social work input. This can cause great tensions for social workers (Postle, 2002) and is in conflict with approaches that place high value on social work input that is about more than providing information and undertaking an assessment (Tibbs, 2001) and that have been shown to be more effective (Kerr, Gordon, MacDonald, & Stalker, 2005).

THE ROLE OF SOCIAL WORK EDUCATION

In many countries, social work with people with dementia is not considered to be high status despite the evidence of the complexity and range of skills that are required (Tibbs, 2001). Helping student social workers develop more positive attitudes to working with people with dementia is seen as one way of increasing the numbers of social workers who are both skilled and effective at working with older people in general and people with dementia in particular (Hughes & Heycox, 2006; Hugman, 2000; Parker, 2001).

CONCLUSION

In their international review of social work, Asquith, Clark, and Waterhouse (2005) identified that social workers have tended to perform one or more of six key roles:

- Counselor (or caseworker) who works with individuals to help them address personal issues.

- Advocate on behalf of the poor and socially excluded.
- Partner working together with disadvantaged or disempowered individuals and groups.
- Assessor of risk or need.
- Care manager who arranges services for users in a mixed economy of care, but may have little direct client contact.
- Agent of social control who helps to maintain the social system against the demands of offenders or other individuals whose behavior is problematic. (p. 3)

Social workers may play all of these roles in different contexts and in various mixes at different times in their career, and there may well be conflict between them. This chapter has shown that welfare systems throughout the world have tended to privilege the roles of care manager or assessor of risk or need but that the roles of advocate or counselor and, to a lesser extent, partner are sometimes carried out.

In many ways, the potential for social work with people with dementia remains underexplored. However, the increase in the numbers of people with dementia across the world and social work's history of seeing a person as a whole and understanding of the systems in which he or she is living mean that this need not continue to be the case. During the coming decades, social workers in the developed world should offer their experiences to those in other countries both to point out what works but also to warn against developments that have not been supportive or successful.

There is also much to learn from developing countries, for example, in approaches based on supporting skills development in families and communities. It is especially important that social workers in the developed world do not assume that what works well in their country will automatically work in another (Coates, Gray, & Hetherington, 2006). Globalization and the constraints on resources resulting from the increase in the numbers of people with dementia will place greater pressures on welfare systems in general. However, there is also the potential to use these changes as a way of rethinking approaches to supporting people with dementia and their caregivers. An important first step in this is to understand the lessons that we can all learn from developments in countries other than our own.

REFERENCES

10/66 Dementia Research Group. (2000). Dementia in developing countries: A consensus statement from the 10/66 Dementia Research Group. *International Journal of Geriatric Psychiatry, 15,* 14–20.

10/66 Dementia Research Group. (2004). Care arrangements for people with dementia in developing countries. *International Journal of Geriatric Psychiatry, 19,* 170–177.

Adams, T. (1996). Kitwood's approach to dementia and dementia care: A critical but appreciative review. *Journal of Advanced Nursing, 23,* 948–953.

Alzheimer Scotland—Action on Dementia. (2003). *Don't make the journey alone: A message from fellow travellers.* Edinburgh: Author. Available at http://www.alzscot.org/downloads/dontmake.pdf

Alzheimer's Disease International. (2002). *ADI's charter of principles for the care of people with dementia and their carers.* London: Alzheimer's Disease International. Retrieved December 7, 2006, from http://www.alz.co.uk/adi/charter.html

Arai, Y., Sugiura, M., Miura, H., Washio, M., & Kudo, K. (2000). Undue concern for others' opinions deters caregivers of impaired elderly from using public services in rural Japan. *International Journal of Geriatric Psychiatry, 15,* 961–968.

Arai, Y., Zarit, S. H., Kumamoto, K., & Takeda, A. (2003). Are there inequities in the assessment of dementia under Japan's LTC insurance system? *International Journal of Geriatric Psychiatry, 18,* 346–352.

Arai, Y., Zarit, S. H., Suguira, M., & Washio, M. (2002). Patterns of outcome of caregiving for the impaired elderly: A longitudinal study in rural Japan. *Aging and Mental Health, 6,* 39–46.

Asquith, S., Clark, C., & Waterhouse, L. (2005). *The role of the social worker in the 21st century—A literature review.* Edinburgh: Scottish Executive.

Bianchetti, A., Scuratti, A., Zanetti, O., Binetti, G., Frisoni, G. B., Magni, E., et al. (1995). Predictors of mortality and institutionalization in Alzheimer disease patients 1 year after discharge from an Alzheimer dementia unit. *Dementia, 6,* 108–112.

Bond, J., Stave, C., Sganga, A., Vincenzino, O., O'Connell, B., & Stanley, R. L. (2005). Inequalities in dementia care across Europe: Key findings of the Facing Dementia Survey. *International Journal of Clinical Practice, 59*(S146), 8–14.

Brodaty, H., Thomson, C., Thompson, C., & Fine, M. (2005). Why caregivers of people with dementia and memory loss don't use services. *International Journal of Geriatric Psychiatry, 20,* 537–546.

Brooker, D. (2003a). Maintaining quality in dementia care practice. In T. Adams & J. Manthorpe (Eds.), *Dementia care* (pp. 240–255). London: Arnold.

Brooker, D. (2003b). What is person centred care in dementia? *Reviews in Clinical Gerontology, 13,* 215–222.

Campbell, J., & Oliver, M. (Eds.). (1996). *Disability politics: Understanding our past, changing our future.* London: Routledge.

Challis, D., von Abendorff, R., Brown, P., Chesterman, J., & Hughes, J. (2002). Care management, dementia care and specialist mental health services: an evaluation. *International Journal of Geriatric Psychiatry, 17,* 315–325.

Chapman, A., & Marshall, M. (Eds.). (1993). *Dementia: New skills for social workers.* London: Jessica Kingsley.

Chung Yan, M., & Ka Tat Tsang, A. (2005). A snapshot on the development of social work education in China: A Delphi study. *Social Work Education, 24,* 883–901.

Coates, J., Gray, M., & Hetherington, T. (2006). An "ecospiritual" perspective: Finally, a place for indigenous approaches. *British Journal of Social Work, 36,* 381–399.

Cox, D., Gamlath, S., & Pawar, M. (1997). Social work and poverty alleviation in South Asia. *Asia Pacific Journal of Social Work, 7,* 15–31.

Cox, D., & Pawar, M. (2005). *International social work: Issues, strategies, and programs.* Thousand Oaks, CA: Sage.

Desai, M., & Narayan, L. (1998). Challenges for social work profession towards people-centred development. *Indian Journal of Social Work, 59,* 531–558.

Di Gioacchino, C. F., Ronzoni, S., Mariano, A., Di Massimo, M., Porcino, R., Calvetti, D., et al. (2004). Home care prevents cognitive and functional decline in frail elderly. *Archives of Gerontology and Geriatrics, 38*(Suppl. 1), 121–125.

Emilsson, U. M. (2005). Recognizing but not acknowledging: On using research information in social work with elderly people suffering from dementia. *British Journal of Social Work, 3,* 1393–1409.

Ferri, C. P., Prince, M., Brayne, C., Brodaty, H., Fratiglioni, L., Ganguli, M., et al. (2005). Global prevalence of dementia: A Delphi consensus study. *Lancet, 366,* 2112–2117.

Gann, D., Barlow, J., & Venables, T. (1999). *Digital futures: Making homes smarter.* York: Chartered Institute of Housing in association with JRF.

Gilliard, J., & Hagen, I. (2004). *Enabling technologies for people with dementia.* Bristol: Dementia Voice. Available at http://www.dementia-voice.org.uk/Projects/Enable FinalProject.pdf

Glendinning, C., Davies, B., Pickard, L., & Comas-Herrera, A. (2004). *Funding long-term care for older people: Lessons from other countries.* York: Joseph Rowntree Foundation. Available at http://www.jrf.org.uk/bookshop/eBooks/1859352065.pdf

Glendinning, C., Halliwell, S., Jacobs, S., Rummery, K., & Tyrer, J. (2000). New kinds of care, new kinds of relationships: How purchasing services affects relationships in giving and receiving personal assistance. *Health and Social Care in the Community, 8,* 201–211.

Gray, M. (2005). Dilemmas of international social work: Paradoxical processes in indigenization, universalism and imperialism. *International Journal of Social Welfare, 14,* 231–238.

Hirakawa, Y., Masuda, Y., Uemura, K., Kuzuya, M., Kimata, T., & Iguchia, A. (2006). End-of-life care at group homes for patients with dementia in Japan: Findings from an analysis of policy-related differences. *Archives of Gerontology and Geriatrics, 42,* 233–245.

Homma, A. (2005). Care for the elderly in Japan in 2015. *Psychogeriatrics, 5,* 69–72.

Hughes, M., & Heycox, K. (2006). Knowledge and interest in aging: A study of final-year social work students. *Australasian Journal on Aging, 25,* 94–96.

Hugman, R. (2000). Older people and their families: Rethinking the social work task? *Australian Social Work, 53,* 3–8.

Inaba, M. (2002). Challenges and issues under long-term care insurance for the elderly in Japan. *Journal of Gerontological Social Work, 36,* 51–61.

Innes, A. (Ed.). (2003). *Dementia care mapping: Applications across cultures.* Baltimore: Health Professions Press.

International Federation of Social Workers and International Association of Schools of Social Work. (2004). *Statement of principles about ethics in social work.* Bern: Author. Retrieved December 7, 2006, from http://www.ifsw.org/en/p38000324.html

Ito, H., Tachimori, H., Miyamoto, Y., & Morimura, Y. (2001). Are the care levels of people with dementia correctly assessed for eligibility of the Japanese long-term care insurance? *International Journal of Geriatric Psychiatry, 16,* 1078–1084.

Ito, Y. (1995). Social work development in Japan. *Social Policy and Administration, 29,* 258–268.

Kat Tat Tsang, A., & Yan, M.-C. (2001). Chinese corpus, western application: The Chinese strategy of engagement with western social work discourse. *International Social Work, 44,* 433–454.

Kerr, B., Gordon, J., MacDonald, C., & Stalker, K. (2005). *Effective social work with older people: A paper prepared for the Scottish Executive by the Social Work Research Centre, University of Stirling as part of the 21st Century Social Work Review.* Edinburgh: Scottish Executive.

Kitwood, T. (1997). *Dementia reconsidered: The person comes first.* Buckingham: Open University Press.

Kümpers, S., Mur, I., Maarse, H., & van Raak, A. (2005). A comparative study of dementia care in England and the Netherlands using neo-institutionalist perspectives. *Qualitative Health Research, 15,* 1199–1230.

Longley, M., & Warner, M. (2002). The national policy context across Europe. In M. Warner, S. Furnish, M. Longley, & B. Lawlor (Eds.), *Alzheimer's disease: Policy and practice across Europe* (pp. 11–27). Oxford: Radcliffe Medical Press.

Macijauskiene, J., & Engedal, K. (2005). Medicosocial care for persons suffering from Alzheimer's disease and related disorders. *Medicina (Kaunas, Lithuania), 41,* 67–72.

Manthorpe, J., & Iliffe, S. (2005). Timely responses to dementia: Exploring the social work role. *Journal of Social Work, 5,* 191–203.

Marshall, M., & Tibbs, M.-A. (2006). *Social work and people with dementia.* Bristol: Policy Press.

Parker, J. (2001). Looking, listening and learning: A rationale for involving student social workers in dementia care. *Social Work Education, 20,* 551–561.

Phillips, J., Ray, M., & Marshall, M. (Eds.). (2006). *Social work with older people.* London: Palgrave Macmillan.

Ponzetto, M., Tibaldi, V., Cavallero, M. L., Fabris, F., Molaschi, M., Aimonino, N., et al. (2004). Home care for demented subjects: New models of care and home-care allowance. *Archives of Gerontology and Geriatrics, 38*(Suppl. 1), 155–162.

Postle, K. (2002). Working "between the idea and the reality": Ambiguities and tensions in care managers' work. *British Journal of Social Work, 32,* 335–351.

Prakash, I. J. (2003). Aging, disability, and disabled older people in India. *Journal of Aging and Social Policy, 15,* 85–108.

Prince, M., Acosta, D., Chiu, H., Scazufca, M., & Varghese, M. (2003). Dementia diagnosis in developing countries: A cross-cultural validation study. *Lancet, 361,* 909–917.

Rimmer, E., Wojciechowska, M., Stave, C., Sganga, A., & O'Connell, B. (2005). Implications of the Facing Dementia Survey for the general population, patients and caregivers across Europe. *International Journal of Clinical Practice, 59*(S146), 17–24.

Rogers, C. R. (1961). *On becoming a person.* Boston: Houghton Mifflin.

Schneider, J., Murray, J., Banerjee, S., & Mann, A. (1999). EUROCARE: A cross-national study of co-resident spouse carers for people with Alzheimer's disease: I—Factors associated with carer burden. *International Journal of Geriatric Psychiatry, 14,* 651–661.

Shaji, K. S., Smitha, K., Praveen Lal, K., & Prince, M. J. (2003). Caregivers of people with Alzheimer's disease: A qualitative study from the Indian 10/66 Dementia Research Network. *International Journal of Geriatric Psychiatry, 18,* 1–6.

Takahashi, M., Tanaka, K., & Miyaoka, H. (2005). Depression and associated factors of informal caregivers versus professional caregivers of demented patients. *Psychiatry and Clinical Neurosciences, 59,* 473–480.

Tibbs, M. A. (2001). *Social work and dementia: Good practice and care management.* London: Jessica Kingsley.

Tsutsui, T., & Muramatsu, N. (2005). Care-needs certification in the long-term care insurance system of Japan. *Journal of the American Geriatrics Society, 53,* 522–527.

Ungerson, C. (1997). Give them the money: Is cash a route to empowerment? *Social Policy and Administration, 31,* 45–53.

Warner, M., & Furnish, S. (2002). Towards coherent policy and practice in Alzheimer's disease across the European Union. In M. Warner, S. Furnish, M. Longley, & B. Lawlor (Eds.), *Alzheimer's disease: Policy and practice across Europe* (pp. 175–192). Oxford: Radcliffe Medical Press.

Wilkinson, D. (2005). Is there a double standard when it comes to dementia care? *International Journal of Clinical Practice, 59*(S146), 3–7.

Wilkinson, H. (Ed.). (2002). *The perspectives of people with dementia: Research methods and motivations.* London: Jessica Kingsley.

Wimo, A., Winblad, B., Aguero-Torres, H., & von Strauss, E. (2003). The magnitude of dementia occurrence in the world. *Alzheimer Disease and Associated Disorders, 17,* 63–67.

Yoshinaga, K., & Une, H. (2005). Contributions of mortality changes by age group and selected causes of death to the increase in Japanese life expectancy at birth from 1950 to 2000. *European Journal of Epidemiology, 20,* 49–57.

CHAPTER THIRTEEN

Caring for Persons With Dementia in Australia

Teorrah Kontos

INTRODUCTION

Australia's population is aging, and the incidence of dementia is growing, bringing with it rising socioeconomic costs and disability burdens. This chapter outlines Australia's dementia policy, service development, and social work models of practice.

AUSTRALIAN DEMOGRAPHICS AND RATES OF DEMENTIA

Australia is a federation of six states and two territories and is comprised by a majority of Anglo-Celtic inhabitants, indigenous Australians, and postwar European migrants. Migrants aged 60 and older make up one-quarter of Australia's population, and 25% of them come from culturally and linguistically diverse backgrounds (Access Economics, 2005). This diversity presents a particular challenge when creating culturally competent services for people with dementia.

Aboriginals and Torres Strait Islanders make up approximately 2% of the total Australian population and 1% of the aged. Indigenous Australians have a heritage dating back many thousands of years, and their unique culture and needs pose a challenge to the Australian health care system. In fact, a specific cognitive assessment tool, the *Kimberly Indigenous Cognitive Assessment,* has been developed to assess cognition in older indigenous Australians (LoGuidice et al., 2006).

Sixty percent of Australia's 20 million residents live in the five state capitals: Melbourne, Sydney, Adelaide, Brisbane, and Perth. However, many others live in rural communities, and meeting the needs of those in remote areas has been yet another challenge facing Australian service providers.

While dementia does not exclusively affect older people, the prevalence of the condition increases exponentially with age, doubling every 5.1 years after the age of 65 years. Among people aged 65 years and over, 6.5% are estimated to have dementia (Australian Institute of Health and Welfare, 2004). Of those aged 85 years and over, the estimate increases to 22% to 24% (Australian Institute of Health and Welfare, 2004).

The new estimates of Access Economics project that, by 2050, the total number of people with dementia will exceed 730,000 (2.8% of the projected population) and that more than 175,000 new cases of dementia will be diagnosed every year. These projections are 25% higher than estimated in 2003 (Access Economics, 2005). There are three main reasons for this:

- Increasing rates of diagnosis of dementia
- More precise (and higher) prevalence rates of dementia for the oldest old
- Revision of Australian Bureau of Statistics demographic projections (Access Economics, 2005)

These significant figures have implications for health and aging care systems and underline the importance of the historic commitment by the federal Australian government in making dementia a national health priority.

Dementia will be the number-one cause of disability burden by 2016. The Australian government is acting in a coordinated way to increase, promote, and understand this growing epidemic. Responsibility for dementia in Australia rests with a range of organizations, including peak bodies such as Alzheimer's Australia, the Department of Human Services, the Council on the Ageing, advocacy groups, researchers, service organizations, and local, state, and federal government.

While more than 162,000 Australians have a reported diagnosis of dementia, there are currently perhaps as many in the early stages who have not yet been formally diagnosed (Australian Institute of Health and Welfare, 2004). In 2004, the cost of Alzheimer's disease alone in Australia was estimated to be $3.6 billion (Access Economics, 2003). Delays in the onset of the disease through prevention would produce substantial reduction in the real costs of dementia.

DEMENTIA PREVENTION METHODS USED IN AUSTRALIA

Although it is not possible to either prevent or cure dementia, Australia is exploring similar ways to those adapted in the United States and Europe to reduce the risk of developing dementia with the hope that such approaches may either delay or prevent onset.

Alzheimer's Australia has promoted positive aging through a primary prevention and social connectedness program titled "Mind Your Mind." Devised in conjunction with a team of Australian geriatricians and psychogeriatricians, the program includes seven signposts to reduce the risk of developing dementia:

1. Mind Your Body—physical exercise encourages blood flow to the brain; people who exercise regularly are less likely to develop heart disease, stroke, and diabetes, which are associated with an increased risk of developing dementia.
2. Mind Your Diet —a good and balanced diet promotes brain health.
3. Mind Your Brain—keeping the brain active is thought to build reserves of brain cells.
4. Mind Your Health Checks—stay healthy by having regular checkups and following medical advice.
5. Mind Your Social Life—Be socially involved and participate in leisure activities.
6. Mind Your Head—protect your head (e.g., use a helmet when cycling) to reduce the risk of dementia.
7. Mind Your Habits—avoid bad habits like smoking and consuming too much alcohol.

Vascular dementia prevention could also be adopted by reducing vascular risk factors, such as hypertension, obesity, and smoking. This will reduce the risk of having a stroke and the possible resultant cognitive impairment.

Effective vascular risk management interventions in the prevention of dementia include treating hypertension as well as the cessation of smoking and normalizing lipids by medication and diet. There is also evidence that a diet high in calories and fat is associated with an increased prevalence of Alzheimer's disease and that fish consumption is associated with a reduced incidence (Grant, 1997). Healthy and active living may assist in preventing or reducing the risk of dementia, and education may protect against cognitive impairment (Ott et al., 1995).

POLICY RESPONSES TO DEMENTIA

Australian governmental policy began to reflect the need for quality dementia care in the 1980s, when a growing appreciation of dementia-related issues was reflected in the Commonwealth's report "States of Confusion" (Howe, 1993) and subsequently the Aged Care Reform Strategy, which initiated a Dementia Grants Program in 1986 (Howe, 1993).

In 1991, as a result of a Mid Term Review of the Aged Care Reform Strategy, a 5-year National Action Plan for Dementia Care (NAPDC) was developed. The NAPDC provided an overview of strategic goals and outcomes for the national development of dementia care services. Its focus was to strengthen aged care programs to respond to the needs of people with dementia and their carers (Howe, 1997). The NAPDC plan outlined the importance of diagnosis and assessment in dementia care. This plan argued that all persons with dementia require a timely and accurate medical diagnosis of their condition, particularly since some presentations were reversible or treatable. It also aimed to provide a framework to address future dementia care in policy and planning.

Since the cessation of the 5-year plan (in June 1997), funding has become available through state government initiatives, leading to notable achievements, particularly in Victoria, which introduced Multidisciplinary Memory Clinics (better known in Victoria as the Cognitive Dementia and Memory Service) (Aged Care Branch Victorian Government, 2006). These are discussed in more detail later in the chapter.

The Commonwealth Government invests more than $2.6 billion per year in dementia care, research, and support. Through the Australian Research Council and the National Health and Medical Research Council, the Commonwealth funds dementia research covering medical, health, and behavioral sciences and social services. The Commonwealth introduced national research priorities in 2002 through the Department of Education, Science and Training; the issue of dementia is being addressed under the health priority "Promoting and Maintaining Good Health."

From 2005 and beyond, the Commonwealth government has committed to helping Australians with dementia and their carers by making dementia a national health priority through the following actions:

- Drawing together dementia research and making it more accessible, helping research institutes work together, and exploring new dementia care and treatment options

- Supporting the primary health sector, including general practitioners, in diagnosing and caring for people with dementia; creating dementia and memory community centers; and setting up dementia study units
- Encouraging prevention and early intervention for people at risk of dementia by promoting healthy lifestyles and providing information and support for people with dementia, their families, and unpaid carers
- Adding more Extended Aged Care in the Home (EACH) packages specifically targeted to people with dementia and complex care needs (EACH packages are discussed later in this chapter) and offering dementia-specific training for residential aged care workers and for people in the community who may have contact with people with dementia, such as police, emergency services, and transport workers.

The Australian Government and State and Territory Governments have responsibilities for providing services for people with dementia and play a key role in the development and implementation of dementia policies and programs. A recent initiative of the Australian Health Ministers Conference led to the development of a "National Framework for Action on Dementia 2006–2010" (Australian Health Ministers Conference, 2006). The Australian Health Ministers identified five key priority areas to improve the quality of life of people with dementia, their families and carers. The following five fundamental areas for action in the Framework are:

1. Care and Support
2. Access and Equity
3. Information and Education
4. Research
5. Workforce and Training (e.g., an appropriately skilled and supported workforce).

(Australian Health Ministers Conference, 2006).

A Health Policy Priorities Principal Committee will oversee the implementation of the National Framework and will be responsible for developing and implementing an evaluation strategy and making future recommendations to Australian Governments that will exceed beyond 2010.

Through the Aged Care Reform Strategy of 1991 and the National Action Plan for Dementia Care of 1992, programs were also established specifically for indigenous people with dementia.

PROGRAMS AND SERVICES

Australia has developed a number of programs and services to assist persons with dementia, their carers, and families.

Multidisciplinary Memory Clinics

Early psychosocial intervention is essential to assist individuals with a diagnosis of dementia to access appropriate supports and services. Multidisciplinary memory clinics, which provide timely educative and psychosocial interventions for individuals with dementia and their caregivers, are well suited to this role.

Cognitive Dementia and Memory Service

The Victorian Cognitive Dementia and Memory Service (CDAMS) clinics were established in 1997. These clinics stemmed from the Victorian state government's Dementia Task Force, which recognized the importance of early diagnosis as well as improvements of services for people with dementia and their carers (1997). Funding was provided for 15 regional CDAMS clinics to cover the entire state of Victoria.

The CDAMS clinics were established to be an accessible, multidisciplinary, specialist service providing early diagnosis, advice, support, and referral for people with cognitive difficulties. Scherer and Kontos (2001) conveyed the opportunities available to this network of clinics. The CDAMS units also provide preventive treatment, advice, consultancy, education, and support to carers and professional service providers throughout the various stages of a person's cognitive impairment. This is a free service available to anyone residing in the state of Victoria.

The Victorian CDAMS constitutes one of the few coordinated efforts in the world to develop clinics across a region. Even within Australia, the approach is unique. As LoGuidice, Flynn, and Ames (2000) highlight, specialised clinics exist in the other capital cities but have no distinct pattern, "each being the brain child of a particular specialist." Outside of Victoria, specialized memory clinics operate without specific state government funding. The CDAMS units are at the leading edge of good practice in early intervention with cognitive impairment and provide opportunity for control and maximize preventive treatment effects for those with dementia (Lincoln Gerontology Centre, 2003).

Individuals targeted for CDAMS services are those (including carers or family members) who are experiencing cognitive, memory, behavioral, and/or personality change. To access services, individuals can be self-referred or be referred by others. A letter of confirmation is sent to all referrals, and subsequently an initial assessment in the home is scheduled followed by service-based appointments. There is no fee for this service.

The CDAMS units assess each person by clinical examination, informal observation of the person's behavior, and an interview with main informants or relatives. These activities are assisted considerably by the use of standard instruments for the assessment of dementia. Following the initial assessment, specialist appointments with a clinical neuropsychologist and either a geriatrician or a psychogeriatrician are arranged. After all three assessments, a case conference is held that involves all multidisciplinary CDAMS team members to discuss the results of the investigation and assessment of each person to formulate a care plan. The case conference is conducted on a weekly basis and may include a decision to obtain further neurological assessments or referral to a neurologist, for example.

The next stage consists of a family feedback meeting; this is held to discuss findings, provide diagnostic feedback and treatment options, assistance, education, counseling, support, and referral to services. A care plan is implemented, documented, and provided to families during the feedback session and to their local medical officer. When warranted, a review of the assessments to determine a diagnosis is rescheduled (generally within 9 to 12 months but within 6 months in more severe cases).

As explained in more detail in chapter 2, the CDAMS assessments incorporates evidence-based screening tools such as the Mini Mental State Examination as well as the Australian developed IQ Code. The Australian Rowland Universal Dementia Assessment Scale (RUDAS) is a multicultural cognitive assessment scale (Storey, Rowland, Conforti, & Dickson, 2004) that is usually performed during the initial psychosocial assessment. The RUDAS provides a reliable indication of whether a person has significant cognitive impairment and whether further investigation needs to be carried out.

COMMUNITY AND RESIDENTIAL CARE SERVICES

In Australia, care is available in various community settings and is also provided in residential facilities. Essentially, aged care services can be thought of as falling into two major groups: community care and residential care. Government-funded community and residential care is widely available for people with dementia and their carers. The following outlines some of the services available.

Community Care

Community care services help people with dementia continue to live in their own homes by offering assistance with home cleaning, showering, or preparing meals, for example.

Aged Care Assessment Teams

Aged Care Assessment Teams (ACATs) are multidisciplinary groups of professionals (doctors, occupational therapists, physiotherapists, nurses, and social workers) who can provide an expert assessment of dementia. They can also help determine the level of care the person with dementia will need and provide information about appropriate services.

ACATs are Commonwealth-funded and are located in all regions across Australia. These teams provide comprehensive assessment of older (usually 65 and older) and disabled people. However, younger people with dementia can also be seen by an ACAT, and anyone can refer to this service for an assessment.

ACATS can assist clients in accessing appropriate residential or community care. For example, ACATS can provide access to community care packages; these packages provide an alternative to low-level care for older people and for people with disabilities in the community.

If increased care and support is required at home, then the ACAT will refer the client to local community services. Some of these services may include the Home and Community Care program, the Community Aged Care Package, or the Extended Aged Care at Home package. All of these are discussed later in this section.

If the person with dementia can no longer manage at home and agrees to residential care, then an ACAT clinician can assess and complete the paperwork required to enable the person to enter government-funded residential care services. This assessment determines whether the person requires low- or high-level care. As this is a federal government funded service, no fee is charged.

Home and Community Care

The main focus of the Home and Community Care (HACC) program is to allow persons with dementia to continue living at home. The HACC program provides a range of basic support services:

- Domestic assistance (also known as home help), which provides people with dementia 1 to 2 hours of cleaning a week
- Personal care: assistance with showering/bathing, dressing, feeding, and personal grooming
- Food services: delivery of hot ready-to-eat meals (Because of recent changes in food safety legislation, the person receiving the meal needs to be at home to accept delivery of these meals.)
- Community respite (as opposed to residential care respite) in the person's own home or at a day center

- Transport to services
- Home maintenance or modification

The HACC program is a joint initiative of both state and territory governments. Jointly, they are responsible for the day-to-day management of the program. Many organizations receive funding to provide HACC services, including local government municipalities or councils and nongovernmental organizations. There is a national fee policy for this program. The fee policy provides protection for those unable to pay in order for people to receive care, regardless of income.

Community Aged Care Packages

Community Aged Care Packages (CACPs) offer a coordinated program of practical support services designed to help people with dementia remain at home. The types of services that make up a package are similar to those provided by the HACC program; however, this package provides a designated case manager to coordinate the services.

The case manager (usually a social worker) assists people with dementia and their carers with accessing supports. The clients have the right to negotiate the types and levels of care to be provided. After the manager and the client have agreed on a plan of care, the manager provides a copy of the care plan setting out the services that will be received. The services provided can change as care needs change. The types of services that may be provided include personal care, social support, transport to appointments, home help, meal preparation, and gardening.

The individual services within a CACP may be provided by a variety of organizations in the person's local area. Those organizations are paid a subsidy per package by the Australian federal government. To be eligible for a CACP, the client must receive an ACAT assessment as requiring low level care.

Clients can be asked to pay a fee for a CACP. The amount charged forms part of the agreement between the person and the service provider. For older people on the maximum basic rate of pension, fees must not exceed 17.5% of that pension. People with higher incomes may be asked to pay higher fees (limited to 50% of any income above the maximum pension rate). The service provider must inform the person and the family of its fees policy. However, no one is denied a service they need on the basis of an inability to pay fees.

The CACP is a highly desirable program, as it provides people with dementia and their carers with a single contact person who can arrange and manage many different types of assistance.

Extended Aged Care at Home Packages

Extended Aged Care at Home (EACH) packages are similar to CACPs but cater to people with higher care needs (better known as *complex care needs*) who would otherwise require a nursing home. These packages are flexible and tailored to individual needs: the types of assistance provided include nursing care, personal care, social support and activities, home help, assistance with oxygen, and/or enteral feeding and allied health care.

Similar to CACPs, the EACH package provider is given a government subsidy with which they purchase services on the client's behalf. Services can be purchased from other government community support programs or from privately funded organizations. The subsidies are sufficient to assist people with multiple or complex care needs to remain in their own homes with maximum support.

To receive an EACH package, a client must be assessed by an ACAT as needing high-level care. The fee service structure is identical to the CACPs package.

Program Activity Groups

Program Activity Groups (previously adult day care centers) provide respite for carers and help improve the quality of life for individuals with dementia who might otherwise sit at home all day.

Department of Veterans Affairs

The Department of Veterans Affairs provides a number of services to war widows/widowers and veterans of the Australian defense forces. This service is similar to the HACC program.

Aged Persons Mental Health Teams

Commonly known as Aged Psychiatry Assessment and Treatment Teams, these teams assist those who have behavioral changes associated with dementia. These services are available in most Australian states or territories; however, they are not federally funded and therefore vary greatly in the services they provide and their availability. This service does not require fees.

Residential Care

Residential care facilities are usually referred to as hostels or nursing homes. Hostels generally provide low-level care, while nursing homes provide more complex or high-level care. However, improvements to aged care arrangements now make it possible for some people with dementia to receive low- or high-level care in the same home. This removes the need to move the patient if his or her needs change and enables the patient to "age in place."

The *Community Visitors Scheme* is a government-funded service that provides a regular friendly visiting program for people living in residential care who do not have friends or family to visit them. Currently, 150,000 visits each year are arranged by the program, and additional volunteer visitors are being assigned to areas in Australia where there have been few or no visitors in the past.

The Community Visitors Scheme was established in 1992–1993 and provides funds for participating organizations to recruit, train, and match volunteer visitors to residents. The Australian government will provide an additional $4.7 million over 3 years to extend the reach of the Community Visitors Scheme and to increase the rate of funding provided to coordinating organizations to support each volunteer visitor.

WORKING WITH CARERS AND FAMILIES

In Australia, there are a wealth of services to assist family carers, including information, resources, referrals and support, respite care, counseling, advocacy, and training workshops. In particular, the Carers Association provides carer advocacy and support services, including research and policy development; the following is an account of government-funded carer support initiatives in Australia.

Carers Australia

The need to support carers in Australia has long been recognized. Carers were recognized in the HACC program in 1984 (Howe, Gray, Gilchrist, Beyer, 1996; Howe, Schofield, Herrman, & Bloch, 1997). Federal government initiatives for caregiver supports have included the following:

- The *carer allowance* and *carer payment* paid to eligible carers by Centrelink
- The funding of Carers Australia (a national advocacy body for the establishment and recurrent funding of Commonwealth Carelink Centres)
- The 1996 National Respite for Carers Program, which established the Carer Respite Centres in every state as well as Carer Respite Centres in each region
- The free call information line

State government initiatives also provide funding for a range of carer support, including the advocacy of carers in each Australian state and Carer Respite Centres in metropolitan and rural regions. Support for carers can be accessed through Carers Australia (which is a national organization advocating for carers of all types, not just those caring for someone with dementia). Carers Australia operates a Carer Resource Centre within each state of Australia and provides carers with information on how to access services specific to carer support. For example, the Carers Association in Victoria was established in 1993. The organization is funded by the Commonwealth and state governments. This is a free service for anyone caring for someone with dementia and other illnesses.

Alzheimer's Australia

The main provider of dementia-related support in Australia is the Alzheimer's Association, which has an array of services available to people with dementia, carers, and/or their family members. Alzheimer's Australia is the national body representing people with all forms of dementia and their families or carers. It is part of a worldwide network of Alzheimer's Associations coordinated through Alzheimer's Disease International and provides the following:

- Information and education about dementia
- The Australian National Dementia Helpline (+61 1800 639 331)
- Support groups for people who have been diagnosed with dementia and their families/caregivers
- Private and confidential counseling (as this is also a major area of Alzheimer's Australia's role).

Alzheimer's support groups provide invaluable assistance for carers. Usually, participation in a support group helps caregivers use professional services appropriately. Often these groups function as an outlet for advocacy and as a safe environment in which people can learn how to cope with dementia.

Although they are labeled "Alzheimer's support groups," they do not exclude caregivers of other dementia types. However, caregivers often exclude themselves from participating. For example, a caregiver whose loved one has vascular dementia, mixed dementias, or dementia with Lewy bodies, which may have somewhat different presentations than Alzheimer's, may be reluctant to join what they perceive to be an Alzheimer's-focused group.

Social workers are encouraged to have partnership strategies with organizations such as the Alzheimer's Australia, which provides a wealth of nonpharmacological programs for people with dementia and their caregivers (such as the Living With Memory Loss groups).

Living With Memory Loss Program

The Living With Memory Loss program is a Commonwealth-funded national service under the auspices of the Alzheimer's Australia. It is a weekly support group for people with early-stage dementia and their families.

The group covers a range of topics, including dementia symptoms and diagnosis, relationship issues, research and treatments, practical caring strategies, community services, and legal issues. Special groups also cater to the needs and issues of early-onset dementia.

Groups are generally held once a week over a period of 6 to 8 weeks. At meetings, participants have an opportunity to obtain information and talk confidentially with others in a similar situation and also explore ways of managing in the present and plan for the future.

CONCLUSION

Working with people with dementia and their carers offers a challenging and rewarding field of social work in Australia. Social work has a distinct role in relation to the provision of support and is inseparable from the assessment and management of dementia. A psychosocial approach to dementia care involves the person with dementia, their family, and the wider social system.

Much of the work in Australia is guided by Kitwood's (1997) personhood model of dementia. This theory enables the experience of dementia to be reconceptualized as an interpersonal experience. It suggests that the primary loss of a sense of self, or one's personhood, results from the ways that others view and treat the person with dementia. Personhood is a term Kitwood associates with self-esteem, which includes the performance of roles, and the integrity, continuity, and stability of the individual's sense of self. Thus, the theory suggests that it is essential to see personhood in relational terms, and the preservation of personhood is a central issue in the care of people with dementia. The work of Kitwood and the Bradford Dementia Group has been particularly influential in Australian social work models of care.

Social workers are in a privileged position and are in the forefront of providing timely assessment, referral, strategies, support, and education for people with dementia and their families. Social workers in Australia are well suited to promote and ensure greater public awareness and understanding about the personal and social dimensions of dementia.

REFERENCES

Access Economics. (2003). *The dementia epidemic: Economic impact and positive solutions for Australia.* Canberra: Alzheimer's Australia.

Access Economics. (2005). *Dementia estimates and projections: Australian states and territories.* Canberra: Alzheimer's Australia.

Aged Care Branch Victorian Government, (2006). Department of Human Services *"Pathways to the Future, 2006 and Beyond,"* Victoria, Australia.

Australian Institute of Health and Welfare. (2004). *Community aged care packages census 2002* (Aged Care Statistics Series No. 17). Canberra: Australian Government Department of Health and Ageing.

Australian Institute of Health and Welfare (AIHW) (2004). *The impact of dementia on the health and aged aged care system.* Canberra, Australia.

Howe, A. L., Gray, L., Gilchrist, J., & Beyer, L. (1996). Survey of access to home and community care services. *Aged and community care service development and evaluation reports.* Report No. 25, Canberra, Australia.

Howe, A. L., Schofield, H., Herrman, S. B., & Bloch, S. (1997). A profile of caregivers in Victoria. *Australian Journal of Public Health, 21, 59–66.*

James, K., & Mackinnon, L. (1986). Theory and practice of structural family therapy: Illustration and critique. Education update. *Australian and New Zealand Journal of Family Therapy, 7*(4), Dec. 1986, 223–233

Kitwood, T. (1997). *Dementia reconsidered: The person comes first.* Philadelphia: Open University Press.

Lincoln Gerontology Centre. (2003). Foreman, P., Davis, S., Gardner, I., & Rosewarne, R. *Review of the Cognitive, Dementia and Memory Services: A report prepared for The Department of Human Services.* Centre for Applied Gerontology, Bundoora Extended Care. Melbourne, Australia.

LoGuidice, D., Smith, K., Thomas, J., Lautenschlager, N. T., Almeida, O. P., Atkinson, D., et al. (2006). Kimberley Indigenous Cognitive Assessment tool (KICA): Development of a cognitive assessment tool for older indigenous Australians. *International Psychogeriatrics, 18,* 269–280.

Ott, A., Breteler, M. M., van Harskamp, F., Claus, J. J., van der Cammen, T. J., Grobbee, D. E., et al. (1995). Prevalence of Alzheimer's disease and vascular dementia: Association with education. The Rotterdam study. *British Medical Journal, 310,* 970–973.

Scherer, S., & Kontos, T. (2001, March). *An overview of a Cognitive, Dementia and Memory Service (CDAMS) in the Central/Outer East of Melbourne.* Conference Proceedings of National Conference of the Alzheimer's Association, Canberra.

Storey, J., Rowland, J., Conforti, D., & Dickson, H. (2004). The Rowland Universal Dementia Assessment Scale (RUDAS): A multicultural cognitive assessment scale. *International Psychogeriatrics, 16,* 13–31.

PART IV

Community Care

CHAPTER FOURTEEN

Care Management With People With Dementia and Their Caregivers

Elizabeth Baxter

INTRODUCTION

"Care management" can be a misleading term for people With Dementia and Their Caregivers because the caregiver is often taking care of everything, especially in the early stages of a progressive dementia, such as Alzheimer's disease. As long as a primary caregiver is in place, there is very little care to "manage," or so it can seem.

This chapter is intended to augment other readings that discuss the basics of care management, the many texts and journals dedicated to care management, and how it overlaps with other disciplines such as social work, nursing, hospital services, long-term care, and others. This chapter does not define care management, tell you what your academic training should be, or provide you with tools or forms that you can use. Instead, this chapter focuses on the one aspect of working with people with dementia that makes care management a bit more complex, challenging, and enriching—how a care manager can evaluate informal caregivers and, in the process, enhance the caregiver's ability to continue in that crucial role.

Almost 20 years ago, I sat with my son's second-grade teacher after school. We spoke briefly about his progress, then somehow began talking about my work. At that time, I was involved with an effort to expand state-funded in-home services to people with Alzheimer's disease. She mentioned that her daughter was on the board of the local chapter of the Alzheimer's Association and wondered if I knew her. This is perhaps interesting only because I missed an opportunity to ask her if someone in her family had Alzheimer's. Several years later, I was working on a research project aimed at studying the impact of care management on people With Dementia and Their Caregivers. This same teacher applied to take part in the research project; it was only then that I realized the opening that she had given me—which I had been unaware of. The next time we saw each other she told me a story that described her typical day taking care of her husband, who had been diagnosed with Alzheimer's disease at age 50.

She got up each morning, would get them each dressed, fix them both breakfast, and then drop him off at an adult day care center before heading to the elementary school where she taught. Her drive to work took her across one of Portland's many bridges. As she crossed on the way to work, she would consciously stop being a caregiver and go about her workday. As she crossed that same bridge on her way home, she would become a caregiver again. The ritual she performed each day of removing her caregiver "hat" allowed her to continue teaching longer than she might have otherwise. The day that we talked in her classroom 20 years ago, she wasn't a caregiver—she was a teacher. By the time she applied for the research project, she had retired from teaching; her husband's dementia had progressed to the point where he could no longer attend the day care program. It was only at that point that she thought she might need help from a "care manager" that she saw herself as a caregiver.

Obviously, the need for care management can exist long before the caregiver identifies the need for an intervention. The challenge we have as professionals is to support people With Dementia *and* Their Caregivers, in part by helping them recognize and acknowledge the amount of care that they provide on a daily basis. The strengths model is based on the premise that all of us have goals and talents, that the environment offers resources, and that there may be perceived barriers keeping us from achieving those goals or seeing our own strengths (Rapp, 1998). It is a model that resonated with me in my early work with caregivers—that each caregiver has an inherent strength and set of resources that professionals can draw on to support them in their caregiving role.

DEFINING "CAREGIVER"

It is estimated that more than 4.5 million Americans have Alzheimer's disease (Hebert, Scherr, Bienias, Bennett, & Evans, 2003). More than

7 out of 10 people with Alzheimer's disease live at home, where almost 75% of their care is provided by family and friends (U.S. Congress Office of Technology Assessment, 1987). On a daily basis caregivers make decisions about housing, finances, medical care, and many smaller decisions—what to wear, how to and when to dress, what or when to eat, and whom to interact with. In short, caregivers are asked to maintain their own lives and support or supervise someone else's too.

In an analysis of caregiver data (National Alliance for Caregiving and the American Association of Retired Persons, 1997), a caregiver was defined as "an adult individual who reports that he or she is now providing, or has provided within the last 12 months, assistance with at least two (2) or more Instrumental Activities of Daily Living (IADL) or at least one (1) Activity of Daily Living (ADL) to someone over the age of 50 years" (Wagner, 1997, p. 2). During that same year, based on focus group discussions, the National Alliance for Caregiving and the American Association of Retired Persons (1997) used a broader definition. A caregiver was defined as someone, "at least 18 years old and either currently providing informal care to a relative or friend aged 50 or older or, to have provided informal care to such a person at some point during the past 12 months" (p. 6). By 2004, the definition had softened to "adults providing unpaid care to relatives or friends 50 and older to help them take care of themselves" (Alzheimer's Association and the National Alliance for Caregiving, 2004, p. 1). For research or eligibility purposes, these definitions are important, but in real life, caregivers vary greatly from one situation to the next.

ASSESSING A CAREGIVER

Understanding the role of the informal caregiver, regardless of his or her relationship to the person with dementia, is critical to any care plan that is developed. The caregiver is often if not usually the central player in carrying out the tasks identified in the care plan. Yet information about the caregiver is more often sought to better understand the care needs of the person with dementia, not to learn about and understand the caregiver. The caregiver should be assessed separately and individually, away from the person with dementia. Instead of viewing the caregiver as part of the environment of the person with dementia, we ought to assess the caregiver as a unique individual with distinct needs that sometimes conflict with the needs of the person with dementia.

We live in a world of scarce resources, and there is pressure to keep active cases open only as long as needed to achieve a tangible outcome. Working with people with dementia is different and requires us to keep our minds open for new models of social work practice (Tibbs, 2001). There are really three essential elements needed to assess a caregiver—patience, time, and a belief that understanding the caregiver is critical to planning, coordinating, and evaluating needed services and resources for the person with dementia. Time, probably our scarcest resource, is critical for care managers working with this population. The care manager may end up with several clients and care plans—the person with dementia (where the caregiver is a resource for care planning) and the caregiver, who may have additional or different needs than the person with dementia.

The fundamental theme that will influence the care manager's role is remembering that the caregiver is much more than a resource to fill the needs of a care plan—the caregiver, while certainly connected, is separate and distinct from the person with dementia. Understanding and meeting the caregiver's needs is as important as understanding and meeting the needs of the person with dementia.

In the early years of care management, the process was often described in linear terms—you started with intake, did an assessment, and completed a care plan. Then you monitored the case, intervening as needed, until it was time for review and reassessment, usually at 3- to 6-month intervals. If your client had dementia, then the person with dementia was the named client for assessment, unless the caregiver was having some distress continuing in the role as caregiver. Rarely was the caregiver the client. Dementia changes the care management process, sometimes in small ways, at other times completely.

Each contact with a caregiver and the person with dementia is part of an evolving, expanding assessment and care planning process. Each contact reveals something new; with each revelation, the pieces of the puzzle fall into another transformed picture. Caregivers—and people with progressive dementia—continue to grow and change over time, as should any clinical assessment of them.

LOCAL AND COSMOPOLITAN KNOWLEDGE

The model I use is based on an article published in the *Journal of Gerontological Nursing* (Harvath et al., 1994). The article provides a framework that can be used for care management, outlining several strategies to form partnerships between health professionals and family caregivers. The framework offers language that defines the caregiver as part of the care management team, the person who has *local knowledge*—history about the individual, family, and available resources—while the professional has the *cosmopolitan knowledge*—information about the disease process and its implications, decision-making assistance, and information about the community and outside resources that can support the caregiver and the care situation. It complements the strengths model used by social workers.

Four key roles were identified by Harvath:

- Acknowledging and affirming local knowledge when it is adequate
- Developing or enhancing local knowledge when it is inadequate
- Assisting family caregivers to apply local knowledge to problem solving
- Blending local and cosmopolitan knowledge

Caregivers carry a wealth of information (the local knowledge), a history of relationship skills, coping strategies, physical and emotional health, and how roles have developed and changed over time. As clinicians assess the caregiver (bringing the cosmopolitan knowledge), they learn what strengths and resources exist and what might need to be added or augmented in a plan of care. In outlining a strategy for caregiver assessment, remember that these assessments occur over time as the relationship between the caregiver and the professional develops (or not).

Throughout the chapter, I refer to care management assuming the established, accepted roles of assessment, planning, care coordination, counseling, and follow-up. I offer questions that could be asked that will move the care manager and caregiver closer to the partnership between local and cosmopolitan knowledge while providing examples of how care management is different when working with caregivers and people with dementia.

CAREGIVER LEARNING AND COMMUNICATION STYLE

Some caregivers go to every support group and classes, starved for information, whereas others never attend one group session, although they might read pamphlets, watch videos, or listen to audiotapes. Some caregivers don't want material sent to their homes with the word "Alzheimer's" on it, reluctant to cause a reaction of the person with dementia. It is important to identify how the caregiver prefers to learn new information (Garity, 1999).

At one caregiver educational session, I asked a daughter caring for her mother how she perceived the level of education she was receiving. She said that, in hindsight, she wished she had not received all her information at once. Her mother was living alone when she was diagnosed, and the family supported that option until it was no longer safe. The daughter said that she did not digest the information that was not relevant to her mother at the time, such as information about incontinence and nursing home placement. It went "right over her head" because it was not part of what they were experiencing at the moment.

She wished that she had been able to zero in on information in a more time-relevant manner. As issues such as agitation, wandering, and incontinence became part of the daily routine, the daughter took many of the educational sessions again. The approach to caregiver education can be personalized and individualized, depending on the caregiver's needs.

It is important to identify any language barriers, including literacy level or availability of information in other native languages. Gaining an understanding of preferred learning styles can help shape options within the care plan. Care plans that are developed collaboratively are more likely to be followed because the care manager spends time with the caregiver discussing the options and shapes the content and approaches that may be offered.

THE COMMUNICATION PLAN

In some cases, communication goes through the primary caregiver; at other times, communication may be delegated to others. Caregivers who use services such as adult day care or in-home care may communicate differently than those who also make financial or legal decisions for the person with dementia. It is important to know whom to communicate with, how to communicate (by phone, in person, or in writing), when to communicate (are mornings better, or are they the most challenging time of day?), and who else you have permission to talk to if the caregiver is unavailable. You need to assess whether there is any conflict around certain decisions, such as placement or medications (Lieberman & Fisher, 1999). Who, if anyone, has the legal authority to make decisions on behalf of the person with dementia? Who else has authority to act (if anyone) on behalf of the caregiver? Is there a plan for sharing information among family members?

Develop a communication plan as part of the assessment and care planning process. Some caregivers share everything with family and friends, and others don't. Does the caregiver wish to have discussions in front of the person with dementia or only in private? An effective care plan takes these issues into account. The plan for communication should be reviewed and revised as the disease progresses and whenever major decisions must be made.

It may not be clear to the caregiver why a communication plan is necessary until there is conflict. If the person with dementia wants to discontinue a service, such as adult day care or in-home respite, who needs to be involved with the decision? Is the primary caregiver the only person involved? If there are adult children, do they have a right to know what is happening with the plan of care? Can they alter the plan? The answers are not always easy and vary from family to family.

THE CAREGIVER'S UNDERSTANDING OF DEMENTIA

An essential component of the assessment of the caregiver is determining the caregiver's understanding of the progression of the disease (Seltzer, Vasterling, Yoder, & Thompson, 1997). Has the caregiver talked to a physician or other health professional about the disease and its current stage? Has there been a diagnostic work-up? What were the results, and how were they communicated to the caregiver?

Does the caregiver understand the information that was given; does the caregiver agree with the diagnosis? Hearing a diagnosis of Alzheimer's disease or any other dementia can be overwhelming. Ascertaining what the caregiver knows, what they understand, and what they still don't understand is important. If a caregiver does not understand the disease, all possible care plan strategies are impacted.

AWARENESS AND ACCEPTANCE OF DEFICITS

Now that the care manager has an idea of how well the caregiver understands his or her own ability and the disease, the next step is to determine how well the caregiver recognizes the abilities and challenges of the person with dementia. Does the caregiver balance reasonable expectations with realistic safety precautions? Do the expectations of the person with dementia match what the care manager has assessed? Does the caregiver sound frustrated? ("Dad just wasn't trying as hard today" or "When my wife decides she is not going to do something, there is no moving her"?)

One daughter caring for her mom supported her mom living alone much longer than many care managers felt was safe. The daughter and her sister-in-law spent time every day in her mother's house. This arrangement made it possible for the mother to live at home for about 5 months, and then she moved in with her daughter. The daughter did not necessarily disagree with the concerns expressed by the care manager but instead chose a different path to address the safety concerns.

On the other end of the spectrum, some caregivers do more for the person with dementia than is necessary. It can cause different stresses if the person with dementia is presumed to be more impaired and less capable than he or she actually is. The caregiver sometimes needs help in balancing information from educational materials with what is known about a specific individual with dementia.

The caregiver requires strategies that will help with a continual assessment of needs while not being overwhelmed by potential changes in the future. It is important to know how the caregiver perceives the person with dementia—whether he or she is still seen as a partner in decision making or as no longer a partner at all. The caregiver's perception of the person with dementia, his or her current skills and deficits, and the caregiver's reactions to those deficits are all important to care planning.

CAREGIVER HEALTH

Caregivers assume both physical and emotional risks by virtue of taking on the caregiving role (Feinberg, 1998). Many studies have noted psychological toils such as depression, increased stress, and burden. As part of assessing the caregiver, it is valuable to assess the risk of depression, perhaps using a tool such as the Geriatric Depression Scale or the Hamilton Depression Rating Scale. If there are symptoms of any mental disorder, this presents an opportunity for introducing formal clinical and community supports to the caregiver. The individual items on the mentioned scales also provide a structure for talking about emotions that can be helpful during caregiver/care manager interactions. Caregivers have expressed that the questions on formal research interview tools were often the first time they had been asked about their emotional health. Asking the questions can sometimes be the beginning of an intervention.

Recent studies have indicated there might also be physiological risks to caregivers. Analyses of changes to the immune system, increased hypertension, and other indications of physiological stress point to the physical burdens that caregiving may add to one's life (Vitaliano, 1997). It is important to find out about the caregiver's physical history and the caregiver's relationship to his or her own primary care provider. Many caregivers spend a lot of time taking the person with dementia to the doctor's office and neglect their own health care. Some caregivers depend on contact with the physician of the person with dementia for incidental evaluation of their own health. Caregivers need encouragement to look after their own health needs, partly because it allows them to continue the activities of caregiving but also because the caregiver's own health has value independent from their caregiving role.

Finding out how the caregiver cares for his or her own health is important:

- Does the caregiver have regular contact with a health provider?
- Does that health provider know that the caregiver is taking care of someone with dementia?
- Does the caregiver seek care when sick or wait until things "get really bad" before getting examined?
- Does the caregiver practice good health habits—eating, sleeping, taking appropriate medications, respite breaks and getting enough exercise?
- Is emergency contact information readily available in case the caregiver has a health emergency?
- Who does the caregiver see (e.g., physician, counselor, naturopath, chiropractor, dentist)?
- What health plan coverage does the caregiver have?
- Does the caregiver's health plan cover the costs of education, respite, and mental health services?

CAREGIVER COPING STRATEGIES

Care managers might assume that becoming a caregiver for someone with dementia is the greatest challenge that a caregiver has taken on. This perception may or may not be true. Caregivers have shared stories about losing children at a young age; caring for and losing a parent, grandparent, or sibling to a disease or accident; or surviving cancer or other life-threatening diseases. Past life events shape our future decisions and the way that we cope (Gonzalez, 1997).

These patterns develop over a lifetime. If the care manager can explore patterns of coping, it can help explain why caregivers make decisions that seem contrary to what is recommended or choose to take an action that seems hazardous to their own health. Sometimes the answer is not in the current relationship or set of conditions but in a past relationship. Understanding how the caregiver came to the decision can help identify and facilitate other options when other needs arise. What role does religion or spirituality play in the caregiver's decision making? Is there support from other sources that help the caregiver cope with challenging times such as support groups, church or volunteer connections, fraternal organizations, or veterans groups? Asking about this can help the caregiver identify potential allies. These are important linkages to identify and foster.

Ask the caregiver what strategies are used when the person with dementia becomes agitated or other behaviors are present. Getting the caregiver to think about what to do when he or she is frustrated, angry, and overwhelmed can be helpful in finding out whether those situations have already taken place. Examples from the past, either from raising children or the workplace, can help elucidate what strategies and techniques the caregiver feels competent in and where help is needed to develop strategies.

For some caregivers, the challenges of caregiving bring about positive changes. During a research study in 1992, several caregivers told us that caregiving had changed the lives of their children and grandchildren, exposing them to caring and supportive activities that were not part of the daily routine previously (Beach, 1997). Does the assessment process allow the caregiver to express the positive aspects of caregiving? Is burden and stress presumed in the questions so that the caregiver does not sense an opportunity to state that he or she feel benefits from the caregiving role?

THE CAREGIVER'S CONTINGENCY PLAN

Caregivers can often think of what needs to be done when the person with dementia is in crisis. Knowing whom to call and how to get urgent needs met can be stressful, but it is part of the caregiving commitment. It is a greater challenge when the caregiver is unavailable, ill, or incapacitated. The information that a typical caregiver carries around "in one's head" is the most valuable component of care planning. Phone numbers, schedules, preferences, what works, what does not work, stressors, and approaches that trigger calm or cause agitation are learned and stored in the caregiver's mind. Getting that information in writing is one of the most valuable assets a caregiver can put together. Joyce Beedle, an expert in caregiving for persons with dementia, developed one strategy.

Beedle (1990) created *The Carebook: A Workbook for Caregiver Peace of Mind,* which fits in a three-ring binder with sections on day-to-day tips, personal history, medical, legal and financial information, care options, and other resources. Over time, the caregivers write their own, individualized resource book. Other family members can use this in an emergency or spend some time gaining an understanding of the complexity of caregiving. It can replace the notes on the refrigerator or the stack of papers by the telephone. Caregivers have expressed surprise when they see physical proof of their knowledge and relief in having all the information in one place, knowing that someone else can step in in an emergency.

But the idea of a contingency plan is not only for emergencies. It has also been a valuable strategy for caregivers who are reluctant to leave the person with dementia with a respite worker, afraid of what might happen in the caregiver's absence. Sometimes, the most valuable information in the contingency plan is the most routine information. Knowing what to do when the person with dementia wants to "go home," not realizing he or she is already home, can be as important as the phone number for the doctor, depending on the situation that arises.

CAREGIVER'S CHOICE OF ROLE

Taking on the role as caregiver of someone with dementia is a long-term commitment. Some caregivers have consciously assumed the role, knowing and understanding the commitment; some have become caregivers by default, being the spouse or adult child within close proximity. Still others reluctantly play a role that they did not want to have. Some have become caregivers so gradually over time that they never realized how much they had taken on until other people identify them as caregivers.

Discerning how someone came to be the caregiver and his or her comfort with that role can help the care manager examine care and service options. These options can help the caregiver either remain in the caregiving role or plan for the day when it may be necessary to leave the role as primary caregiver. Is the caregiver employed outside the home? Was the caregiver employed before, and how was the decision made to decrease or cease employment? Were there important plans that the spouse had after retirement that have now been put aside?

Sometimes a person becomes a caregiver but should not have done so. There may be several reasons for this: perhaps he or she does not provide good care, or there is a financial conflict of interest, or they truly do not want to be the primary caregiver. Questions need to be asked about how someone took the role of caregiver in order to assess if the caregiver is prepared, capable, and appropriate to be the primary caregiver. It is important to offer support and services to caregivers who want to be the caregiver but may also need help becoming adequately prepared. What reward does the caregiver perceive from taking on this role? The caregiver may find meaning in the tasks he or she does for another person or simply in the role as caregiver.

Find out what the relationship was like between the caregiver and the person with dementia before the onset of the dementia. Was the person with dementia a caring, loving, and demonstrative person? Was the relationship good or not? Asking the caregiver these questions can be difficult, but the care manager can gain insight into perceived duties, responsibilities, and tasks by probing about the prior relationship. Society's desire to have a family member as the primary caregiver can sometimes blind us to a difficult family history. Although the majority of caregivers have positive memories of the person with dementia and take on the role out of love and loyalty, sometimes the memories are not so pleasant. A care manager once shared a story about a wife who was caring for her husband. He had been physically abusive to her throughout their marriage. She had conflicted feelings caring for him and described times when she wanted to hurt or injure him, knowing he could not fight back. The care manager could never have discussed appropriate service options without knowing her story.

CAREGIVER'S KEY CONFIDANTS

Does the caregiver have others to confide in? The caregiver may rely on health or social services professionals, neighbors, support group members, or other family members. Do these confidants have an understanding of the disease, its progression, the level of caregiving needed, and what types of help the caregiver may need routinely or even once in a while? It is hard to rely on someone for help who does not understand the disease or what caregiving entails. One of the most common quotes of caregivers is that they felt isolated until they became connected to community resources and supportive services.

An effective care plan will identify who the supports are and develop strategies for communication among that network to support the caregiver so that the caregiver does not always have to "ask" for help. Friends and family will often say "I have offered to help, but she always says there is nothing that needs to be done." Sometimes "helping the caregiver" needs to be redefined. Caregivers have suggested mowing the lawn, sweeping sidewalks, planting flowers in the spring, taking trash cans to and from the street, washing the car, or getting the oil changed. Note that these do not involve cleaning the house, doing personal care, or providing respite, which is often more difficult for the caregiver to accept help with. These tasks can be done without interrupting the flow of day-to-day caregiving.

Find out how the caregiver's pattern of close relationships has changed over the years. It may be that the caregiver has always been solitary, with few if any intimate relationships, or it may be that the disease and caregiving role have diminished the ability to stay connected with people who are important in his or her life. The care planning process can help a caregiver find time to spend with people or activities that were once part of his or her routine, begin new relationships, or find time for solitude.

THE CARE MANAGER INFLUENCE

In addition to all the caregiver's attributes, there is also some indication that the style of the care manager can make a difference in measurable outcomes such as caregiver stress, depression, and burden. In a national Medicare demonstration carried out in eight sites from 1989 to 1994, the training of the care management staff and the focus of the interventions varied from site to site. There were some differences in outcomes among the groups of caregivers at each site. Arnsberger (1997) identified factors that can affect care management outcomes: routine service monitoring, caregiver education and training, crisis intervention model, clinical nursing/caregiver support, mental health and advocacy, and focus on client safety and placement. The six factors were predictive of the level of service use and caregiver outcomes, while they were least predictive of how the person with dementia functioned or his or her level of health care usage.

CONCLUSION

In addition to the traditional assessment process that often includes questions about demographics, health history, financial and legal infor-mation, and informal and formal support systems, care managers should assess the primary caregiver, and that assessment takes time. There is a need to build a relationship—and a partnership—with the caregiver.

The questions mentioned throughout this chapter don't easily fit on a preprinted form, but they are crucial to understanding the caregiver, who is the center of most care plans of people with dementia. The care-giver has a lot to teach care managers about the person with dementia, and learning about the caregiver will shape and reshape the care planning process over time. Someone with dementia is not a reliable historian, and the caregiver's perspective is essential to formulating a plan of care. The caregiver's history and perspective about him- or herself is critical because the caregiver can help identify untapped resources, benefits, and challenges to the caregiver in relation to his or her caregiving role.

The person with dementia and the caregiver are both separate *and* joined in the assessment and care planning process. Care managers should assess the caregiver as they would any individual in need, coming to them for help. The caregiver both plays the role of client and can be a resource in developing a care plan. Evaluation of the caregiver's history, needs, preferences, strengths, and challenges provides valuable information to the care manager in understanding the needs and resources to develop the care plan.

According to Alexopoulos, et al., (1998), "Living with Alzheimer's means learning to 'bend without breaking'" (p. 9). The phrase evokes what is asked of caregivers every day—to allow their lives to be out of their control, without giving up or losing sight of their own lives. Alzheimer's disease places enormous burdens on caregivers, intertwining their present (and foreseeable future) with the life of another person. Caregiving is a role that is taken on, but care managers must both remember and remind caregivers that it does not represent their entire identity. Assessment will enable the care manager to learn about the caregiver as a unique individual and to partner with caregivers to coordinate care for the person with dementia.

Care management with people With Dementia and Their Caregivers is about building relationships and partnerships. The caregiver brings a life commitment and a set of strengths to the partnership, while the care manager brings the knowledge of what is available in the community and who can help support the care plan that has been set in place. The evolving and growing relationship opens the doors, allowing the care manager to see the strengths and challenges of the caregiver and trusting the care manager to find ways that will enhance and support the caregiver's chosen role.

REFERENCES

Alexopoulos, E. S., Silver, J. M., Kahn, D. A., et al. (1998). The expert consensus guideline series: Agitation in older persons with dementia. A postgraduate medicine special report. Minneapolis: McGraw-Hill Healthcare Information Programs.

Alzheimer's Association and the National Alliance for Caregiving. (2004). *Families care: Alzheimer's caregiving in the United States.* Chicago: Alzheimer's Association.

Arnsberger, P. (1997). Case management styles for people with AD: Do the differences make a difference? *Geriatrics, 52*(Suppl. I2), S44–S47.

Beach, D. L. (1997). Family caregiving: The positive impact on adolescent relationships. *Gerontologist, 37,* 233–238.

Beedle, J. (1990). *The carebook: A workbook for caregiver peace of mind.* Portland, OR: Ladybug Press.

Feinberg, A. W. (1998). Caregivers' health is top priority, too. *Health News, 4*(12), 3.

Garity, J. (1999). Gender differences in learning style of Alzheimer family caregivers. *Home Healthcare Nursing, 17,* 37–44.

Gonzalez, E. W. (1997). Resourcefulness, appraisals, and coping efforts of family caregivers. *Issue of Mental Health Nursing, 18,* 209–227.

Harvath, T., Archbold, P., Stewart, B., Gadow, S., Kirschling, J., Miller, L., et al. (1994). Establishing partnerships with family caregivers: Local and cosmopolitan knowledge. *Journal of Gerontological Nursing, 20,* 29–35.

Hebert, L., Scherr, P., Bienias, J., Bennett, D., & Evans, D. (2003). Alzheimer disease in the U.S. population: Prevalence estimates using the 2000 census. *Archives of Neurology, 60,* 1119–1122.

Lieberman, M. A., & Fisher, L. (1999). The effects of family conflict resolution and decision making on the provision of help for an elder with Alzheimer's disease. *The Gerontologist, 39*, 159–166.

National Alliance for Caregiving and the American Association of Retired Persons. (1997). *Family caregiving in the US: Findings from a national survey.* Bethesda, MD: Author.

Rapp, C. A. (1998). *The strengths model: Case management with people suffering from severe and persistent mental illness.* New York: Oxford University Press.

Seltzer, B., Vasterling, J. J., Yoder, J. A., & Thompson, K. A. (1997). Awareness of deficit in Alzheimer's disease: Relation to caregiver burden. *The Gerontologist, 37*, 20–24.

Tibbs, M. A. (2001). *Social work and dementia: Good practice and care management.* London: Jessica Kingsley.

U.S. Congress Office of Technology Assessment. (1987). *Losing a million minds: Confronting the tragedy of Alzheimer's disease and other dementias.* Washington, DC: U.S. Government Printing Office.

Vitaliano, P. P. (1997). Physiological and physical concomitants of caregiving: Introduction. *Annals of Behavioral Medicine, 19*, 75–77.

Wagner, D. L. (1997). *Comparative analysis of caregiver data from caregivers to the elderly 1987 and 1997.* Bethesda, MD: National Alliance for Caregiving.

CHAPTER FIFTEEN

Community Mobility and Dementia

Nina M. Silverstein and Lisa R. Peters-Beumer

INTRODUCTION

Social workers are well positioned to assist individuals, their families, and their communities in understanding the critical components of safe mobility and in working with others to develop community and individual strategies for transitioning from the driver's seat to the passenger's seat. The goal for social workers in addressing this issue is to keep people engaged in their communities in a meaningful way and to get them where they want to go when they need or want to go there.

Life expectancy significantly exceeds safe driving expectancy, with the average man outliving his safe driving ability by 6 years and the average woman by 10 years (Foley, Heimovitz, Guralnik, & Brock, 2002). It is important that the general aging population plan for a time when driving is no longer safe for them. It is even more critical for the person with dementia that discussions about driving and community mobility occur often and early on in the disease process and that such conversations be respectful, sensitive, and inclusive.

This chapter reviews the current practices in community mobility and dementia from driving to cessation counseling to community mobility options and concludes with recommendations for social work intervention. A comprehensive resource list is included in the resource section at the end of this book to assist social workers in accessing the best available options in their communities and to become informed advocates where such options are limited or nonexistent.

WHY IS COMMUNITY MOBILITY IMPORTANT?

Transportation is a vital issue that impacts quality of life for people with dementia, their families, and their communities. By 2030, 70 million Americans will be 65 or older (AARP, 2004). Approximately 80% of this group will likely be driving themselves. And without appropriate interventions or breakthroughs in treatment, many with Alzheimer's disease are likely to be driving. As the number of persons with dementia increases with the aging of the population, community mobility becomes a major public health issue.

People with dementia often feel less and less in control and involved in their own decision making as the disease progresses. "Giving up the keys," for many, is tied to losing their last thread of independence. For decades, the primary concern around dementia and community mobility was "When should Mom give up the keys?" or "How do we get Mom to stop driving?" Although these issues are important for communities, families, and persons with dementia, more global questions have come into focus, such as "How will Mom safely transition from driving?" and "How will Mom continue to get around and maintain her connections to family, friends, and community life?" In other words, how can we as professionals help the individual transition from the driver's seat to the passenger's seat? And how can we ensure that that transition be as smooth and as empowering as possible?

Continued connectedness in the community and productivity in daily life are no less important to people with dementia than they are to the rest of us. Community mobility options for people with dementia who no longer drive are essential to sustain connectedness. While in some cases families and friends provide much of the necessary transportation, at other times "non-drivers may be hesitant to ask for transportation from family for 'non-essential' or social/quality of life appointments" (Vanderbur & Silverstein, 2006), and in others still, the person with dementia may have been the primary transportation provider for a nondriving spouse.

A person with dementia might be less resistant to driving cessation if he or she is familiar with or has had experience with alternative community mobility options such as public transportation, specialized senior transportation, taxis, and volunteer transportation programs. Further, he or she may be willing to use such options if the services met the criteria of "senior-friendly" transportation, that is, available, acceptable, affordable, accessible, and adaptable (Beverly Foundation, 2001a). However, alternative modes of transportation in many areas are not likely to be very "senior-friendly" let alone "dementia-friendly." Figure 15.1 explains the five key aspects of senior-friendly transportation.

DRIVING AND DEMENTIA

Every person with dementia will reach a point in their disease process when driving is no longer safe. Dementia is believed to affect many critical skills needed for driving, including perception and visual processing, selective attention, inability to divide attention, inability to make accurate decisions (such as which drivers have the right of way), and inability to control impulses when pressured to act in a traffic situation (Janke, 1994; Uc, Rizzo, Anderson, Shi, & Dawson, 2004).

Although individuals with dementia may be capable of driving during the early stages of the disease because the mechanisms of operating a vehicle are well established within their long-term memories, this skill will eventually become compromised. The glaring question is "When?" During the early stages, driving may continue safely under normal driving conditions, but serious concern exists in that the driver may have difficulties responding to new or challenging circumstances. Early-stage individuals may stop scanning their surroundings and instead focus on looking straight ahead and may become lost while driving (Hunt, 2003; Silverstein, Flaherty, & Tobin, 2002).

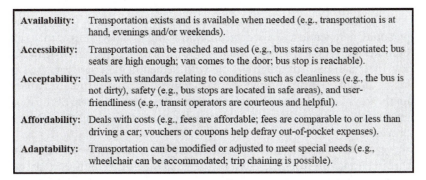

Availability:	Transportation exists and is available when needed (e.g., transportation is at hand, evenings and/or weekends).
Accessibility:	Transportation can be reached and used (e.g., bus stairs can be negotiated; bus seats are high enough; van comes to the door; bus stop is reachable).
Acceptability:	Deals with standards relating to conditions such as cleanliness (e.g., the bus is not dirty), safety (e.g., bus stops are located in safe areas), and user-friendliness (e.g., transit operators are courteous and helpful).
Affordability:	Deals with costs (e.g., fees are affordable; fees are comparable to or less than driving a car; vouchers or coupons help defray out-of-pocket expenses).
Adaptability:	Transportation can be modified or adjusted to meet special needs (e.g., wheelchair can be accommodated; trip chaining is possible).

FIGURE 15.1   The five As of senior-friendly transportation (developed by the Beverly Foundation, 2001a).

As an individual becomes more impaired, the ability to drive competently is highly compromised, as is the ability to have insight into the impairment of his or her own driving skills (Anstey, Wood, Lord, & Walker, 2005; Janke, 1994).

The inability to drive and the resulting reduction in community mobility for persons with Alzheimer's disease can have varying effects on an individual's ability to stay active in the community, continue to engage in routine activities, and attend medical and other appointments and would thus ultimately increase the risk of social isolation for the individual (Adler, Rottunda, & Kuskowski, 1999).

Transportation is indeed a big part of caregiving. A 2004 report from the National Alliance for Caregiving and AARP shows that family members provide the majority of transportation and that this is the primary type of assistance offered by caregivers (National Alliance for Caregiving & AARP, 2004). However, to have one's entire transportation plan dependent on the family caregiver is not advisable. Transportation can be a taxing and time consuming task, and concerns exist that caregivers may become increasingly isolated, just as persons with dementia may, because transportation can become more challenging as the disease progresses and can adversely impact family relationships. Programs such as the Easter Seals' Administration on Aging–funded Transportation Solutions for Caregivers developed materials to address this issue and help decrease caregiver stress around transportation. (To learn more about Transportation Solutions for Caregivers, visit http://www.easterseals.com/transportation.)

IMPORTANCE OF THE COMMUNITY MOBILITY ISSUE TO SOCIAL WORKERS

As a social worker and advocate for your clients, the line between personal independence/self determination and public safety can easily become blurred—especially when working with people with dementia and their families. Although people with dementia experience a series of losses and often a diminished sense of control, the move toward "giving up the keys" and the inability to drive oneself seems to be one of the most emotionally charged losses that they will experience during their disease process.

It is also difficult for the family members or close friends who find themselves involved in the often heart-wrenching decision/process to encourage someone to stop driving because of safety concerns. The person with dementia will frequently lack insight into his or her unsafe driving behaviors in spite of recommendations from family, friends, and clinicians to cease driving. Unlike the majority of older adults who gradually and responsibly withdraw from driving when physical limitations make it difficult to drive safely, those with cognitive impairment are less likely to judge their driving abilities correctly (Adler & Kuskowski, 2003).

For this reason, and to provide solution-oriented support for your clients with dementia, it is essential that we, as advocates, reframe the community mobility issue as a continuum of needs and services. In other words, the point at which someone with dementia must stop driving and make the move to the passenger seat can no longer be framed as the "end" of the continuum—or of independence—but rather the center of the continuum. It is important to note that impairments in critical driving skills may likely be early signs of dementia that has not yet been diagnosed, and thus the individual will not self-define as a "patient," nor will the family self-identify as a "caregiver" or "care partner." Considering driving cessation as one step along a pathway to supportive transportation may help the entire family unit "mobilize" toward finding creative solutions to meet community mobility challenges at each stage of the disease process.

Planning and preparation in the area of transportation are as vital to one's control and independence as planning for one's financial needs or end-of-life care. This is particularly important when advising individuals and families about housing in retirement decisions for the general aging population and specifically those with chronic conditions such as dementia. Often these decisions are made without consideration of community mobility options. During the planning process, information on community resources and the variety of mobility options for different stages of the continuum can be gathered, and preferences can be expressed. For instance, your client may share that for as long as possible, it is important to him or her to go to synagogue on Saturdays and to play bridge at the senior center on Wednesdays and go for a haircut once a month on Thursdays. These quality-of-life trips should be considered as "essential" to well-being as medical appointments and food shopping. Yet, given scarce resources, such life-enhancing trips are often not recognized as necessities.

Social workers have long understood that nondrivers are particularly vulnerable to social isolation. Those who are transportation dependent may feel burdensome and much more likely to ask for transportation to essential activities such as medical appointments and grocery shopping and to participate less in social and quality-of-life enhancing activities (AARP, 2005).

CURRENT PRACTICES IN DRIVING ASSESSMENT

While working with clients with dementia and their families, social workers may see issues such as "When is driving no longer safe?" and

"How do we determine driving safety?" Although research provides insights about why driving is difficult for those with dementia, the level of cognitive impairment associated with an unacceptable driving risk is yet to be determined (Vegega, 1990). Myriad tests are used to measure a variety of domains known to affect driving safety and fitness. However, with the exception of the on-road test, currently held by researchers as the "gold standard," to date no test or combination of tests has been conclusive and validated to determine driving safety directly. (For a summary of current tests, see Table 15.1.)

An additional and perhaps equally important issue is the time frame regarding how often someone with cognitive impairments who is still

TABLE 15.1   Selected Driving Assessment Tests

Test	Domain Measured	Cited in the Literature
Mini Mental Status Exam (MMSE)—often used in conjunction with neurological measures	Cognitive ability and driving fitness	Adler, Rottunda, and Kuskowski (2000); Lincoln, Radford, Lee, and Reay (2004) Dobbs, McCracken, Carstensen, Kiss, and Triscott (1998); Fox, Bowden, Bashford, and Smith (1997); Lincoln et al. (2004); Shua-Haim and Gross (1996) Reger et al. (2004); Vegega (1990)
Clinical Dementia Rating Scale	Disease severity; categories that include memory, judgment, problem solving, and personal care; American Academy of Neurology recommended that individuals with a CDR of 0.5 have a driving evaluation, as they may pose a serious traffic safety problem	Dubinsky, Stein, and Lyons (2000)
Useful Field of View Test (UFOV)—may be used in conjunction with neurological measures	Detect cognitive impairment—measures speed of processing when attention is divided	Rinalducci, Mouloua, and Smither (n.d.)

Assessment of Driving-Related Skills (ADRes). Battery includes the Snellen E Chart; Visual Fields by Confrontation Testing; Trail-Making Test, Part B; Clock Drawing Test; Rapid Pace Walk; Manual Test of Range of Motion; Manual Test of Motor Strength	Vision, cognition, and motor function	Wang, Kosinski, Schwartzberg, and Shanklin (2003)
Maze Test	Cognitive screening: indicates the likely competence of drivers with mild cognitive impairment or early dementia; correlates with known measures of attention, visuoconstructional skills, and executive functions	Snellgrove (2005)
On Road driving assessments—"gold standard"	Evaluate driving abilities	Wang et al. (2003)
Simulators	Score safety errors	Szlyk, Myers, Zhang, Wetzel, and Shapiro (2002)
Trail-Making Test, Part B, plus Clock Drawing Test (CDT) (with Freund Clock Scoring for Driving Competency)	Useful in identifying individuals who should be referred to a specialist for more in-depth screening	Wang et al. (2003)

driving must be reevaluated. Of concern for individuals with dementia, their families, and the driving evaluators is the assertion that those who need driving evaluations must be assessed multiple times in multiple settings (Lococo & Staplin, 2005), believed necessary to counteract the "good day/bad day" effect of Alzheimer's disease. Some recommendations involve multiple on-road evaluations in diverse geographic areas with a frequency of every 3 to 6 months. Such assessment intervals have significant implications for persons with dementia and their families—especially with regard to the cost of assessment and the time necessary for multiple-day testing (Lococo & Staplin, 2005).

Specialized driving assessment programs are beginning to emerge that are specifically designed to address impairments in critical driving skills associated with the aging process. Some of the programs address impairments related to cognitive skills. The DriveABLE Program, directed by Dr. Allen Dobbs, is an example of a driving evaluation program based on extensive research surrounding the driving abilities of those with mental impairments (Dobbs, Triscott, & McCracken, 2004). The program consists of two phases, starting with in-office testing of cognitive abilities and proceeding to in-car testing when necessary. DriveABLE is based in Edmonton, Alberta, Canada.

DriveWise, codirected by neuropsychologist Dr. Margaret O'Connor and social worker Lissa Kapust, is a comprehensive evaluation of the performance of individuals who may have compromised driving skills because of impairments in motor, cognitive, perceptual, and/or sensory abilities. DriveWise is located at Beth Israel Deaconness Medical Center in Boston. The DriveWise team includes clinicians from behavioral neurology, social work, and occupational therapy. Together, they work with families to bring objectivity to the issue, conducting a thorough evaluation that includes a clinical social work assessment, in-clinic occupational therapy assessment, on-road driving assessment with an occupational therapist and driving instructor, and patient/family feedback meetings with the clinical social worker.

Driver rehabilitation specialists are emerging as important resources in specialized driving assessment for older drivers who are concerned about safe mobility and for monitoring the critical driving skills of persons with dementia. The American Occupational Therapy Association has taken a strong lead in recognizing the need to build capacity and have occupational therapists certified in specialized driving assessment through their Older Driver Initiative. Their Web site also has the nation's most comprehensive and searchable database of driver rehabilitation specialists (http://www.aota.org/olderdriver).

Who Conducts the Assessment?

Whereas a lack of agreement exists among researchers around how to determine driving safety and fitness to drive, likewise there is a lack of consensus in terms of who should be responsible for conducting driving assessments. A physician is generally responsible for basic cognitive tests surrounding dementia and driver's licensing. However, physicians are often adverse to playing the role of "licensing gatekeeper" (Skinner & Stearns, 1999) and have expressed concern for disrupting established rapport with their patients as well as for a lack of time to discuss driving (Silverstein & Murtha, 2001).

Where there are no strict regulations in place, the responsibility shifts between the Department of Motor Vehicles and licensed medical practitioners (Skinner & Stearns, 1999). When asked, individuals with dementia mentioned both themselves and their family members as better evaluators of their driving abilities than their physicians (Adler & Kuskowski, 2003).

This raises much concern for those with dementia in particular since they often lack the insight to evaluate their own abilities, and caregivers may be unaware of the impact on driving safety (Silverstein & Murtha, 2001). In a 1999 study, 43% of caregivers surveyed believed that the driver with dementia would be able to continue driving throughout the course of the disease (Adler et al., 1999). While it is true that many older adults begin to self-regulate their driving as their abilities decline (Brayne et al., 2000), individuals with Alzheimer's disease are often unable to recognize the loss of their abilities (Molnar, Eby, & Dobbs, 2005; Wild & Cotrell, 2003).

In 2003, the American Medical Association (AMA), in conjunction with the National Highway Traffic Safety Administration, published *Physician's Guide to Assessing and Counseling Older Drivers* (see Wang, Kosinski, Schwartzberg, & Shanklin, 2003). The importance of driver evaluation is discussed, including what the AMA sees as the ethical obligation of the physician to assess drivers for the safety of society. It states that, in the case of a known unsafe driver, the threat to the public safety is seen as more important than the health of the doctor–patient relationship.

However, although physicians may make assessments, research also shows that only experienced neurologists who conducted full patient evaluations were able to predict driver safety with accuracy comparable to that of the driving evaluator (Brown, Ott, et al., 2005; Brown, Stern, et al., 2005).

In addition to the AMA assessment of the physician's ethical obligations, the manual recommends two quick tests to administer when conducting a driving evaluation: the Trail-Making Test, Part B (only), and the Clock Drawing Test with the Freund Clock Scoring for Driving Competency are considered useful in identifying those individuals who should be referred to a driving rehabilitation specialist for more in-depth screening (Wang et al., 2003).

When an evaluation involves in-depth screening, patients are often referred to a driver rehabilitation specialist or occupational therapists who provide similar driving evaluation and counseling services. These individuals specialize in assessing driver ability and implementing devices to increase driver safety. They also make recommendations surrounding when and how often individuals should drive, including the need for cessation (Wang et al., 2003).

Monitoring

Like screening and assessment, the responsibility for monitoring currently falls to the primary care physician. Ideally, people with dementia will be reevaluated on a routine basis during physician visits throughout the progression of the disease. Such reevaluations should include referrals for follow-up specialized driving assessment that include on-the-road testing by driver rehabilitation specialists. Advocating for routine reevaluation for your clients with dementia is even more vital because of the serious coexisting medical conditions that they may experience in addition to dementia (Maslow, 2004). Many of the coexisting medical conditions such as diabetes, arthritis, glaucoma, and macular degeneration are known to impact critical driving skills.

Compliance With Assessments

Unfortunately, studies indicate that many with dementia are reluctant to discontinue driving on the basis of a physician's advice (Adler et al., 1999). The majority believe it is the individual with dementia's responsibility to make that determination. There is also concern that even if individuals do initially comply with the results of driving assessments, the disease progression might cause them to forget the recommendations (Sainz, 2004).

There is also concern regarding the lack of conformity of driving regulations. It is thought that those retiring may relocate to states with less stringent licensing procedures in an effort to maintain community mobility longer (Bener, 2005). This would be an especially dangerous practice for drivers with dementia because of the need for the periodic reassessment of driving skills (Vanderbur & Silverstein, 2006).

Policy Concerns

In addition to concerns surrounding state-to-state discrepancies in screening and reporting policies, funding for specialized driving assessment is an equally challenging barrier for many people with dementia. Medicare, Medicaid, or private insurance companies often do not cover the costs of driver evaluation or rehabilitation services. In 2006, the cost of an initial evaluation session was, on average, between $300 and $500. Adding to that the cost of providing the recommended complete medical history to the examiner, privacy or patient cooperation issues may also occur (Marottoli, 1998).

In the United States, driver screening and reporting policies vary from state to state. Some states require age-based mandatory screening, while in others screening is triggered by reports from physicians, family, or others. However, generally, the responsibility of recognizing driver impairment continues to fall to the impaired drivers themselves and their family members (Silverstein & Murtha, 2001).

Reporting Practices

The AMA guide (Wang et al., 2003) has an appendix of state-by-state licensing and renewal requirements. More up-to-date summaries may be found on the Web site of the American Association of Motor Vehicle Administrators (http://www.aamva.org). It is important to know the reporting and screening policies and requirements in your own state.

Currently, the range of reporting requirements varies from state to state, and these requirements are often a challenge for physicians, professionals, families, and persons with dementia to navigate. Age-based testing has been implemented in some states to screen high-risk drivers.

The Department of Motor Vehicles sees drivers periodically at the time of license renewal (unless renewal can be done by mail or through the Internet). Many departments report that they train their licensing personnel on how to observe impairing conditions. However, only a few others provide additional specialized training (Lococo & Staplin, 2005; Szlyk, Myers, Zhang, Wetzel, & Shapiro, 2002).

Where Counseling May Help

The power of the disparity of public safety versus individual independence and risk versus autonomy—especially between social worker and other advocates for vulnerable populations and public health and community planners—often causes conflict (and sometimes a stalemate) during assessment and decision-making processes surrounding the issue of dementia and driving. This conflict often spills over into the more global issue of community mobility and dementia. As a social workers, you advocate for personal autonomy and independence for your clients. As a responsible practitioner, it is important that you consider public safety and risk not only to your client but to the community as well.

To encourage a smooth transition from driving to nondriving, planning and counseling are essential for people with dementia and their families. Planning for the nondriving years is as important to independence and community involvement and a sense of control as financial planning and should begin long before alternative transportation is needed. Theoretically, if one has planned for the nondriving years, has been involved in the decision-making process, and is familiar with alternatives, the transition from driving to nondriving may be less difficult (Stephens et al., 2005).

Effective planning before the onset of more advanced cognitive impairment is a proactive way to support personal autonomy. In the case of dementia and driving (and nondriving), thoughtful planning can be a source of personal control and independence. It is important to encourage a person with mild cognitive impairment to make an agreement with his or her family or friends about when to stop driving, to gather resources about existing alternative transportation options before they are needed, and to craft a transportation plan for the nondriving years.

The Hartford Financial Services Group, Inc., and the MIT AgeLab together developed two guides that are useful to help families start proactive conversations about driving safety (*We Need to Talk: Family Conversations With Older Drivers*) and about driving and dementia (*At the Crossroads: A Guide to Alzheimer's Disease, Dementia, and Driving*). Both guides are available free of charge through the Hartford Web site noted in the resource section at the back of this book.

Counseling is important during the planning process. Effective counseling includes emotional support for people with dementia and their families and access to resources around perceived loss of independence. In addition, ongoing education on the continuum of transportation services available and guidance toward alternatives that will best meet one's needs are critical (Stephens et al., 2005).

Although it is advisable to encourage a gradual transition to alternative transportation options while still an active driver, it is important to make the most informed and objective decision regarding when driving is no longer safe. Identifying resources and encouraging the most objective evaluation possible are best practices when there is concern about driving safety and fitness for someone with cognitive impairments.

CURRENT COMMUNITY MOBILITY OPTIONS

That driving expectancy is significantly less than life expectancy and that men outlive their ability to drive by 6 years and women by 10 (Foley et al., 2002), in conjunction with findings suggesting that more than 600,000 people age 70 and older stop driving each year and become dependent on others to meet their transportation needs, compels us to take a hard look at the availability of alternative transportation options. Creating transportation options that truly meet the community mobility needs of people with dementia and their families, allowing them to stay active in their communities for as long as possible, may be an even greater challenge.

Although some communities offer a spectrum of transportation services from public transportation with flexible routes so that people can be picked up at or near their homes, to specialized senior transportation, to paratransit for people with disabilities and special needs and medical transportation, to volunteer transportation, many communities lack these resources. The situation becomes more poignant as we consider where elders reside. It is expected that the majority of the growth of the 85-and-older population will occur in rural areas and recently established suburbs that have yet to set up reliable and easy-to-use public transportation (Koffman, Raphael, & Weiner, 2004). Other growth will occur in frontier communities that are completely removed from direct services such as respite care and adult day care services. They are classified as being at least 60 miles and/or 60 minutes from the nearest market center and where many critical health and social services are located. As such, many older individuals often live in extremely isolated areas where community mobility is unavailable.

When helping people with dementia plan for their transportation needs after they cease driving, identify the transportation services that do exist in their area and consider the supportive assistance that will be needed as the disease progresses. For instance, while those in the very early stages of the disease may, in fact, be able to find their way on public transportation with clear maps and some minor assistance (Sterns, Sterns, Sterns, & Naidoo, 2006), as they experience increased confusion, they will require additional support to arrange and utilize transportation services. In most cases, those who become lost or easily confused or who cannot navigate complex situations while driving are usually unable to find their way in complicated public transportation systems that involve maps, routes, and schedules. Rosenbloom (2003) observed that those unable to drive are often unable to use public transit services as well.

Special transit services currently have very limited availability. They are generally for use only during regular transit services hours, and there are residential distance requirements (within three-quarters of a mile) to be considered for services. Many of those who live near existing bus routes remain ineligible for services because of service providers' strict eligibility requirements (Rosenbloom, 2003).

The requirements of the Americans for Disabilities Act place a large financial burden on urban paratransit services without providing for any funding of the projects. Many service providers are forced to restrict eligibility to keep down the cost of the service (Rosenbloom, 2003). Such paratransit services will likely not provide a viable strategy for addressing the community mobility needs of older individuals in general and the person with dementia specifically (Vanderbur & Silverstein, 2006).

According to a case study by Adler, Rottunda, Bauer, and Kuskowski (2000), transportation for those with dementia must involve as little waiting as possible as well as very unrestricted hours and routes. Traditional public transportation has none of these options. Applying the concepts of travel training and mobility management, such as is done for disabled populations, might be a useful strategy for persons with dementia, particularly in the early stages of the disease process.

In addition to a spectrum of transportation options to consider when identifying services for your clients, there is also a continuum in terms of how the services are provided, which fall into categories such as (a) stop-to-stop, (b) curb-to-curb, (c) door-to-door, (d) door-through-door, (e) arm-to-arm, (f) chair-to-chair, and (g) arm-through-arm. Stop-to-stop is the least supportive because one has to be able to get to a bus stop or station and wait for services. Curb-to-curb service may, in fact, pick people up and drop them at their homes but does not assist them to the door or ensure that someone is home to receive them. As an individual with dementia increasingly requires assistance, door-to-door, door-through-door, and even arm-through-arm service may be required (Figure 15.2). Westat and the Beverly Foundation have produced an Administration on Aging–funded report entitled, "How to Establish and Maintain Door-Through-Door Transportation Services for Seniors," which addresses the need for increased levels of transportation assistance among the aging and those with chronic illnesses such as dementia (Burkhardt & Kerschner, 2005).

CALL TO ACTION

To meet the needs effectively of people with dementia and their families throughout the disease, transportation options must offer door-to- or door-through-door and arm-to- or arm-through-arm services. In addition to providing the five As of "senior-friendly" transportation (as noted in Figure 15.1, those options also must incorporate "dementia-friendly" qualities. The national Alzheimer's Association (1997) has defined agencies that serve elders as dementia specific, dementia capable, or dementia friendly. Dementia-specific agencies are those that serve individuals with Alzheimer's disease or a related disorder exclusively. Dementia-capable agencies are those that have staff trained in dementia care and also serve elders who are not cognitively impaired. Dementia-friendly agencies are agencies that serve all elders but do not have staff members specifically trained in dementia care.

An assessment of your client's needs can help determine the types of transportation services from which your client would benefit as well as the flexibility required to meet those needs. An inventory of the services offered in your community by a variety of transportation providers is recommended to help align needs and services.

Curb-to-curb: Driver picks passenger up at the curbside or in the driveway. Organizational policy will articulate the extent of assistance provided to the passenger while entering and exiting the vehicle.

Door-to-door: Driver retrieves passenger from door of pickup location to door of destination, often including assistance into and out of the vehicle.

Door-through-door: Driver may enter passenger's home, often providing assistance (i.e., tying shoes, help donning jacket, ensuring that the home is locked, etc.) at pickup and drop-off locations.

Arm-through-arm assistance: Driver physically assists passenger with getting in and out of vehicle.

Arm-to-arm or Chair-to-chair: Driver receives the passenger from a responsible person and delivers the passenger to a "responsible arm" when the destination is reached. Chair-to-chair implies that the driver assists the passenger from the chair in his or her home to the chair at the destination, for example, the doctor's office.

Transferring assistance: Driver physically assists passenger in transferring to and from wheelchair when getting into and out of vehicle.

Escort:
First definition— Volunteer or paid driver drives passenger to and from appointment, and accompanies and stays with him during appointment or event—providing companionship and emotional support regarding information or news given at appointment.
Second definition— Volunteer or paid escort accompanies care receiver to and from appointment or event on public transit, para transit, taxicab, etc. rather than driving and stays during appointment—providing companionship and emotional support regarding information or news given at appointment.

Nurse escort: Same as above; however, escort is a working or retired nurse who helps interpret medical information for care receiver and family.

While some programs provide rides only for medical appointments, many others transport for shopping, personal business, picking up medications, social events, religious services/events, and other purposes.

FIGURE 15.2   Types of transportation services.
Source: Adapted from Easter Seals' *A Solution Package for Volunteer Transportation Programs*, 2003.

We are using the concept of dementia-friendly as a first step toward envisioning transportation that incorporates elements of dementia-capable and dementia-specific services. Building awareness among transportation providers that the individuals they serve may now or may in the future have cognitive impairments and providing increased recognition through support-ive environments and staffing could make a difference not only in addressing safety concerns but in keeping people mobile later in life as well.

In our vision, dementia-friendly supportive transportation provides trained dispatchers and drivers with understanding of the disease and a capacity to provide services in a sensitive manner. Such a transportation system designs services to be flexible and prompt in order not to leave passengers waiting or unattended or traveling too long on the vehicle. Trained attendants are in the vehicle when necessary to ensure the safety of the passengers and someone (other than the driver) to escort passen-gers to/through the door of his or her residence. The vehicle environment is soothing to discourage agitation; however, agitation in itself will not disqualify riders from the transportation service.

Although it is currently challenging to identify supportive transpor-tation options meeting these criteria, the responsibility of transportation for people with dementia will likely remain solely on the shoulders of family and friends. Persons with dementia without functional kin will take fewer trips and will likely be at risk for increased isolation, depres-sion, and premature institutionalization.

Determining existing transportation options that might meet needs and arranging such transportation options are often initial barriers that people with dementia and their families must overcome in maintaining community mobility. Currently, few tools exist to assist people in over-coming these obstacles. An additional factor in the decrease in commu-nity mobility among people with dementia may bring about increased stress among family caregivers. Figure 15.3 includes questions to ask when arranging transportation for someone with dementia.

Moving the Transportation Agenda Forward

To eliminate duplication of services in order to lower per-trip operating costs and enhance transportation for those in need of transportation services, including people with dementia, President Bush initiated the United We Ride Program in February 2004 (http://www.unitedweride. gov). United We Ride and the Interagency Transportation Coordinating Council on Access and Mobility are charged with coordinating the 62 different federal programs across nine departments that provide funding in support of human services transportation. In addition to this initiative, the transportation authorization bill titled Safe, Accountable, Flexible, Efficient, Transportation Equity Act: A Legacy for Users (SAFETEA-LU), which passed in 2006, includes mandates for locally developed coordinated plans for all human services transportation funded under the legislation.

Whether you are looking for transportation for a client or are a caregiver in search of transportation for a loved one with dementia, use the following questions to gather more detailed information from the transportation provider:

1. What is the service area?

2. Is there a limitation on distance?

3. How much will the service cost?

4. Will insurance pay for rides provided by the service?

5. Are there requirements to qualify for the service? If so, what are they?

6. Is there an evaluation that must take place before the first ride?

7. Is there a membership fee that must be paid before scheduling rides with the service?

8. How far in advance must reservations be made?

9. Are rides provided in the evenings, on weekends, or on holidays?

10. Are rides provided to social as well as medical or shopping appointments?

11. Are door-to-door, door-through-door, or arm-through-arm services provided?

12. Are rides provided to people who use wheelchairs? If so, do riders stay in their wheelchairs, or are they transferred to seats during the ride?

13. Are drivers trained specifically to work with people with dementia?

14. Is there an escort or attendant in the vehicle with the driver?

15. Does someone stay with the passenger during appointments?

16. Can a family member serve as an escort? If so, is there an extra cost associated?

17. Will there be a wait when picked up from home? If so, how long?

18. Will there be a wait when picked up for the return trip? If so, how long?

19. Will the driver or attendant come into the office/building pick up for the return trip?

20. Will other passengers be riding? If so, what is the maximum length of time of the ride while others are being picked up/dropped off?

FIGURE 15.3   What you should know about transportation services (modified from the Beverly Foundation and Easter Seals' Senior Transportation Options Template, 2003).

Easter Seals and the National Association of Area Agencies on Aging have partnered to spearhead the National Center on Senior Transportation, funded by the Federal Transit Administration. The center will provide technical assistance, develop materials, and build a national clearing house specifically to assist local communities and states in the expansion and provision of transportation services for older adults.

Although the Americans for Disabilities Act mandates that public transportation operators must also provide demand-responsive paratransit services where fixed-route transportation is available, this mandate accounts only for areas that have public transportation and in many cases does not impact suburban, smaller metropolitan, or rural areas that have no or limited public transportation. Initiatives like United We Ride are attempting to address these shortcomings.

Medical appointments certainly are not the only or even the most important need for which people with dementia require transportation. However, Medicaid does provide health care coverage that includes transportation to medical appointments. Approximately $1.8 billion is spent annually to provide about 110 million rides. States take a wide variety of approaches to the provision of Medicaid transportation. The good news is that the new emphasis on home and community-based services has encouraged creativity among states with Medicaid waiver programs. As many as two-thirds of these states have implemented programs that will pay for essential trips, such as grocery shopping, with Medicaid dollars.

Medicare, on the other hand, does not pay for medical or any other transportation with the exception of emergency transportation in an ambulance. This has sparked a twofold growing controversy among transportation and elder advocates in that not only are expensive emergency trips—and vehicles—being used inappropriately when less expensive nonemergency vehicles would be adequate, but many expensive emergency trips could be avoided.

Supplemental Transportation Programs

In 2000, the AAA Foundation for Traffic Safety and the Beverly Foundation of Pasadena, California, gathered information and studied the effectiveness of community-based transportation programs for seniors in the United States. It was in this project that the term *supplemental transportation programs* was coined to encompass both formal and informal transportation programs outside public transportation (Beverly Foundation, 2001b). The project identified over 400 such programs across the nation.

The Independent Transportation Network (ITN), a promising supplemental transportation model that is both community based and consumer oriented, originated in Westbrook, Maine. The ITN is a non-profit organization that provides transportation services for seniors and people with visual impairments. It utilizes shared rides (both volunteer and paid drivers) and advance planning to provide seniors with quality, efficient, door-to-door, and if needed, an arm-through-arm service 7 days a week, 24 hours a day (see www. itnamerica.org).

Public–private partnerships have held the key to success for some communities addressing the ever-growing need—and in some cases desires—for senior-friendly, supportive transportation among older non-drivers, people with dementia, and their families. One such example is in Annapolis, Maryland, where a public–private partnership was cultivated between public transit officials and Partners in Care, a local nonprofit volunteer organization. Whereas public transit did not have the resources to develop services for frail elders and people with disabilities but recognized the unmet need, they applied for an AmeriCorps volunteer to do so. Through this volunteer, Partners in Care was identified as having the capacity to provide rides in addition to other assistance (Hensley-Quinn & Hardin, 2006).

The state of Florida, too, is approaching the issue of dementia and driving with a statewide comprehensive program. The Florida model encompasses policy development, community network involvement, education and services for seniors, and collaboration between public agencies and service providers (see the Florida Department of Highway Safety and Motor Vehicles Web site at http://www.hsmv.state.fl.us/ddl/atriskdrivers.pdf). The Florida program is unique in that it considers important ethical issues under consideration, such as the determination of acceptable risk, the balance of autonomy and personal safety, individual rights and confidentiality versus public safety, participatory decision making wherever possible, informed consent versus beneficence, and responsibilities of professionals (Carlin Rogers, 2006). The program has published articles for drivers with dementia and their families, including the booklets *Is Driving Your Best Choice?* and *Is It Time to Stop Driving?* developed in collaboration with Florida Atlantic University (see http://www.fau.edu/memorywellnesscenter/stopdriving.pdf and http://www.fau.edu/memorywellnesscenter/driving.pdf).

Getting Involved

At some point, all people with dementia who are currently driving will face the difficult, independence-threatening, and often heart-wrenching decision to give up the keys. This builds a compelling case for social workers to identify community and other resources to help support clients through the transition from driving to nondriving. These resources can be equally valuable in working with family caregivers since it often falls to families to enforce driving restrictions, especially when their loved one is confused and forgetful and perhaps not even aware of lapses in driving safety. Consider the following steps to better equip yourself, your colleagues, your clients, and your community and to better support the transition of people with dementia from drivers to passengers and to enable them to remain active in the community for as long as possible:

- Identify local transportation services that meet your clients' needs.
- Obtain planning materials such as the Hartford guides listed in the resource section at the back of this book.
- Play an active role in transportation planning in your community and in the communities you serve and join—or form—senior transportation consortiums to do the following:
  - Raise awareness
  - Improve safety for older drivers and pedestrians
  - Help coordinate service
  - Advocate for transportation programs and services that do not exist in order to fill current gaps
  - Advocate for and provide training toward dementia-friendly supportive services
- Work with and advocate for existing transportation providers to adapt their services to become more dementia friendly.
- Expand your network of resource people to include the following:
  - Occupational therapists
  - Driver rehabilitation specialists
  - Transportation providers
  - Representatives from departments of motor vehicles and their medical review boards

A framework for action can be found in the vision laid out for a future transportation system in the document *Safe Mobility for a Maturing Society: Challenges and Opportunities* (U.S. Department of Transportation, 2003). Working toward safe mobility for all elders will certainly benefit persons with dementia as well.

Social workers can have a role in sharing this responsibility and truly making a difference. Social workers are natural catalysts for change and are especially skillful at working with groups to solve problems. Getting people talking together from federal agencies, Congress, states, counties, municipalities, health and social service agencies, and the private sector is a necessary strategy for sustainable community interventions.

REFERENCES

AARP. (2004, January). *Enhancing mobility options for older Americans: A five-year national action agenda*. Washington, DC: AARP Public Policy Institute.

AARP. (2005). *Beyond 50.05: A report to the nation on livable communities creating environments for successful aging*. Washington, DC: AARP Public Policy Institute.

Adler, G., & Kuskowski, M. (2003). Driving cessation in older men with dementia. *Alzheimer Disease and Associated Disorders, 17*, 68–71.

Adler, G., Rottunda, S., Bauer, M., & Kuskowski, M. (2000, July/August). Driving cessation and AD: Issues confronting patients and family. *American Journal of Alzheimer's Disease, 15*, 212–216.

Adler, G., Rottunda, S., & Kuskowski, M. (1999). Dementia and driving: Perceptions and changing habits. *Clinical Gerontologist, 20*, 23–34.

Alzheimer's Association. (1997). *Community assessment workbook for dementia services*. Chicago: Author.

Anstey, K. J., Wood, J., Lord, S., & Walker, J. G. (2005). Cognitive, sensory and physical factors enabling driving safety in older adults. *Clinical Psychology Review, 25*, 45–65.

Bener, L. (2005, April). *Closing the gap: A comprehensive, multidisciplinary approach to the older driver*. Paper presented to the White House Conference on Aging Officially Designated Event, Transportation Solutions for an Aging Society, Massachusetts Institute of Technology, Cambridge, MA.

Beverly Foundation. (2001a). *On the road to senior friendly transportation: The 5 A's*. Pasadena, CA: Author.

Beverly Foundation. (2001b). *Supplemental transportation programs for seniors*. Washington, DC: AAA Foundation for Traffic Safety.

Brayne, C., Dufouil, C., Ahmed, A., Dening, T. R., Chi, L.-Y., McGee, M., et al. (2000). Very old drivers: Findings from a population cohort of people aged 84 and over. *International Journal of Epidemiology, 29*, 704–707.

Brown, L. B., Ott, B. R., Papandonatos, G. D., Sui, Y., Ready, R. E., & Morris, J. C. (2005). Prediction of on-road driving performance in patients with early Alzheimer's disease. *Journal of the American Geriatrics Society, 53*, 94–98.

Brown, L. B., Stern, R. A., Cahn-Weiner, D. A., Rogers, B., Messer, M. A., Lannon, M. C., et al. (2005). Driving Scenes test of the Neuropsychological Assessment Battery (NAB) and on-road driving performance in aging and very mild dementia. *Archives of Clinical Neuropsychology, 20*, 209–215.

Burkhardt, J. E., & Kerschner, H., (2005, September). *How to establish and maintain door-through-door transportation services for seniors*. Washington, DC: Administration on Aging.

Carlin Rogers, F. (2006, January). *Florida's roadmap for drivers with dementia*. Paper presented at the 85th annual meeting of the Transportation Research Board, Human Factors Workshop, Washington, DC.

Dobbs, A. R., McCracken, P. N., Carstensen, B. A., Kiss, I., and Triscott, J. A. C. (1998). *The evaluation of competence to drive*. Canadian Consensus Conference on Dementia.

Dobbs, A. R., Triscott, J. A. C., & McCracken, P. N., (2004). Consideration of assessment of medical competence to drive in older patients. *Geriatrics and Aging, 7*(1), 42–46.

Dubinsky, R. M., Stein, A. C., & Lyons, K. (2000). Practice parameter: Risk of driving and Alzheimer's disease (an evidence-based review). Report of the Quality Standards Subcommittee of the American Academy of Neurology. *Neurology, 54,* 2205–2211.

Easter Seals. (2003). *Transportation Solutions for Caregivers: A Solutions Package for Volunteer Transportation Programs.* Chicago, IL: author.

Foley, D. J., Heimovitz, H. K., Guralnik, J. M., & Brock, D. B. (2002). Driving life expectancy of persons aged 70 years and older in the United States. *American Journal of Public Health, 92,* 1284–1289.

Fox, G. K., Bowden, S. C., Bashford, G. M., & Smith, D. S. (1997). Alzheimer's disease and driving: Prediction and assessment of driving performance. *Journal of the American Geriatrics Society, 45,* 949–953.

Hensley-Quinn, M., & Hardin, J. (2006, January). *Innovative practices in community transportation.* Paper presented at the 85th annual meeting of the Transportation Research Board, Human Factors Workshop, Washington, DC.

Hunt, L. (2003). Driving and dementia. *Generations, 27,* 34–38.

Janke, M. K. (1994, July). *Age-related disabilities that may impair driving and their assessment* (RSS-94-156). Sacramento: Research and Development Section, Program and Policy Administration, California Department of Motor Vehicles.

Koffman, D., Raphael, D., & Weiner, R. (2004, October). *The impact of federal programs on transportation for older adults (2004–17).* Washington, DC: AARP Public Policy Institute.

Lincoln, N. B., Radford, K. A., Lee, E., and Reay, A. (2004). *The assessment of fitness to drive in people with dementia.* Unpublished manuscript, University of Nottingham and Walton Hospital, Chesterfield, UK.

Lococo, K., & Staplin, L. (2005). *Strategies of medical advisory board licensing (HS 809 874).* Washington, DC: U.S. Department of Transportation, National Highway Traffic Safety Administration.

Marottoli, R. A. (1998). The assessment of older drivers. In W. R. Hazzard, J. P. Blass, J. B. Halter, J. G. Ouslander, & M. Tinetti (Eds.), *Principles of geriatric medicine and gerontology* (4th ed., pp. 267–274). New York: McGraw-Hill.

Maslow, K. (2004). Dementia and serious coexisting medical conditions: A double whammy. *Nursing Clinics of North America, 39,* 561–579.

Molnar, L. J., Eby, D. W., & Dobbs, B. M. (2005). Policy recommendations to the 2005 White House Conference on Aging. *Public Policy and Aging Report, 15,* 24–27.

National Alliance for Caregiving & AARP. (2004, April). *Caregiving in the U.S.* Bethesda, MD: Author. Retrieved August 28, 2005, from http://www.caregiving.org/data/04finalreport.pdf

Reger, M. A., Welsh, R. K., Watson, G. S., Cholerton, B., Baker, L. D., & Craft, S. (2004). The relationship between neuropsychological functions and driving ability in dementia: A meta-analysis. *Neuropsychology, 18*(1), 85–93.

Rinalducci, E. J., Mouloua, M., & Smither, J. (n.d.). *Cognitive and perceptual factors in aging and driving performance* (Report No. VPL-03-01). Orlando: Visual Performance Laboratory, Department of Psychology, University of Central Florida.

Rosenbloom, S. (2003, July). *The mobility needs of older Americans: Implications for transportation reauthorization* (Transportation Reform Series). Washington, DC: Center on Urban and Metropolitan Policy, Brookings Institution. Retrieved August 28, 2005, from http://www.brookings.edu/dybdocroot/es/urban/publications/20030807_Rosenbloom.pdf

Sainz, A. (2004, June 11). Alzheimer's sufferer who won't stop driving ordered to state care. Associated Press.

Shua-Haim, J. R., & Gross, J. S. (1996). The "co-pilot" driver syndrome. *Journal of American Geriatrics Society, 44*, 815–817.

Silverstein, N. M., Flaherty, G., & Tobin, T. S. (2002). *Dementia and wandering behavior: Concern for the lost elder.* New York: Springer.

Silverstein, N. M, & Murtha, J. (2001, April). *Driving in Massachusetts: When to stop and who should decide?* Boston: Gerontology Institute and College of Public and Community Service, University of Massachusetts Boston.

Skinner, D., & Stearns, M. D. (1999, January). *Safe mobility in an aging world.* Washington, DC: John A. Volpe National Transportation Systems Center, Research and Special Programs Administration, U.S. Department of Transportation.

Snellgrove, C. A. (2005). *Cognitive screening for the safe driving competence of older people with mild cognitive impairment or early dementia.* Canberra: Australian Transport Safety Bureau.

Stephens, B. W., McCarthy, D., Marsiske, M., Shechtman, O., Classen, S., Justiss, M., et al. (2005). International older driver consensus conference on assessment, remediation and counseling for transportation alternatives: Summary and recommendations. *Physical and Occupational Therapy in Geriatrics, 23*, 103–121.

Sterns, A., Sterns, H., Sterns, R., & Naidoo, L. (2006, January). *Designing maps and schedules for older adults.* Paper presented at the 85th annual meeting of the Transportation Research Board, Washington, DC.

Szlyk, J. P., Myers, L., Zhang, Y. X., Wetzel, L., & Shapiro, R. (2002). Development and assessment of a neuropsychological battery to aid in predicting driver performance. *Journal of Rehabilitation Research and Development, 39*, 483–496.

Uc, E. Y., Rizzo, M., Anderson, S. W., Shi, Q., & Dawson, J. D. (2004). Driver route-following and safety errors in early Alzheimer disease. *Neurology, 63*, 832–837.

U.S. Department of Transportation. (2003, November). *Safe mobility for a maturing society: Challenges and opportunities.* Washington, DC: Author. Retrieved August 28, 2005, from http://www.eyes.uab.edu/safemobility/SafeMobility.pdf

Vanderbur, M., & Silverstein, N. M. (2006). *Community mobility and dementia: A review of the literature.* Report prepared for the Alzheimer's Association and National Highway Traffic Safety Administration. Washington, DC: Alzheimer's Association and the National Highway Traffic Safety Administration.

Vegega, M. (1990, November). *The effect of aging on the cognitive and psychomotor abilities of older drivers: A review of the research.* Washington, DC: U.S. National Highway Traffic Safety Administration, Office of Driver and Pedestrian Research.

Wang, C. C., Kosinski, C. J., Schwartzberg, J. G., & Shanklin, A. V. (2003). *Physician's guide to assessing and counseling older drivers.* Washington, DC: National Highway Traffic Safety Administration. Retrieved August 27, 2005, from http://www.ama-assn.org/ama/pub/category/10791.html

Wild, K., & Cotrell, V. (2003). Identifying driving impairment in Alzheimer disease: A comparison of self and observer reports versus driving evaluation. *Alzheimer Disease and Associated Disorders, 17*, 27–34.

CHAPTER SIXTEEN

Social Work and Dementia Care Within Adult Day Services

Jed Johnson and Marilyn Hartle

INTRODUCTION

The social work profession has and will continue to play a vital role in preparing for and responding to what has been often referred to as the "graying of America." The burgeoning population of older adults has been well documented. As of 2001, there were more than 34.7 million individuals age 65 and over in the United States representing approximately 13% of the population. The U.S. Census Bureau expects this figure to double by 2030 (Kinsella & Velkoff, 2001, pp. 128–129).

This social work role is particularly important when working with persons with dementia and related diagnoses. Since increasing age is the greatest risk factor for Alzheimer's disease, it is anticipated that there will be a commensurate increase in persons diagnosed with Alzheimer's and other dementias, a group of conditions that gradually destroy brain cells and lead to progressive decline in mental function. The national Alzheimer's Association indicates that currently 1 in 10 individuals over age 65 and nearly half of those over age 85 are affected.

A number of authors have highlighted the fact that the diagnosis of dementia impacts not only the individual themselves but also the vast constellation of family members, friends, and others who may at some point become involved in the caregiving role (Fazio, Seman, & Stansell, 1999; Hoffman & Kaplan, 1996). It is estimated that there are more than 44 million Americans age 18 and over providing unpaid care. One-quarter of the caregivers assisting someone age 50 or older report that the person they care for is suffering from Alzheimer's disease, dementia, or other mental confusion (National Alliance for Caregiving & AARP, 2004).

Over the past 25 years, adult day centers have emerged as a viable long-term care option providing support and respite for persons with dementia and their caregivers (Dziegielewski & Ricks, 2000, pp. 51–64; Gaugler et al., 2003, pp. 37–58; Smyth-Henry, Cox, Reifler, & Asbury, 2001). This chapter emphasizes the important roles that social workers can and should play within this often-perceived nontraditional setting.

DEFINITION OF DAY CARE

The National Adult Day Services Association defines an adult day center as

> community-based group programs designed to meet the needs of functionally and/or cognitively impaired adults through an individual plan of care. These structured, comprehensive programs provide a variety of social and other related support services in a protective setting during any part of a day, but less than 24-hour care. Adult day centers generally operate programs during normal business hours five days a week. Some programs offer services in the evenings and on weekends.

The National Study of Adult Day Services identified three primary types of adult day centers: social model, medical model, and combination model programs (Adult Day Services Program, 2001–2002). The *social model* focuses on recreational activities and social interactions, while the *medical model* most often integrates nursing, rehabilitative, and personal care components into the array of services offered.

A number of organizations house both types of programs under one roof, forming the combination model. An emerging trend within the social model genre targeting those persons with early-stage dementia has been "club-model" programs (Bosky, 2003; Zarit, Femia, Watson, Rice-Oeschger, & Kakos, 2004, pp. 262–269).) Within these programs, persons with mild memory loss play a leadership role in program development and ongoing operations.

DEMENTIA AND DAY CARE

While the spectrum of care within adult day services runs from younger adults with developmental disabilities, multiple sclerosis, or human immunodeficiency virus to physically frail older adults and those post-stroke, the vast majority of persons served within adult day centers are individuals with a dementia diagnosis. In fact, the National Study of Adult Day Services conducted in 2001–2002 found that across all three types of centers highlighted previously, dementia (all forms) was by far the most prevalent participant diagnosis/condition, representing more than 50% of all those enrolled. The top four conditions/diagnoses were dementia (52%), frail elderly (41%), developmental disability (24%), and physical disability (23%). The total exceeds 100%, as many of those enrolled in adult day programs have multiple diagnoses.

Those persons enrolled in adult day programs who experience memory loss range from persons with early-stage dementia in a social model program through those in the final stages of Alzheimer's disease attending a medical model center. In the latter case, in spite of their potential eligibility for nursing home–level care, an adult day program affords them the opportunity to remain at home with family and/or other caregivers throughout the entire course of the disease process.

Of the estimated 3,400 centers across the United States from the 2001–2002 National Study, approximately 20% are identified as being "dementia specific." There has been a marked increase in these specialized centers over the past 20 years. In a 1984 survey of the adult day services industry, Mace and Rabins (1984) identified only 20 dementia-specific programs out of nearly 800 programs. This enormous increase reflects both the ever-increasing need and the demand for these services. Little is known, however, about the prevalence and interventions of social workers within adult day centers serving persons with dementia. The 2001–2002 National Study did indicate that 85% of centers provided some form of social services.

The unique aspects of social work within adult day services are many: the social worker as sole practitioner, challenges in defining who the client is, the luxury (and challenge) of having the time to build long-term relationships with clients and their carers, the opportunity to work within an interdisciplinary team, and the blurring of roles that often happens within many adult day centers.

These dynamic factors require a strong grounding in social work principles and self-directed work skills for practitioners. The remainder of this chapter focuses on these unique elements and discusses the roles for social workers to fulfill within the context of working with people with dementia within adult day services.

UNIQUE ASPECTS OF SOCIAL WORK IN
ADULT DAY SERVICES

Work with persons with dementia presents unique challenges to the social worker. Ascertaining the needs, wants, and interests of a person who may not logically, accurately, or rationally be able to communicate because of their disease process can present many dilemmas.

A common dilemma is deciding who is the client. Adult day service practitioners actually balance the needs, interests, and wants of various client subsets (Johnson, Sakaris, Tripp, Vroman, & Wood, 2004, p. 12). The family/caregiver may initiate admission to adult day services for the purpose of respite, yet the person with dementia may perceive no need to attend. The family may request the person be kept active while at the center, but the person may have no interest in being active. The person may query, "What's wrong with me?" but the family has told staff they do not want the diagnosis shared with the person. How does one honor the expressed desires of the client who has lost the ability for rational thought?

Core social work values such as self-determination and the rights of the individual may also be challenged. The client may seek sugary snacks yet staff knows the client is diabetic. The client may attempt to go outside the facility during inclement weather that is deemed unsafe by staff. What are the ethical implications of imposing the practitioners' or family members' views of what is appropriate over that of the person affected by dementia? There are no easy answers. Fundamentally, however, it is important to remember the *person* who has the disease rather than focus on management of symptomology (Kitwood, 1997, p. 7).

The social worker needs to be clear in his or her own mind and in their interaction with others who the client is, and this is dependent on the situation. In many situations, it is the adult day center participant who is the client; at other times, it is the caregiver(s). The social worker may have to help colleagues understand this dynamic—that, at different times, different people are the client within the care system.

To understand the person, one must build relationships. Adult day services often afford social work practitioners the time needed to build relationships with clients. The average length of time that a person attends adult day services is 2 years (Adult Day Services Program, 2001–2002). This far exceeds the brief encounters of time-limited interventions of many other social work settings. The time for relationship building also applies to the support network of clients including their family members and others, suggesting that social workers within adult day services will have the opportunity to fulfill multiple roles over the course of the person's experience of dementia.

Typically, social workers within adult day services are the lone social work practitioner within the multidisciplinary team. This calls for practitioners who are characterized by a strong sense of personal and professional definition as well as having initiative, creativity, and flexibility in evolving their roles. Persons requiring a well-defined structure may not be well suited for work within adult day services or for work with people with dementia.

The ever-changing status of persons experiencing the progressive effects of dementia affords an opportunity for practitioners seeking diversity of interventions and continuous learning. There is also diversity in focus and approach to care dependent on the model of adult day services followed, such as the club model versus the medical model. This diversity and flexibility also provides opportunity to expand social work roles beyond those traditionally found within the long-term care arena as in admissions processing, support group facilitation, and "handling" problem behaviors.

The definition of who is client, the long-term nature of the relationship, being the sole clinician within the setting, and the interdisciplinary focus all contribute to the rather unique environment for social work within adult day programs serving persons with dementia (Beaver & Miller, 1985, pp. 65–70; Johnson et al., 2004, pp. 5–6). Previous works have expounded on the variety of roles that social workers fulfill within various settings. For the purposes of this chapter, the focus is on social worker as educator, counselor, broker, advocate, and researcher.

Cast within the nontraditional setting of adult day services, the social worker often has great flexibility in defining how to fulfill these various roles. In part, the definition of roles and the type of interventions will be defined by the model of adult day services in which the practitioner works. This chapter now explores in some detail five specific social work roles within the adult day setting.

Social Worker as Educator

Found by the police wandering in a shopping center parking lot, Paul M. was unable to provide any information to the officers. Suspecting alcohol consumption, Paul was transported to a local hospital. The emergency room social worker realized that Paul's confusion was the result of dementia and was skillfully able to discern his identity and contacted the family. She took the opportunity to educate the officers about signs and symptoms of dementia. When his daughter-in-law arrived at the hospital, the worker was able to educate her about a variety of home and community-based options to support Paul and the family's caregiving efforts, including adult day services.

The role as educator for social workers within adult day services requires a multifaceted approach. The intended audience for the message suggests the content and method of delivery. For instance, the social worker in varied employment settings has a role in educating the greater community to the services and benefits of adult day services. This may involve developing educational pamphlets or brochures, speaking to community and professional groups, or exhibiting at local health fairs. Funders and potential funders may also need heightened understanding of the unique aspects of caring for persons with dementia as well as the vital role adult day services can play within the continuum of care.

Individual clients may need education on understanding diagnosis or self-care skills. As not all adult day services centers have nurses or other medical staff, health and wellness education may fall to the social worker. Family members/caregivers may also need information on diagnoses and caregiving skills. An issue unique to caregiving of people with dementia is gaining insights into how to stay connected to the individual as they lose their memory and other cognitive skills. Education on person-centered approaches to interventions and relationship building may benefit family members, staff, and other caregivers.

Additionally, education on cultural, ethnic, lifestyle preferences, and other issues related to uniqueness must be addressed to effectively uphold and support individuals experiencing dementia. The social worker also has a responsibility to educate coworkers, including direct care staff, on diagnoses, symptoms, and effective interventions that support the well-being of the client.

A function that needs to be the responsibility of all social workers is to educate the business community to an awareness of adult day services and the important roles it plays in the care of persons with dementia and their caregivers. Often employers are unaware of the high costs of caregiving. "Alzheimer's disease costs American businesses $33.16 billion a year . . . the figure is probably a low estimate as many factors cannot be measured . . . on average, a full time employed caregiver of a person with Alzheimer's is absent 12.66 days or partial days per year and is interrupted an average of 50 hours per year" (Koppel, 1998, pp. ii–iii). Social workers, whether within adult day centers or employee assistance programs, can use these compelling statistics to educate and encourage corporations to address caregiving issues and promote adult day services.

Another important aspect of education is the opportunity to provide supervised fieldwork experiences for social work students. As the need for community-based long-term care services expands, increasing numbers of social workers will be required. Ensuring that students have a meaningful and valuable placement in adult day settings is critical for the future development of competent and caring practitioners.

Social Worker as Broker

John B., a 78-year-old accountant diagnosed with midstage dementia, had begun attending a local day center 3 days per week. His spouse of more than 50 years, Marge, had never written a check and was extremely frightened when the utility companies threatened to disconnect services. The social worker at the day program was able not only to negotiate with the various utilities to forestall collections but also to set up an appointment with a bank trust officer to assist Marge on an ongoing basis.

People all too often do not know what services are available in the community or how to access them. The traditional social work role as broker links individual or groups who need help with services to support them. This process involves assessing need and interests, providing information about what services are available, and linking with supportive organizations. Within the realm of the broker role, the social worker may also provide case management that develops a care plan, assist clients with navigating institutional processes, evaluate outcomes in terms of client satisfaction, monitor progress, and review the care plan.

The Dementia Care and Respite Services Program showed that adult day centers could serve people with dementia and be the locus of care by arranging or providing other needed respite and personal care services (Robert Wood Johnson Foundation, 2000). The adult day services center becomes a "one-stop shop" where clients and families can have coordination of what often is fragmentation of services by a practitioner with whom they have built a relationship.

Social Worker as Counselor

Earline was a 58-year-old housewife recently diagnosed with early-stage Alzheimer's disease. While her family was concerned about her ability to stay home alone, they were resistant to talk collectively about the diagnosis and to seek any outside assistance. The social worker who facilitated a local "Memory Club" program 2 days a week was able to help both Earline and her family better understand Alzheimer's disease and the therapeutic value of the structured, person-centered socialization that the day program offered.

A core skill for working with persons with dementia is that of empathy—skills that very few people have developed highly, including those who regard themselves as carers (Loveday, Bowe, & Kitwood, 1998, pp. 23–24). "Good care requires a very highly developed person: one who is open, flexible, creative, compassionate, responsive, inwardly at ease" (Kitwood, 1997, p. 120). These characteristics become even more critical when counseling persons with dementia. At this juncture, training that is specific to working with people with dementia is evolving but still not ideal. Students "may have been given little more than a simplistic induction in the medical model, which offers very little help with the practice of care" (Kitwood, 1997, p. 112; Loveday et al. p. 16).

A carryover from the medical model is the focus on the professional role with the expectation of suppressing the p315ersonal self—personal feelings and reactions (Shulman, 1984, p. 14). Yet the literature indicates that those individuals most effective in working with people with dementia are those who are emotionally available (Kitwood, 1997, p. 5). Additionally, it has been noted that "we are at our best in work when we are able to synthesize the two—that is, integrate our personal self into our professional role" (Shulman, 1984, p. 14).

People in early stages of dementia may need support in coming to terms with the diagnosis; dealing with grief and loss issues, depression, and anger; redefining roles; and financial and legal planning. As the disease progresses and the individual loses verbal skills, rational thought, orientation, and reasoning abilities, the social work role as counselor relies more on being psychologically available. This calls on active listening skills and a stronger reliance on nonverbal communication. It requires the practitioner to develop a genuine relationship with the client. For persons in later stages of dementia, this calls for the practitioner to "be present with and for another person without distraction from outside or disturbance from within; perceiving the other with far less of the distortions, projections and judgmental reactions that so often get in the way of real meeting" (Kitwood, 1997, p. 119).

The setting of adult day services is often structured programmatically to enhance the ability of workers to develop genuine relationships with participants. There is usually flexibility within structure to adapt quickly to the needs of participants. As the average length of time a participant is enrolled in adult day services is 2 years (Adult Day Services Program, 2001–2002), long-term relationships evolve, and consequently the social worker is able to engage in both extensive and intensive counseling, often with both the individual and the family.

Social work practitioners within adult day services are in a strategic position within the continuum of care to facilitate support groups of many types. Persons with dementia are often overlooked as being good candidates for support groups. Yet early-stage support groups have been found to have positive outcomes for participants (Jones, Cheston, & Gilliard, 2002). Additionally, the National Institutes of Health report results of a study conducted at New York University that show short-term intensive counseling in combination with readily available support can significantly reduce the long-term risk of depression among spouses caring for a husband or wife with Alzheimer's disease (Mittelman, 2004, pp. 850–856). The positive impact of these interventions was also found to have continued more than 3 years postcounseling (Mittelman, 2004, pp. 850–856).

Counseling with family caregivers is multifaceted. Support is merely one dimension of the social work counseling role. A survey conducted by the MetLife Foundation found that Alzheimer's disease is the second most feared illness in America (20%) behind cancer (38%). However, adults aged 55 and older fear getting Alzheimer's disease even more than cancer (Harris Interactive Inc., 2006). The survey found that while most of those surveyed were aware of the disease (93%), 74% said they knew only a little or nothing about the disease. From a financial standpoint, 8 out of 10 Americans think it is important to plan for the possibility of getting Alzheimer's disease, yet 9 out of 10 have taken no steps to create a safety net for themselves or their family (Harris Interactive Inc., 2006). This lack of preparedness highlights the need for social workers to step forward with new counseling interventions.

Social Worker as Advocate

Mario was an 82-year-old day center participant who relied on the local paratransit system to transport him to and from the facility. Because of his dementia diagnosis, Mario often became confused and agitated on his rides and at one point while the vehicle was in motion attempted to unbuckle his seat belt and exit. When the transportation provider threatened to discontinue their service, the center's social worker was able to advocate on Mario's behalf assigning a volunteer "buddy" to escort him on each trip. In addition, the social worker was able to advocate on a macrolevel for the creation of a volunteer program to assist others with similar situations.

Advocacy is something one person does in support of another. It is about the following:

- Safeguarding people who are in situations where they are vulnerable
- Speaking up for or standing alongside people who are not being heard
- Enabling people to make informed choices about and remain in control of their own social and health care (Glasgow City Council, 2004)

This definition of advocacy seems specifically designed to reflect work with persons with dementia. As the disease progresses and the individual markedly loses skills and rational thought, the person becomes increasingly vulnerable in society. Well-meaning carers step forward to take over the care (and life) of the affected person "for their own good." What is lost sight of is "the person," who is much more than a collection of symptoms and who still has hopes and desires, can still experience fear, sadness, joy, and contentment and still has the essence of being human. As such, the social worker has an obligation to advocate for the individual to still be in control as much as possible, to make informed choices that they can still make with appropriate support.

Within adult day services, this advocacy takes place on both the micro- and the macrolevel. Principles of person-centered dementia care as developed by Kitwood (1997) and the Bradford Dementia Group provide supporting tenets for advocating for the affected person to still be involved in their care planning and to still guide their life course. This process may require persistence in advocacy efforts both with other staff and with family caregivers.

The medical model of care suggests that "others" know what is in the best interest of the person. Person-centered care suggests that "the person" is the authority on his or her own life. It is the responsibility of the carers to support and facilitate this process, even until late stages, through skillful interventions. This approach often meets resistance from seasoned carers and uninformed family members. However, a body of evidence is growing to suggest that with good psychosocial care, persons with dementia can experience relative states of well-being and have their personhood remain intact until death (Bradford Dementia Group, 1997, p. 1; Kitwood, 1997, p. 1).

As previously noted, adult day services generally care for individuals an average of 2 years. This enables practitioners to have the time to establish trusting relationships with participants and families. These relationships in turn should assist in ascertaining the desires of the affected person and advocating on their behalf.

Social workers are change agents, and their goal "is to bring about positive changes, either directly in the client's functioning or in environmental factors immediately impinging upon the client's functioning" (Fischer,

1978, p. 12). The psychosocial environment of care for persons with dementia is increasingly identified as critical to their state of well-being. "A person's state of being is affected by other factors ... such as personality, life history, physical health and—perhaps the most crucial of all—the nature of the social psychology with which he or she is surrounded" (Loveday et al., 1998, p. 10).

With regard to the physical environment, the social worker in the adult day setting should also advocate for changes in the center's design to support people with dementia. As Diaz Moore (2005) asserts in his *Design Guidelines for Adult Day Services,* "From a design perspective, adult day service facilities should promote if not maximize the therapeutic intentions of the adult day services program" (p. 82).

The social work advocate role is directed toward changing systems, influencing policy changes or changes within communities. Societal response to dementia care is evolving. This evolution translates to change with ample opportunities for social work practitioners to advocate with and for persons with dementia.

An example of effective macrolevel advocacy that resulted in policy change is that of the Medicare interpretation of rehabilitative services for persons with dementia. In the past, physical and occupational therapy was rarely a service authorized by insurance to be covered for persons with dementia. As of September 2001, the Medicare regulations state,

> Throughout the course of their disease, patients with dementia may benefit from pharmacologic, physical, occupational, speech-language, and other therapies.
>
> Contractors may not use ICD-9 codes for dementia alone as a basis for determining whether a Medicare covered benefit is reasonable and necessary because these codes do not define the extent of a beneficiary's cognitive impairment. For example, a claim submitted with only a diagnosis of Alzheimer's Disease (ICD-9 code 331.0) may entitle a beneficiary to evaluation and management visits and therapies if the contractor determines that these therapies are reasonable and necessary when reviewed in the context of a beneficiary's overall medical condition. (Centers for Medicare & Medicaid Services, 2001)

This change in approach to care at a federal level is the result of persistent advocacy efforts.

There is ample opportunity for social work practitioners within adult day services to join the advocacy efforts for persons with dementia. Chapter 5 provides an overview of several national advocacy groups that partner with persons with dementia to address advocacy issues.

Social Worker as Researcher

Gladys L., a social worker for a local adult day program, has facilitated their monthly support group for nearly 5 years. It wasn't until the MSW field placement student she was supervising tabulated the results of annual assessments and satisfaction surveys that she was able to document the significant and positive impact of her interventions. Her organization was then able to use this information as part of a successful United Way grant proposal to further support their work.

The paucity of research available from the field of adult day services suggests that there is a critical need for social workers to engage in research in day care settings. "There is little evaluation evidence available on which to base opinions of the effectiveness of service . . . most research on day services is small scale and/or relies on secondary sources" (Clark, 2001, pp. 31–32). Compounding the issue for participants with dementia is the fact that measuring their well-being and satisfaction is not straightforward. The "cognitive impairments experienced as a result of the dementia make interpretation of emotions, appraisal of satisfaction with life, and recall of experiences over time, increasingly difficult" (Loveday et al., 1998). The scarcity of baseline data impedes the ability to measure efficacy of interventions at all levels: the individual, the specific adult day services center, and adult day services collectively.

Practitioners may believe that the formal process of research is too daunting to tackle, especially if the social worker is the sole practitioner within the adult day services program. However, in the normal reporting cycles of most adult day services centers, various data are already collected. The previous vignette is an example. Satisfaction surveys are often a standard process within centers. These results may be used to formulate changes in programming or the structure or breadth of services offered or to improve processes. In effect, this is a simple research process already in place that can have a major impact on service development.

Thoughtful consideration should be given to outcomes measurement and/or research related to the effectiveness of interventions with persons with dementia within adult day services. There are constructs such as dementia care mapping (DCM) that may be useful tools in this process. Dementia care mapping consists of a set of observational tools that have been used in formal dementia care settings for developing person–center care practice and as a tool for research. In DCM, the level of relative well-being or ill-being that individual participants experience is assessed through direct observation (Loveday et al., 1998, p. 35). Quality-of-life surveys are available, both self-report and proxy report, to ascertain satisfaction with life. Using results of these types of surveys and observational methods can influence the evolution of practice standards.

Adult day services also need formal research projects to establish baseline measurements, test hypotheses, and ascertain the efficacy of methodologies within these nontraditional settings. It is only with the results of these types of efforts that the role of social work in adult day services can hope to expand and thrive. Additionally, the contributions this body of knowledge can contribute to upholding the quality of life for persons with dementia may be immeasurable.

CONCLUSION: WHERE DO WE GO FROM HERE?

The role of social work in adult day services is not clearly defined. Adult day services is widely considered a nontraditional setting for social work practice. This requires social work practitioners within the setting to possess the abilities to be self-directed, identify with the profession of social work, articulate the contribution of social work practice within the setting, and assist in defining and evolving the roles of the social worker. Fulfillment of one role often overlaps with other roles, as illustrated in the vignettes throughout this chapter. Advocacy often contains elements of education, counseling may involve education and advocacy, and brokering may require education and advocacy. Interventions with issues of suspected abuse and neglect call on all roles. As the professional training related to dementia care is still often minimal, the social worker needs to seek information to build a strong knowledge base of current and best practices for care with and for persons with dementia.

The Dementia Care and Respite Services Program showed definitively that adult day centers could serve people with dementia and be the locus of care by arranging for or providing other needed respite and personal care services (Robert Wood Johnson Foundation, 2000). Given the many opportunities and challenges faced by persons with dementia and their caregivers, social workers can play a definite social work role throughout this journey, be it as an educator, a broker, a counselor, an advocate, or a researcher. However, despite the need for social work within adult day centers serving persons with dementia, many issues remain that can limit their involvement.

Unfortunately, many trained social work professionals are unaware of the important role that adult day centers play in the long-term care continuum for persons with dementia. Schools of social work do not consistently include education about adult day services in their curriculum or offer field placement opportunities at local facilities. Those social workers employed within settings other than adult day centers do not consistently make appropriate referrals to day services for their clients.

Meanwhile, the American system of care for persons with dementia remains significantly out of balance, with a much greater proportion of resources supporting institutional alternatives as opposed to home and community-based care. "Overall, spending for community-based long term care services ... are now almost one-third of all Medicaid long term care costs. Reported community-based services expenditures were 33% of long-term care spending in FY 2003, with 67% spent on institutional services" (Burwell, Sredl, & Eiken, 2004).

Few state licensing or certification processes for adult day centers require social work involvement within these programs, and even fewer require that the person performing the social work role have an actual professional degree in social work. Additionally, as was mentioned previously, the social worker within adult day services is most often a "department of one," and few formal professional networking opportunities exist.

Finally, there is little if any research documenting positive outcomes for persons with dementia and/or their caregivers resulting from social work–related interventions within the adult day services arena. Most research on day services is small scale and/or relies on secondary sources (Clark, 2001). Clearly, there is much work yet to be done.

On the other hand, victories are being won at the local, state, and federal levels in the policy arena. The tide is shifting to promote more home and community-based alternatives such as adult day services. "This distribution continues to change by one to three percentage points each year, as Medicaid programs continue to invest more resources in alternatives to institutional services" (Burwell et al., 2004). For the first time in its history, the Medicare program is exploring funding for adult day centers (Medicare Prescription Drug, Improvement, and Modernization Act of 2003).

Additionally, an ever-increasing number of social work students are seeking specialized training in dementia care and/or gerontological social work. For example, the John A. Hartford Foundation provides funding to infuse the study of gerontology into the curricula of social work schools throughout the United States. Even the inclusion of the present chapter in this book can be seen as a positive and significant stride forward. As a result, the social work profession's knowledge and awareness of adult day centers continues to grow, forming a basis for increased involvement.

Perhaps most important, however, each and every day literally thousands of lives of persons with dementia and their caregivers (who are past, present, or future users of adult day services) are touched by dedicated, caring, and knowledgeable social work professionals. These interventions continue to have a profound and often life-changing impact.

REFERENCES

Adult Day Services Program, PMD Advisory Services LLC, & Seniors Research Group (Comps.). (2001–2002). *National Study of Adult Day Services: Adult Day Center Survey.* Available at http://www.rwjf.org/newsroom/featureDetail.jsp?featureID=183&type=3&pageNum=3&gsa=1

Beaver, M. L., & Miller, D. (1985). *Clinical social work practice with the elderly: Primary, secondary, and tertiary intervention.* Homewood, IL: Dorsey Press.

Bosky, B. (2003). *Morning Out Club: A program of the Alzheimer's Association of San Diego serving individuals with mild memory loss and their families.* San Diego, CA: Alzheimer's Association.

Bradford Dementia Group. (1997). *Evaluating dementia care the DCM method* (3rd ed.). Bradford, UK: Bradford Dementia Group, University of Bradford.

Burwell, B., Sredl, K., & Eiken, S. (2004, May 25). *Medicaid long term care expenditures in FY 2003.* Available at http://www.hcbs.org/files/35/1720/2003LTCExpenditures.doc

Centers for Medicare and Medicaid Services. (2001). *Medical review of services for patients with dementia* (Program Memorandum AB 01-135). Baltimore, MD.

Clark, C. (2001). *Adult day services and social inclusion: Better days.* Philadelphia: Jessica Kingsley.

Diaz Moore, K. (2005). *Design guidelines for adult day services.* Available at http://www.aia.org/SiteObjects/files/Diaz_Moore_color.pdf

Dziegielewski, S. F., & Ricks, J. L. (2000). Adult day programs for elderly who are mentally impaired and the measurement of caregiver satisfaction. *Activities, Adaptation, and Aging, 24,* 51–64.

Fazio, S., Seman, D., & Stansell, J. (1999). *Rethinking Alzheimer's care.* Baltimore: Health Professions Press.

Fischer, J. (1978). *Effective casework practice.* New York: McGraw-Hill.

Gaugler, J. E., Jarrott, S. E., Zarit, S. H., Parris Stephens, M. A., Townsend, A., Greene, R. (2003). Respite for dementia caregivers: The effects of adult day services use on caregiving hours and care demands. *International Psychogeriatrics, 15,* 37–58.

Glasgow City Council. (2004). *Advocacy.* Available at http://www.glasgow.gov.uk/en/YourCouncil/CustomerInvolvement/ServiceDepartments/SocialWork/Advocacy.htm

Harris Interactive Inc. (2006, May 11). *MetLife Foundation Alzheimer's survey: What America thinks.* Available at http://www.metlife.com/WPSAssets/20538296421147208330V1FAlzheimersSurvey.pdf

Hoffman, S. B., & Kaplan, M. (1996). *Special care programs for people with dementia.* Baltimore: Health Professions Press.

Johnson, J., Sakaris, J., Tripp, D., Vroman, K., & Wood, S. (2004). The role of social work in adult day services. *Journal of Social Work in Long-Term Care, 3,* 3.

Jones, K., Cheston, R., & Gilliard, J. (2002). *Group psychotherapy for people with dementia: Development, facilitation and evaluation of psychotherapeutic support groups.* Available at http://www.dementia-voice.org.uk/Projects/psychotherapyreport.pdf

Kinsella, K., & Velkoff, V. A. (2001). *An aging world: 2001.* Washington, DC: Superintendent of Documents. U.S. Census Bureau, Series P95/01-1, U.S. Goverment Printing Office.

Kitwood, T. (1997). *Dementia reconsidered: The person comes first.* Philadelphia: Open University Press.

Koppel, R. (1998). *Alzheimer's cost to U.S. business.* Alzheimer's Association. Washington, DC.

Loveday, B., Bowe, B., & Kitwood, T. (1998). *Improving dementia care: A resource for training and professional development.* London: Hawker Publications.

Mace, N. L., & Rabins, P. V. (1984). *A survey of day care for the demented adult in the United States.* Washington, DC: National Council on the Aging.

Medicare Prescription Drug, Improvement, and Modernization Act of 2003. Public Law No. 108–173, S 1860D-42, 703.

Mittelman, M. S. (2004). Sustained benefit of supportive intervention for depressive symptoms in caregivers of patients with Alzheimer's disease. *American Journal of Psychiatry, 161,* 850–856.

National Alliance for Caregiving & AARP. (2004, April). *Caregiving in the U.S.* Available at http://www.caregiving.org/pubs/data/04finalreport.pdf

Robert Wood Johnson Foundation. (2000, September). *Partners in caregiving: The Dementia Services Program grant results.* Available at http://www.rwjf.org/portfolios/resources/grantsreport.jsp?filename=partnerse.htm&iaid=142#int_grantinfo

Shulman, L. (1984). *The skills of helping: Individuals and groups.* Itasca, IL: F. E. Peacock.

Siebenaler, K., O'Keeffe, J., O'Keefe, C., Brown, D., & Koetse, B. (2005, August 26). *Regulatory review of adult day services: Final report.* Available at http://aspe.hhs.gov/daltcp/reports/adultday.htm

Smyth-Henry, R., Cox, N. J., Reifler, B. V., & Asbury, C. (2001). Adult day centers. In S. L. Isaacs & J. R. Knickman (Eds.), *To improve health and health care 2000.* San Francisco: Jossey-Bass. Available at http://www.rwjf.org/files/publications/books/2000/index.html?gsa= 1

Zarit, S. H., Femia, E. E., Watson, J., Rice-Oeschger, L., & Kakos, B. (2004). Memory Club: A group intervention for people with early-stage dementia and their care partners. *The Gerontologist, 44,* 262–269.

CHAPTER SEVENTEEN

Support Groups: Meeting the Needs of Families Caring for Persons With Alzheimer's Disease

Edna L. Ballard

In the middle of the night while most of America sleeps, they are awake—wives and daughters, husbands and sons—doing things they never imagined they would have to do. A woman in her seventies struggles out of bed to change her husband's diaper for the third time.

A husband in his eighties dresses his wife, who has been wandering around the house for hours, and walks her to the car—driving seems to be the only thing that will calm her down. Daughters and sons sit by the bedsides of their elderly parents and talk to them, holding their hands or gently brushing their hair. For a fortunate few, parents still know and call them by name.

Bradford (1999, p. 21)

INTRODUCTION

Simple, ordinary tasks, such as taking a bath, driving a car, or holding an intimate conversation with family and friends, become increasingly difficult for persons with Alzheimer's disease. Insidious and subtle in its presentation, individuals may look healthy and have periods of such clarity in the early stages that family and friends wonder if indeed anything is wrong. This can create confusion, frustration, and even anger in family members who may decide the person is being manipulative or "just

321

not trying hard enough." Changes in personality, unexplainable new behaviors, unreasonable demands, and losses in cognitive function and abilities that may have previously defined the person become reasons for caregiver concern. This is a progressive illness where the person eventually becomes dependent for his or her most basic needs.

Described as "a journey behind closed doors," many caregivers feel isolated and alone in what they often believe is a journey unique to them as they struggle most with the behavioral symptoms of the disease— that is, managing eating problems, incontinence, aggressive behaviors, apathy, coping with cursing or taking things that belong to others, and helping the person with personal care tasks, such as bathing, dressing, and dental hygiene—all of which can make for prolonged physical and emotional distress. Often referred to as "caregiver burden," it is defined by George and Gwyther (1986) as "the physical, psychological or emotional, social, and financial problems that can be experienced by families caring for impaired older adults" (p. 253).

As Gwyther (1996) writes, "This is no ordinary illness—and the patient won't respond to ordinary measures. Confronting, ignoring, rationally explaining, arguing, and reminding the person of old promises won't work" (p. 251). Caregiving is very hard, complex work that includes both an instrumental and an emotional dimension (MacRae, 1998). It often involves caring for someone (in the sense of servicing their needs) and caring about someone (in the sense of feeling affection about them). Thus, some behaviors that require little in the way of physical effort or attention, such as repeatedly asking to go home when the person is already at home or asking "what time is it?" every 5 or 10 minutes, become extremely stressful.

Feelings of depression, fear, frustration, and anger are common in both the patient and the caregiver with the realization that this is an illness that will continue to get worse. Without education about the disease and its behavioral symptoms, tips on care management, and social and emotional support, the caregiver is at risk of becoming "the hidden patient." One unfortunate consequence is that caregivers may adapt negative coping strategies, including, for example, the following behaviors:

- Denial—choosing to believe that other reasons (e.g., retirement, recent illness, depression, or normal aging) account for changes in the individual
- Insisting that the person "try harder," that is, insisting the spouse or parent maintain the checkbook when he or she is no longer able and then becoming angry or resentful when the person fails
- Doctor shopping, hoping for an acceptable diagnosis

Caregivers who are successful are able to distinguish between behaviors brought on by the disease and those choices of the patient that appear to deliberately annoy or manipulate the caregiver. Most caregivers need help in assessing the situation and responding appropriately.

THE ROLE OF SUPPORT GROUPS IN HELPING CAREGIVERS

Much of the support in attending group sessions has to do with learning to accept and manage situations that are fixed in their progression. These are situations that no matter how hard the caregiver tries, the core pathology and progression of the disease cannot be changed in any permanent way. What can be changed and what is exceedingly crucial to patient and caregiver is (a) enabling the patient to function at his or her highest level whatever the disease status and (b) ensuring that caregivers provide that support while also caring for self. In support groups, these lessons most often come from others who have been through the typical stages of caregiving and are willing to share lessons learned along the way.

"Self-help and support groups have become an integral part of mainstream culture.... Such groups are available for almost any situation or concern and are accessible to a growing number of people in the United States and around the world" (Kurtz, 2004, p. 139). Even families who are reluctant to attend in the beginning report that support groups become an important resource in their ability to care for their family member and their ability to cope emotionally. As discussed by a participant, "Early on, I attended several Alzheimer's support groups. I soon learned that sharing experiences was much more valuable than having someone simply tell me how to cope with a particular problem" (quoted in Castle, 2001, p. 82).

Most families do not have the ability to evaluate the quality or effectiveness of resources accessible to them in caring for their family member. They may need specific guidelines on choosing and evaluating a program or resource best suited to the family's need or preference. This is not always an easy task. It is time consuming and difficult to put together an appropriate mix of services. Many support groups address the problem of fragmented community services by searching out resources and compiling lists or directories that may also contain contact persons or resources not found in the formal network, such as an individual respite worker, sitter, or a church program offering limited short-term respite or emergency financial help.

SUPPORT GROUPS HELP NORMALIZE
THE CAREGIVING EXPERIENCE

Support groups, perhaps more than any other venue, normalize patient and family reactions to the disease. Caregivers report finding help in managing feelings like anger, resentment, fear, and other debilitating emotions. "The understanding, practical experience, and unconditional availability of individuals who share a common problem . . . provide new opportunities to learn practical coping skills, and redefine oneself through involvement with others" (Gwyther, in Ballard & Poer, 1999, Preface, para 1). Families learn they are not alone, that the most bizarre behaviors or incidents may be normal expressions of this disease.

Caregivers also learn from support group facilitators and other participants that caregiving approaches that may seem strange are acceptable: "The caregiver who lets her mom get in the tub with her clothes on because for reasons of propriety, she refuses to let the daughter undress her; the caregiver who supports the person's use of eating with his hands by preparing finger foods, or the caregiver who lets the patient sleep with a doll for comfort and security all benefit and feel more confident in their choices when supported by professionals who work with them" (Ballard, Gwyther, & Toal, 2000, p. 21).

The cost of caregiving is high: chronic fatigue, depression, family conflict, decreased personal time, anger, fear, and other negative emotions. (See Figure 17.1 for a list of common caregiving stressors.) Yet most caregivers elect to care for their family member in the community. Many experience rewards and even pleasure in giving care. "In sickness and in health. . . . It is a covenant we make not only with spouses, but with parents, children, siblings, and perhaps even friends and neighbors" (Giorgianni, 1997, p. 4). The commitment is strong. Providing encouragement and support may prolong the ability of these caregivers to continue, particularly where caregiving tasks are unrelenting, exhaustive, and a constant reminder of the care receiver's growing dependence.

The support group ideally becomes a place where it is safe to share difficult feelings such as anger, fatigue, regret, and frustration without shame or guilt; where it is safe to express disappointment in professionals, providers, and family who do not live up to expectations or standards; where you do not feel like a failure when things do not go well for the patient; and, most important, where participants share areas of growth—whether it's the mastering of a new caregiving technique or learning to control emotional responses in a more constructive way" (Ballard & Poer, 1999, Preface, para 1). Caregivers learn that there are *no saints, no superwomen or men, no perfect answers to every problem*. This is significant because many caregivers report doubts and recriminations about much of what they do for their care-dependent family member. Moreover, despite the known

Examples of Caregiving Stressors

- Difficult, unpleasant caregiving tasks: incontinence, brushing the person's teeth, giving instructions repeatedly, etc.

- Little or no appreciation for efforts: "What are the reciprocity rules? She was never there for me."

- Insufficient emotional or concrete support: "Even in the beginning state when I was so enraged and resentful, feeling all alone, not knowing what to do next, I still knew there were logical, humane, and intelligent solutions to every problem I faced with Hughes. But I had to get beyond my rage and self-pity before I could see them" (Shanks, 1996).

- Family conflict or questioning the diagnosis, what and how care should be given: "I just didn't see the problems my sister complained about. I thought she was exaggerating."

- Ineffective caregiving or coping skills: arguing, scolding, becoming impatient—"I wish someone had told me. I was always yelling at him, trying to get him to do it right."

- Feeling captive to an old promise: "Promise me you will never put me in a nursing home."

Source: Excerpted from Ballard, Gwyther, and Toal (2000, pp. 10–12). Used with permission.

FIGURE 17.1   Examples of caregiving stressors that may compromise caregivers' effectiveness.

risk factors for prolonged caregiving, caregivers are often reluctant to seek or accept help that could ease some of the crises they face:

> Many caregivers, regardless of place of residence, income, ethnic background, or education may be reluctant to seek help for a relative with Alzheimer's disease. The reasons are legions and may be as different as the caregivers themselves. There is the caregiver who feels the need to protect her husband's "image" in the community, the husband who refuses to believe that there is anything wrong with his wife—if she just tried harder, the mother who wants to protect her children from what's happening to their dad, the caregiver who has sought help before and has been disappointed at every turn, and so on. (Ballard, Cook, Gwyther, & Gold, 1996, p. 19)

THE MANY FACES OF ALZHEIMER'S SUPPORT GROUPS

There are many university support groups for families, generally associated with Alzheimer's Disease Centers or Alzheimer's Disease Research Centers. Duke University offers more than 50 university and community support groups, three of which are Alzheimer's specific and are discussed here.

The Durham Evening Support Group

One of the earliest support groups and a prototype for many that subsequently developed around the country, the Durham Evening Support Group had its beginnings in what was first a model for galvanizing community resources to support families of dementia-impaired individuals.

In 1955, the Duke University Center for the Study of Aging and Human Development (Center for Aging) was mandated by the university to develop multidisciplinary research and training that would eventuate in family-centered care of adults, including geriatric evaluation, treatment, education, and research (Gwyther, 1982). It became increasingly clear to clinicians that the majority of patients presented problems related to irreversible dementia. Family members—spouses, children, daughters-in-law, nieces, and occasionally friends and neighbors—began to meet and discuss with staff their need for current information on dementia and its management at home (Gwyther, 1982).

Interest quickly increased, and by 1980 almost 2,000 families had evolved into a network of mutual help. The Duke Family Support Program, the service arm of the Center for Aging, began helping local communities develop support groups that would be accessible and helped communities train facilitators to lead the groups.

The National Alzheimer's Association, first incorporated as the Alzheimer's Disease and Related Disorders Association in 1980, has had as one of the primary goals the development of support groups to assist families. It is an extremely effective national resource for family caregivers of persons with Alzheimer's and other dementias. The Durham Evening Support Group is part of a local chapter under the National Alzheimer's Association administrative umbrella. With minor exceptions, it is like many other support groups around the country.

The Durham Evening Support Group, one of the longest-running groups for Alzheimer's families, continues today. The meeting format generally has an "expert" speak on a topic relevant to caregiving techniques, coping with the caregiving role, or evaluating and using local resources. Typical support group topics include the following:

- How Your Ombudsman Can Help With Nursing Home Concerns
- How to Handle Anger, Grief and Other Difficult Feelings
- Activities: Things to Do When the Day Gets Too Long
- When Working Saves Your Sanity: Meeting Your Needs and Your Relative's Needs
- Advanced Directives: Health Care Power of Attorney and Living Wills

There are also "sharing" or open discussion meetings where there is no set topic. This seems to be especially helpful after an extended break, such as following a holiday when caregivers have more issues or crises to discuss. It is a free open monthly meeting for family and friends of persons with Alzheimer's. By request of family members who wish to be free to talk about any topic, some of which may be upsetting to the person with Alzheimer's, it is not open to persons with the disease.

The group is facilitated by two social workers. All groups aim to provide a safe, secure environment where individuals respect differences and the rules of confidentiality. In sharing, individuals give and receive help in the form of information, new skills, and strategies to try. An important benefit for participants is that occasionally they have the opportunity to examine attitudes and behaviors that have both negative and positive effects on caregiving.

Contrary to what is often reported, we have had periods over the years where there were more male participants than female. We surmise that the university setting may be a factor.

The Daughters and Daughters-in-Law Support Group

This group began as a forum addressing general concerns of women—daughters and daughters-in-law—of aging parents. Although it is free and open to the community, it consists primarily of university faculty and staff. Typical questions include the following:

- What are the signs that a parent needs assistance?
- How do I get my family to work together?
- How do I manage from a distance?
- How do I balance caregiving, work, and family responsibilities?

Most participants have an issue or concern that is dementia related. Facilitated by two social workers, this group meets monthly at noon in a comfortable hospital conference room. Parking and complexity in finding the meeting place are frequently noted as barriers for non–university persons driving in from the community.

Women participants vary widely in education and positions at the university. Participants may include a scientist who is struggling with being a long-distance caregiver or an executive in hospital administration feeling the pressure of work coupled with caring for young children and the needs of an aging parent. Notably absent are women from lower-status jobs (i.e., housekeeping, cafeteria workers, and so on) whose caregiving concerns are often complicated by fewer financial resources and less freedom or knowledge to effect help they need in the care of a dependent family member. One explanation for the lower participation of these women, as reported by the women themselves, is that they have less discretion for taking the time to come to a meeting that is not directly job related. This barrier may be reflected in the larger communities when caregivers have less discretionary time and/or resources.

The Duke Family Support Program offers free elder care consults for all university staff and faculty regarding elder care issues. This can be an office visit, telephone, or e-mail contact. This program appears to reach across all categories of staff and faculty. Telephone support offers special advantages for caregivers. Many of the Daughters and Daughters-in-Law Support Group participants also take advantage of the Employee Eldercare Consult, and most consults revolve around dementia care. The support group and the consult service are supported by the university, which recognizes elder care responsibility and its impact on employee on-the-job effectiveness.

The Cary and Ruth Henderson Patient and Caregiver Support Group

Diagnosed with Alzheimer's at the age of 55 in 1992, Cary Henderson, a history professor from Virginia, decided while visiting the Duke Memory Disorders Clinic that his time could be well spent if he could talk with others like himself who were also having memory problems. The clinic responded by helping to establish a support group for patients and their caregivers that continues to meet.

It is a monthly meeting, sometimes numbering as many as 40 caregivers and patients. The group meets for an hour and a half; the first 30 minutes, caregivers and patients meet together to share news bits. A few caregivers have patients who now reside in nursing homes. Several have spouses who are deceased. One person who is an original member of the group, beginning 14 years ago, continues to participate even though his wife has been in a nursing home for more than 5 years. Members say the group provides them with a sense of community, with help in making sense of the trauma of dealing with this disease, with a safe place to express anger and grief that other family and friends find uncomfortable, and with a forum for helping others as well as help dealing with their own grief and healing. Following are comments from caregivers on how the group serves them:

> "Where else can I say how I feel and have 'fellow travelers' understand?"

> "I had to learn new things, take control. It was a time of devastation, being overwhelmed. When I found the group it was like finding a foundation for a lost soul."

> "My friends didn't understand. If your voice breaks they don't want to hear it. At the group everybody understands and listens. You realize they've been there."

Facilitated by three social workers, one social worker remains with family caregivers to discuss issues pertinent to their concerns. The patient group is facilitated by two social workers both of whom are generally present for all meetings. The most successful format for the patients' meeting is letting each participant introduce him- or herself and talk about their past careers (work and/or military). Sharing the past seems to validate the individual and his or her contributions to family and community. These stories repeated at each meeting bring a sense of satisfaction to the storyteller and the listeners. Interest is enhanced in that several of the participants grew up together and have known each other for many years. Other things in common include military service, related work areas, and playing musical instruments. One individual whose dementia is getting progressively severe will occasionally agree to play his harmonica. He retains the ability to play a few renditions well and is always rewarded by the appreciation of everyone in the group.

Over the past year, the patient group has generally been all men with only one woman who, though quiet, appears to be at ease and enjoys the group activity. Most participants have a college education or more. The group composition changes as the patients' health status and needs change; they die or are placed in a long-term care facility, or the caregiver stops attending because of increased care tasks or related problems.

Meeting in a university community has an advantage for the support groups. The group facilitators have access to a rich source of Alzheimer's researchers and other professionals with Alzheimer's knowledge, including physicians, chaplains, social workers, and psychologists. Family members who participate in the support groups also offer their expertise. Some share their experience and subsequent knowledge of the disease at training seminars for medical students, community seminars and workshops, and the Annual Joseph and Kathleen Bryan Alzheimer's Conference, which began 20 years ago.

In addition, many have participated in producing written and audiovisual materials on Alzheimer's for lay and professional audiences. Cary Henderson, aware of quickly losing his cognitive capacity, wanted to record what it was like to have Alzheimer's from the patient's perspective. A widely circulated article, "Musings"; a book, *The Partial View* (Henderson, 1998); and a number of interviews for national media poignantly define the agonizing odyssey of Alzheimer's disease. He writes,

> With Alzheimer's people, there's no such thing as having a day which is like another day ... and you don't know what's going to happen in any one day or any other thing like that—it's as if every day you have never seen anything before like what you're seeing right now. It just never will be the same again. (Henderson, 1992, p. 6)

GUIDELINES FOR RUNNING SUCCESSFUL SUPPORT GROUPS

Once you have established the need for a support group in your community, whether it is a small, rural community with limited resources or an urban area with ease of access to materials and expertise, these guidelines increase the likelihood of success:

Have very clear goals about the purpose of your group. Focus on one problem or a limited number of related problems (i.e., a support group for men caregivers or support groups for adult children of aging parents).

Choose sponsorship by community organizations that are widely accepted. This lends credibility and legitimacy to your group.

Choose leaders who are committed and enthusiastic about the goals of the group. The will to succeed is a necessary ingredient in developing successful support groups.

Decide on the kind of group you wish to develop. Will it be a closed group with a limited number of persons, an open group where members come and go at will, or a time-limited group with a set number of sessions? The goal or purpose of your group will help determine the kind of group that will be most effective.

Be flexible about group size. Typically the most effective group is small in size (from 5 to 12 persons). However, many support groups are larger. When the group is too small, participants may feel pressure to share before they are ready; when the group is too large, the feeling of intimacy necessary for support may be lost. (There are exceptions. A local Alzheimer support group regularly had more than 40 participants. When asked to divide into two separate groups, they refused, explaining that they all knew and enjoyed each other and did not want to separate. One person commented that it was the skill of the facilitator that made the group exciting and relevant to their needs. The group meets once a month and has a potluck dinner after the meeting, the only social event for many of the caregivers.)

Logistics should meet the needs of participants. Meeting time, location, physical setting, and so on should all be considered in light of the participant's needs. Do most participants work during the day, necessitating a night meeting? Are potential participants older persons who are unable or unwilling to drive at night? Is there easy access to community transportation? Do people feel safe or comfortable coming to the meeting site? All are factors important in planning your meetings.

Meetings must be relevant and interesting. Some meetings are self-sustaining because the need is great; others require more attention to programming to maintain interest. Consider carefully the agenda for the year. Will you have formal speakers? Will part of the agenda be devoted to discussion and sharing among participants? What are the skills of the facilitators in maintaining positive, helpful interactions among members? Are special needs of the participants factored in the decisions: education, cultural beliefs, or traditions? One person writes,

Some members of the community tried to organize a caregiver's support group without success. . . . This community is primarily a rural farming and lumber area. The older generation, raised during the 30s—days of the depression and even up to World War II—had to work in the fields and could not afford to go to school. . . . They can not use written materials that can help, and they don't want anyone to know that they are unable to read or write. I hope to start discussion meetings using speakers, videos, and tapes on Alzheimer's disease. It is my hope that this will allow us to have a caregiver's support group much closer home.

You'd be amazed even at eighty plus years of age what [we] can accomplish!

—An older resident in a rural Florida community

(There is an increasing availability of materials for low-literacy individuals, such as "Understanding Alzheimer's Disease" [U.S. Department of Health and Human Services, 2006a] and "Understanding Memory Loss" [U.S. Department of Health and Human Services, 2006b]).

Canvass participants for suggestions about topics they would like information or education on. Be sensitive to the fact that some caregivers learn better by hearing presenters—some by viewing video programs, others by exchanging ideas and experiences with other caregivers. Support group topics tend to fall in the following areas:

- *Alzheimer's disease and dementia:* Diagnosis, types of dementia, progression of the illness, medications, research update, participation in research, and end-of-life issues.
- *Caregiving strategies:* Communication, behavior management, positive physical approach, helping with physical needs, nutrition issues, and organizing the day.
- *Systems of care:* Residential care (nursing facilities, assisted living) adult day programs, home care (home health, hospice, private duty), respite care, and hospitalization.
- *Legal/financial/insurance:* Advanced directives, financial and estate planning, social security/disability, Medicare/Medicaid, and long-term care insurance.
- *Coping strategies:* Caregiver stress; emotion (denial, grief, guilt, anger, depression); making decisions; "when others won't help;" asking for help; and developing positive coping strategies (Alzheimer's Association, Eastern North Carolina Chapter, 2005 [used with permission]).

REASONS CAREGIVERS DON'T PARTICIPATE IN TRADITIONAL SUPPORT GROUPS

Many reasons are given for not attending support groups. A surprising but powerful reason for many is that they do not recognize themselves as caregivers or resist the label. This is significant in its implication for reaching and assisting caregivers who might benefit from services, resources, and support. "Most families do not view their role as caregivers—they are wives, husbands, sons, and daughters, daughters-in-law—fulfilling their obligations of care out of loyalty, love, and commitment to the dependent person" (Ballard & Poer, 1999, para 2).

Two caregivers comment,

> I couldn't understand. I had given birth to three children. I had performed all the same functions for them that I had for my mother. I fed them, diapered them, bathed them, helped them to walk, and helped them to dress. In that case, my job title was "mother." Why then did I lose my relationship with my mother when I performed the same care for her? She is still my mother, I'm still her daughter, and I'm not a "caregiver." (Mrs. E. Ennis, *Don't Call me 'Caregiver,' I'm Her Daughter!* in Ballard & Poer, 1999, para 1)

> I am proud to be a caregiver, but it is something I do, not who I am. (Hill, 2004, p. 16)

Other reasons include the following:

- Caregiver views participating in a support group as betrayal to spouse.
- Caregiver feels uneasy sharing personal problems. "He would be so embarrassed . . . "
- Male caregiver views support groups as "something women do."
- Caregiver fears dreadful predictions regarding the progression of the disease.
- Caregiver cannot find a support group in his or her immediate area.
- Caregiver feels overwhelmed by caregiving responsibilities: "Where would I find the time?"
- Caregiver faces a lack of respite: no one else can stay with the care receiver.

THE GROWING DIVERSITY OF ALZHEIMER'S SUPPORT GROUPS

The support group is not a panacea for every caregiver. There are other options that offer varying albeit often unpredictable levels of support: friends, family, various sources of information (physicians, Web sites, journals, lay magazines, and Alzheimer's chapter newsletters), and resources and services, such as adult day care and adult day health programs that address specific caregiver and patient needs.

There are also barriers or restraints in choosing support groups: the need to fit the schedule, location, or agenda of a particular support group meeting. There may be time constraints for the caregiver who cannot predict the patient's behavioral or physical needs that require the caregiver to remain at home. Finding substitute care or supervision of the care receiver may be an issue. Salfi, Ploeg, and Black (2005), in a study exploring the use of the telephone to empower caregivers of dementia-impaired family members, write, "Each caregiving situation is unique, and the perceived level of burden experienced by each dementia caregiver varies. Each situation requires a unique combination of supports based on the individualized needs of the caregiver" (p. 716).

With increasing focus on caregiver well-being as a necessary component of patient care and our current knowledge of those characteristics and behaviors important for caregiver health, support groups continue to evolve to meet the focused needs of the participants, that is, male caregiver groups and groups specifically for children and adolescents, spouses, and adult children caregivers.

With early diagnosis and increased information about early stages of Alzheimer's, patients benefit from support group participation as well:

> An early-stage support group, for example, can help people with Alzheimer's disease understand, adjust and cope better with their illness. . . . They have the opportunity to share experiences with others facing similar challenges. Groups help offset the sense of isolation and stigma that often comes with this type of chronic illness. (Yale & Rochmes, 2005, p. 21)

TECHNOLOGY-BASED SUPPORT GROUPS

Perhaps the greatest change and value in support group participation results from the vast expanse and rapid access to information. "Technology-based groups, including groups on the Internet and over the telephone, provide useful resources for people who are unable to find local face-to-face groups for their condition or who are not able or willing to travel to the sites where they meet" (Kurtz, 2004, pp. 144–145). These groups will continue to grow in usefulness as the population of elders increase and the need for information in their care grows. Online groups offer the advantage of allowing the caregiver to connect with others from home.

For many individuals, this may be the only way to connect with others sharing a similar concern or problem. Examples of online groups include the following:

- Bulletin boards—Caregivers can discuss problems and receive feedback from their peers.
- Chat sessions—Caregivers can share information and stories in real time with others on the chat line.
- E-mail–based support and discussion group for family caregivers and health professionals.

Access to the Internet and online support groups represent a tremendous resource otherwise not available to some families. There are, however, some families who may have difficulty accessing or interpreting information or simply be overwhelmed by the vast amounts of information. "Nearly half of all American adults—90 million people—have difficulty understanding and using health information" (Institute of Medicine, 2004). Other research findings show that "literacy skills predict an individual's health status more strongly than age, income, employment status, education level, and racial or ethnic group" (Wilson, 2003, p. 875).

Consequently, many elders and their families will continue to need help in accessing services appropriate for their relative and themselves. Given the uneven availability of services, social workers and other professionals can help families identify, recommend, access, and evaluate relevant health, social, and financial programs.

CONCLUSION: THE CONTINUING NEED FOR SOCIAL WORK INVOLVEMENT

Over the long haul of caring for someone with Alzheimer's, individuals also need help accepting and coping with the unpredictable, unfamiliar, sometimes bizarre behaviors that can be more distressing than the cognitive symptoms or the need for nursing or personal care. A recent survey of 539 adult caregivers for the Alzheimer's Foundation of America (2006) found that almost half (45%) were more distressed from "the emotional toll" of seeing a family member ravaged by Alzheimer's. Social workers and other health professionals are a vital link for both practical and emotional support.

The primary caregiver may need support in making difficult decisions—especially when the care recipient and other family members object. Caregivers are easily mired in the everyday minutiae of caring for the person with Alzheimer's. Pragmatic suggestions on how to pace themselves, how to care for themselves as well as the patient, and how to consider long-term planning, including legal and financial planning for what may be an extended caregiving period, are critical to being successful in the caregiving role. Early judicious planning may make the difference in having sufficient resources to provide for long-term care (Ballard, 1989). Social workers can play roles in helping families develop these plans, ensuring that the plans are implemented.

ACKNOWLEDGMENTS

Supported by the Bryan ADRC's grant *P50 AG05128 from the National Institute on Aging.

REFERENCES

Alzheimer's Association, Eastern North Carolina Chapter. (2005, June). *Handbook for Alzheimer's support group facilitators.* Raleigh, NC: Author. Available at http://www.alznc.org

Alzheimer's Foundation of America. (2006, March). *I CAN: Investigating caregivers' attitudes and needs* (Survey conducted by Harris Interactive, Inc.). New York, N.Y.: Author.

Ballard, E. L. (1989). Support systems: Meeting the needs of patients and family caregivers coping with Alzheimer's disease. In M. C. Singleton & E. F. Branch (Eds.), *The geriatric patient: Common problems and approaches to rehabilitation management* (pp. 41–52). New York: Haworth.

Ballard, E. L., Cook, G. M., Gwyther, L. P., & Gold, D. (1996). *Alzheimer's disease: Reaching the reluctant and underserved patient: The physician's role.* Durham, NC: Duke University Medical Center.

Ballard, E. L., Gwyther, L. P, & Toal, T. P. (2000). *Pressure points: Alzheimer's and anger.* Durham, NC: Duke University Medical Center.

Ballard, E. L., & Poer, C. M. (1999). *Lessons learned: Shared experiences in coping: Participants of Duke University Alzheimer support groups.* Durham, NC: Duke University Medical Center.

Bradford, R. (1999, Winter). Miles to go. *Duke Medical Perspectives,* 21–29.

Castle, E. (2001). A couple's journey with Alzheimer's disease: The many faces of intimacy. *Generations, 25,* 81–86.

George, L., & Gwyther, L. (1986). Caregiver wellv-being: A multidimensional examination of family caregivers of demented adults. *The Gerontologist, 26,* 253–259.

Giorgianni, S. (1997). A profile of caregiving in America. *Pfizer Journal, 1*(3), 4.

Gwyther, L. P. (1982). Caring for caregivers: A statewide family support program mobilizes mutual help. *Center Reports on Advances in Research, 6,* 1–8.

Gwyther, L. P. (1996). Ask the Expert. *Journal of Practical Psychiatry and Behavioral Health,* 2(4), 251–255.

Henderson, C. S. (1992, Summer). Musings. *The Caregiver,* 6–11.

Henderson, C. (1998). *Partial view: An Alzheimer's journal.* Dallas: Southern Methodist University Press.

Hill, S. (2004, Fall). Zen Alzheimer's. *The Caregiver, 23*(2), 16–17.

Institute of Medicine. (2004, April 8). *Report: Health literacy: A prescription to end confusion* [Press release].

Kurtz, L. F. (2004). Support and self-help groups. In C. D. Garvin, L. M. Gutierrez & M. J. Galinsky (Eds.), *Handbook of social work with groups* (pp. 139–159). New York: Guilford.

MacRae, H. (1998). Managing feelings: Caregiving as emotional work. *Research on Aging, 20,* 137–160.

Salfi, J., Ploeg, J., & Black, M. E. (2005). Seeking to understand telephone support for dementia caregivers. *Western Journal of Nursing Research, 27,* 701–721.

Shanks, L. K. (1996). *Your name is Hughes Hannibal Shanks.* Lincoln: University of Nebraska Press.

U.S. Department of Health and Human Services. (2006a, March). *Understanding Alzheimer's disease* (NIH Publication No. 06-5441). Washington, DC: U.S. Government Printing Office. Available at http://www.nia.nih.gov/Alzheimers/Publications/UnderstandingAD/

U.S. Department of Health and Human Services. (2006b, March). *Understanding memory loss* (NIH Publication No. 06-5442). Washington, DC: U.S. Government Printing Office. Available at http://www.nia.nih.gov/Alzheimers/Publications/UnderstandingMemoryLoss/

Wilson, J. F. (2003). Current clinical issues: The crucial link between literacy and health. *Annals of Internal Medicine, 139,* 875–878.

Yale, R., & Rochmes, A. (2005, Fall). *The benefits of togetherness: Early-stage support groups.* careADvantage. New York: Alzheimer's Foundation of America.

CHAPTER EIGHTEEN

Respite

Rhonda J. V. Montgomery and Jeannine M. Rowe

INTRODUCTION

An estimated 5.8 to 7 million people provide care to a person aged 65 or older who needs assistance with everyday activities. Another 5 million people provide care for someone aged 50 or older with dementia. Eighty-nine percent of this care is provided informally within the family by relatives (Alzheimer's Association and the National Alliance for Caregiving, 2000).

According to a report published by the Agency for Healthcare Research and Policy, informal caregiving is the most prevalent source of care for the elderly receiving long-term care in the community, with two in five elderly care recipients receiving all care informally and two in three receiving some informal care (Spector, Fleishman, Pezzin, & Spillman, 2000). In 1994, there were 5.9 million informal caregivers or 23 million households providing care for the 3.6 million elderly in the community. The number of households that provide care is expected to rise to 39 million by 2007 (Family Caregiver Alliance, 2005).

Older adults prefer to receive care from family members because they are familiar with them and their assistance enables older adults to continue to reside in their own homes and communities. It is also generally believed by many people that family members know best how to provide care. The decision by family members to assume caregiving responsibilities often reflects the affection that the caregiver has for the care recipient, but it is also made in response to a sense of obligation by most caregivers. Therefore, caregiving entails more than meeting the physical needs of the elder, as it often involves managing feelings and maintaining relationships. The collision between caring about the elder and caring for the elder, or what Hooyman and Gonyea (1995a) call the fusion between love and labor, often intensifies the stress that is experienced by family caregivers.

Family caregiving is not only a concern for families; it is also a concern for policymakers. From a public policy perspective, family members as providers of care save public funds. There is a general belief that by keeping older adults in their homes and communities, we delay the need for publicly funded services. Not surprisingly, then, there has been extensive movement in public policy arena to support family members who care for relatives. The array of support services that have been created for family caregivers includes respite services, educational programs, support groups, counseling, and care management. Despite the range of services available to caregivers, respite care has historically been—and continues to be—the most widely requested and used service (Kagan, 2001) and the source most frequently prescribed by practitioners (Montgomery, 2005; Montgomery & Rowe, 2003).

The majority of support programs for family caregivers have been created and supported at the state and local levels. Consequently, the availability and composition of respite programs have been inconsistent across communities. The authorization in 2000 of National Family Caregiver Support Program (NFCSP) as Title IIIE to the Older Americans Act (Administration on Aging, 2000) was the first public policy that officially recognized the contributions and needs of family caregivers who care for older adults. The NFCSP provides resources for all states working in partnership with local area agencies on aging, faith- and community-based service providers, and tribal organizations to offer services that meet caregiver needs. While notable for its recognition of the needs of family caregivers, the NFCSP has not provided uniformity in structure or access to support services. This is due largely to the flexibility for implementation that the program allows the states and the limited amount of dollars that are associated with the program. In most states, however, a substantial portion of the Title IIIE monies has been directed toward respite services.

WHAT IS RESPITE?

The term *respite care* refers to a range of services designed to give caregivers a break from caregiving responsibilities (Gaugler, Jarrott, et al., 2003;

Montgomery & Kosloski, 1995; Sorensen, Pinquart, & Duberstein, 2002). The concept of respite care was developed in the United States as part of the early 1970s deinstitutionalization movement for developmentally disabled children and adults. The need for temporary relief from caregiving responsibilities created a demand for respite services as families assumed primary responsibility for the developmentally disabled. Recognition in the United States of a parallel need by family members who were caring for frail and disabled relatives did not emerge until the mid-1980s, when formal respite services were developed as demonstration projects (Montgomery, 1996; Montgomery & Kosloski, 1995).

Types of Respite

The word *respite* means a "break," and in the realm of elder care, the term is associated with informal help or formal support services that afford a caregiver a break from normal caregiving obligations. Although there is general consensus that respite means "time away from caregiving responsibilities," there are a wide range of services and programs that are considered respite services. These include informal help provided by family members or a volunteer, paid in-home services, adult day care services, and overnight stays in institutions. Respite services usually provide direct care for the care receiver, but the primary goal is to provide the caregiver time away from the caregiving responsibilities.

Informal respite refers to unpaid assistance with care that is typically performed by family members, relatives, friends, or volunteers. Formal respite refers to care that is provided by individuals who are paid for their services. The operative words here are *unpaid* and *paid*. While the majority of families rely on family and friends to assist in caring for the older relative, many families also seek the services from volunteers or from agencies where paid employees perform the needed services.

Formal respite services can be categorized by the location or setting in which the service is delivered and the level of care that is provided. *Out-of-home* services include nonresidential care delivered in group settings such as adult day care centers and care provided in residential facilities such as group homes, nursing homes, and, although rare, hospitals. *In-home* services include companion programs and personal care services offered in a recipient's home. Many respite programs offer multiple levels of assistance and may also offer services in multiple settings.

Out-of-Home Respite Services

Throughout the country, there are a small number of organizations that offer respite care through family cooperatives and adult foster homes and in nursing home settings. The most common form of out-of-home respite, however, is provided through adult day care centers (ADCs). Historically, ADCs were best able to serve clients who needed minimal assistance, and these centers often did not enroll elders who were incontinent or wandered (Montgomery, 1996). Today, however, ADC programs are viewed as a realistic way to provide respite to caregivers of individuals suffering from Alzheimer's disease or other forms of dementia (Dziegielewski & Ricks, 2000).

Adult day centers vary widely in their hours of operation and the types of services they provide. At one extreme there are programs that operate 8 to 10 hours per day for 5 days a week. These comprehensive programs are most often located in urban areas. At the other extreme, there are adult day programs that operate only 1 or 2 days a week for 3 to 4 hours. Between these extremes are ADC programs that are open for 5 to 6 hours a day. Some of these programs are restricted to 2 or 3 days a week, while others operate daily.

Just as there is variation among ADCs in their hours of operation, there is also great variation in the level of care that is provided within day centers. Broadly defined, ADCs provide services such as personal assistance, meals, social activities, and transportation with the goal of allowing families to relinquish care responsibilities for several hours during the day (Gaugler, Jarrott, et al., 2003). Many ADCs also perform a range of health-related services and some forms of skilled nursing care (Montgomery, 1996). Differences in the level of care are predicated largely on the type of model adopted within individual facilities.

Adult day care centers that follow the social model offer a range of social activities, such as games, arts and crafts, discussion groups, and some personal assistance and attention from staff. In addition, ADCs that operate using a *medical model* offer various health-related services. In many states, the costs of care provided by ADCs that employ a medical model are covered by Medicaid as part of Medicaid waiver program for home and community-based services.

In-Home Respite Services

In-home respite services include companion programs, homemaker services, and personal care services delivered in the care recipient's home. These are the services that are most frequently requested and used. Most often, in-home respite services are offered through agencies that provide home health or homemaker services, but they are sometimes offered as part of senior companion programs funded through the Older Americans Act. Like ADC programs, in-home programs vary widely in terms of the levels of care and the amount and duration of service available. Some programs limit their services to short periods of 2 to 4 hours, while others only provide in-home respite for periods of 24 hours or more. To a large degree, the availability of services is linked to payment sources. Private pay clients can usually obtain services in any quantity; the hours of services available through publicly funded programs, however, are often capped in terms of the number of hours per day or number of hours per month. Some programs offer emergency respite services, but most programs require advanced notice (Montgomery, Marquis, Schaefer, & Kosloski, 2002).

Comprehensives Respite Care Models

Comprehensive respite programs offer multiple levels of care in multiple settings for a variety of time periods. Programs of this type are often better able to meet the needs of a wider range of clients as well as provide the flexibility necessary to adapt to changing needs of clients (Montgomery et al., 2002).

THE BENEFITS OF RESPITE CARE

An underlying assumption about respite services is that by providing caregivers with a temporary break from care responsibilities, they will also reduce the stress associated with caregiving and, thereby, enable caregivers to continue in the caregiving role longer. In short, policymakers and service providers believe that respite care can prevent or delay of nursing home placement (Gaugler, Kane, Kane, Clay, & Newcomer, 2003). The notion that respite services will prevent or delay institutionalization has been the driving force among advocates of respite programs.

The Caregiver Stress Model

The potential influence of caregiver stress on caregiving behaviors is best understood within the context of the stress model articulated by Pearlin and his colleagues (Pearlin, Mullan, Semple, & Skaff, 1990). The model provides a conceptual framework that identifies four domains that make up the stress process: the background and the context of stress, the stressors, the mediators of stress, and the outcomes or manifestations of stress.

The background and the context factors include the demographic and ascribed characteristics of the caregiver, the relationship between the caregiver and the care receiver, and aspects of the social and service delivery environment that frame the context in which care is provided.

As individuals become caregivers, they are exposed to primary stressors and secondary stressors. Primary stressors are conditions and characteristics of the care receiver that translate into the care tasks and responsibilities that are assumed by the caregiver. These include the care receiver's cognitive status, problematic behaviors, and the need for assistance with activities for daily living (ADLs) and instrumental activities of daily living (IADLs). Primary stressors may impact negatively on the caregiver and lead to secondary role and intrapsychic strains. These secondary strains on the caregiver include constraints on other aspects of the caregiver's life, including family and occupational roles, social and recreational activities, and intrapsychic strains such as loss of self-esteem, loss of self, role captivity, and lowered sense of competence.

The outcomes of the caregiving stress process may include caregiver depression and a subjective sense of stress or anxiety, change in caregiver physical and mental health, and/or abandonment of the caregiving role. Pearlin, Turner, and Semple (1989) hypothesized that social supports and positive coping mechanisms may buffer the effects of the primary and secondary stressors and thereby reduce the sense of strain and prevent or reduce the negative outcomes associated with caregiving responsibilities. For example, caregiver role captivity and loss of self may be offset by assistance with personal care from other family members, which may reduce the objective demands on the primary caregiver and the level of anxiety or depression experienced by a caregiver (Montgomery & Williams, 2001).

From the perspective of the stress model, respite services may operate as a buffer between primary stressors (e.g., the care tasks) and secondary stressors (e.g., role conflict or role loss) and, thereby, prevent negative outcomes such as depression, poor health, or placement of a care recipient in a long-term care facility.

The Impact of Respite

Although the potential benefits of respite for relieving caregiver stress and reducing the public costs of long-term care have been widely touted, evidence to support these assertions has been somewhat limited. The most consistent finding from studies of respite programs is that clients are satisfied with the services they receive (Baumgarten, Lebel, Laprise, Leclerc, & Quinn, 2002; Dziegielewski & Ricks, 2000; Townsend & Kosloski, 2002; Warren, Kerr, Smith, Godkin, & Schalm, 2003).

Impact of Respite on Stress

With respect to the impact of respite services on stress or burden, the findings have been inconsistent. Based on a meta-analysis of 13 studies of respite care, Sorenson and her colleagues (2002) concluded that respite interventions have been effective at reducing caregiver burden and depression and improving well-being. Indeed, a small number of studies have successfully documented a link between the use of respite services and improved psychological conditions, including decreased burden and stress and increased well-being among caregivers (Dellasega & Zerbe, 2002; Gaugler, Jarrott, et al., 2003; Kosloski & Montgomery, 1994a; Levesque, Cossette, & Laurin, 1995). Conversely, Baumgarten and her colleagues (2002) found that respite had no (or a mild) effect on caregiving outcomes. Similarly, an earlier meta-analysis of 18 articles published between 1980 and 1990 on psychosocial interventions and respite care concluded that respite services had a moderate effect (Knight, Lutzky, & Macofsky-Urban, 1993).

The Impact of Respite on Nursing Home Placement

There is some, albeit limited, evidence to support the notion that respite, when provided in an appropriate manner and used in sufficient quantity, may reduce institutionalization. Although most early studies of respite provided little evidence to support the prevention or delay of nursing home placement, findings from a small number of large studies are more encouraging. In a reanalysis of data from a study of 541 caregiver and care receiver dyads, Kosloski and Montgomery (1994a) found evidence to support the utility of respite as an intervention to delay or decrease the likelihood of nursing home placement. More recently, Gaugler and his colleagues (2000) found that caregivers were far less likely to institutionalize their relatives when family members provided overnight help and assisted with ADLs.

Our understanding of the link between respite care and positive outcomes for caregivers is incomplete because of several conceptual and methodological limitations. Unfortunately, previous research has given little attention to the wide variation in the composition of respite services. It is very likely that not all forms of respite are of equal value. Similarly, little attention has been given to the inconsistent patterns of service use and the way in which service use may change over the caregiving experience. To adequately assess the merits of respite, it is necessary to first understand the patterns of service use and factors that influence these patterns.

PATTERNS OF SERVICE USE

Both researchers and service providers have frequently lamented the tendency for respite services to go unused or underused (Kosloski,

Montgomery, & Karner, 1999; Montoro-Rodriguez, Kosloski, & Montgomery, 2003; Spector et al., 2000; Zarit, Stephens, Townsend, Greene, & Leitsch, 1999). All too often, caregivers seek respite care too late or receive services in the wrong setting or insufficient quantity. Indeed, the issues of appropriate timing for use of respite services and the most effective intensity and duration of services remain a challenge for researchers and social work practitioners. An examination of patterns of respite use and nonuse and the factors that are associated with these patterns provides important insights for guiding practice.

Three general patterns of respite service use have been observed among caregivers. First, a significant number of caregivers who have been identified by service providers as being in need of respite care do not use services. Second, among those caregivers who do use respite services, about 30% can be classified as brief users. These are clients who use respite for relatively short periods of time. The third group of caregivers includes those who use respite for an extended period of time (Cox, 1997; Montgomery et al., 2002). Yet, even among this group, there is significant variation in the intensity and duration of use.

For most social workers, nonuse or delayed use of respite care by families who are judged to be in need of respite is difficult to understand. A small number of studies that have examined patterns of respite use provide some important insights into the reasons that caregivers fail to use services (Cox, 1997; Kosloski & Montgomery, 1994b; Kosloski, Montgomery, & Youngbauer, 2001).

Nonusers

Nonusers include people who are simply unaware of the availability of a service and persons who know about the services but still do not use them (Kosloski et al., 2001). For the group of caregivers who are simply unaware that respite services exist, outreach efforts on the part of service providers are critical to foster service use. Among those who have knowledge of service availability, nonuse appears to be related to their perception of need. Caregivers do not seek help unless they perceive a need for it (Cox, 1997). Two factors that have been linked to perceived need are high levels of stress and the absence of an alternative caregiver in an individual's informal network of family and friends (Kosloski et al., 2001).

Clearly, the perception of need is subjective, and many caregivers do not make a decision about need solely on the basis of the functional level or care needs of the person for whom they care. The costs associated with using respite influence caregivers' perceptions of need. These costs can include money as well as the time and effort that caregivers must exert to arrange for transportation and groom the care recipient to attend a respite program. The perception of need is also tempered by culturally based attitudes and beliefs about personal obligations to provide care. For example, caregivers have reported not using respite because of guilt or the sense of failure that they incur when they abdicate care tasks to others. Other caregivers have expressed a reluctance to leave their older relative with a stranger, believing that a respite program may be too upsetting for the care recipient (Cox, 1997; Gwyther, 1989; Hooyman & Gonyea, 1995b; Kosloski et al., 2001).

In part, normative expectations and cultural beliefs about familial responsibility may account for differences in patterns of service use among ethnic groups. Several studies have noted a strong sense of filial responsibility among African Americans, Asian Americans, Latinos, and other minority groups that includes direct care (Clark & Huttlinger, 1998; Cox, 1993; Delgado & Tennstedt, 1997; Henderson & Gutierrez-Mayka, 1992; Ishii-Kuntz, 1997). These beliefs about family responsibility may prevent some caregivers from perceiving themselves to be in need of services and thereby prevent them from using services (Kosloski et al., 1999). Differences among ethnic groups in use of respite services may also be linked to differences in family structures and the availability of alternate caregivers. Several studies reported that caregivers from minority groups draw on a wider circle of helpers than do Whites (Forester, Young, & Langhorne, 1999; Ishii-Kuntz, 1997; Laditka & Laditka, 2001). These findings suggest that race and culture play a significant role in how minority groups view the utility of services and consequently their judgment of need for respite services and, ultimately, their use of services.

Brief Users

In contrast to caregivers who do not use respite services, there are care-givers who use respite services but for only a brief period of time. Brief users have been shown to comprise from 24% to 30% of all respite users (Cox, 1997; Kosloski et al., 2001; Montgomery et al., 2002; Zarit et al., 1999). Knowledge about this last group of caregivers is particularly important for two reasons. First, this group may be more costly to serve because of the inefficiencies created by the expense associated with initial assessment and enrollment processes and the need to orient staff to the client's needs and preferences. Second, brief users have, by their behavior, indicated a need for respite services, yet they discontinued using these services. Whereas nonusers and seekers may simply not have perceived a need for outside assistance, the same cannot be said for brief users. In fact, it is hard to escape the impression that the respite program has somehow failed these individuals. If brief users are indeed dissatisfied customers, then information about factors leading to brief use may be valuable for improving services.

The most pervasive reasons given by caregivers for discontinued use of respite services are related to the impairment level of the care receiver and the capacity of provider organizations to meet the needs of highly impaired individuals. When Zarit and colleagues (1999) conducted a study on brief users, they found that 35% of caregivers stopped using the ADC program because their relative's health had declined to the point of not being able to attend and/or benefit from ADCs. Another 25% of their sample reported that their relative had become acutely ill, and 20% reported that their relative's behavior problems led to discharge.

When Montgomery and her colleagues (2001) observed similar links between brief use of adult day care and high levels of functional impairment and problem behaviors, they concluded that families continue to use day care services until the elder's impairment level becomes too high, at which point families seek in-home services or place the older adult in a long-term care facility. Day care was most often used as a support system when caregivers needed to be away from home or when caregivers had other obligations that required their attention. When the impairment level of the elder increased to higher levels, adult children who could not leave a parent home alone were more likely to cease caregiving. Clearly, the link between brief use of respite services and high levels of disability is consistent with other reports that caregivers often delay formal services until their relatives' problems are quite severe. By that point, respite may be of little help to overburdened caregivers (Zarit et al., 1999).

Patterns of Long-Term Use

Among caregivers who use respite services for an extended time, there is a great variation in the patterns of use. Families vary in the *intensity* or number of hours they use, the *consistency* of service use, and the *duration* of time over which they use services. Differences in patterns of use reflect the characteristics of both the clients and the respite programs themselves (Montgomery et al., 2002). Client characteristics linked to use include race and ethnicity, functional level, and income of the care recipient. Additionally, the gender and familial relationship of the caregiver are associated with patterns of use.

After examining longitudinal data for almost 5,000 caregivers, Montgomery and her colleagues (2002) noted that African Americans, as a group, used day care for a longer period of time than any other group. However, they used fewer hours of service each week. In contrast, ADC was used by the Hispanic/Latino clients more intensely for a shorter length of time. As a consequence, the total amount of service used did not differ significantly between the two groups. However, both groups used more services than did Whites. These patterns of use draw into question widely held beliefs that minority groups will not use services because of cultural values. In fact, the observed patterns support the notion minority groups will use services—and will continue to use services—if they are offered in a manner that is consistent with clients needs and culture.

In a similar manner, spouse caregivers differ from adult children in their use of services. Although spouses tend to be more frequent users of in-home services, Montgomery and her colleagues (2002) found that spouses used fewer hours of respite each month than did adult children or other more distant relatives. Elders with male caregivers used more respite services of both types.

Generally, use of in-home respite is associated with higher levels of need for help with ADLs and with more problem behavior (Montgomery et al., 2002). In contrast, the level of need for help with IADLs is associated with use of respite in day care settings. Interestingly, Montgomery and her colleagues (2002) found that while a higher need for assistance with IADLs was associated with a shorter duration of day care use, it was also associated with more consistent use and a greater number of hours of use on each occasion. Moreover, the number of hours of respite use during a month increased with duration. This pattern of associations underscores the fact that adult day care programs serve a different segment of the caregiving population than do in-home respite programs.

Dual users, or those caregivers who used multiple forms of respite, tended to use each service for shorter periods of time. This pattern of use suggests that clients who have the option of using multiple services shift from using day care to using in-home care when there are significant changes in the elder's level of functioning or their caregiving context.

When considered as a whole, research findings regarding variations in the pattern of respite use underscore the differences in the kind of support that is afforded by each type of respite service. Day care is most often used as a support system when caregivers must be away from the home or when caregivers have other obligations that require their attention. In this capacity, day care allows caregivers to retain responsibility for the care of the impaired elder while meeting other work and family obligations. When, however, the impairment level of the elder increases, caregivers must make an important lifestyle decision. For adult children who cannot leave a parent at home alone, that decision may be to cease caregiving. Clearly, a greater number of spouses continue to provide care when day care is no longer appropriate for their level of need. Consequently, spouses are more frequent users of in-home respite care.

Finally, the association between income and service use that was observed by Montgomery and her colleagues is of particular interest because it is not linear. Rather, middle-income elders used more service than either low- or high-income groups. This pattern may reflect the fact that for middle-income elders, in-home respite is probably the most economical solution for long-term care. This group of elders has little discretionary money, is not eligible for Medicaid, and, consequently, is least likely to place an elder in the nursing home.

PRACTICE IMPLICATIONS

Current knowledge regarding the use and benefits of respite services suggests that respite services will be most beneficial when the type and amount of service provided for a family are appropriately matched to a caregiver's perceived need and when services are offered in a timely manner. Moreover, for maximum impact, it is important that respite services be made available in each community in multiple forms to ensure that services are able to meet the needs of different segments of the client population and to provide support for families as needs change over time. Unfortunately, minimal research has been completed that can provide definitive guidance for social workers to identify the correct type of service or the most appropriate time for initiating respite use (Coon, Gallagher-Thompson, & Thompson, 2003; Pillemer, Suitor, & Wethington, 2003). Recently, however, Montgomery and Kosloski (in press) have articulated a theory of caregiver identity that may be useful to social workers working with family caregivers.

Caregiver Identity Theory

The *caregiver identity theory* is an extension of the caregiver marker framework, which has been advanced as a tool useful for guiding the design and delivery of support services (Montgomery & Kosloski, 2000, 2001). The theory also builds on research that indicates that caregivers will not use services that they do not "perceive as needed or useful" (Kosloski et al., 2001) and is grounded in an extensive body of literature concerned with identity (Burke, 1991; Stryker, 1994).

Central to the theory is the notion that caregivers will perceive a need for services (i.e., respite, education, or support groups) when there is a substantial discrepancy between their care-related activities and their personal identity in relation to the care recipient. Essentially, the model argues that caregivers will experience distress when they are engaged in care activities that are inconsistent with their views of self. Subsequently, this distress will prompt caregivers to seek help. These points of distress may be viewed as periods in the caregiving process at which a caregiver is "servable." This model suggests that caregivers will be most apt to use and benefit from respite services at these "servable moments." Although the caregiver identity theory is quite complex, important elements of the theory and their implication for guiding the delivery of respite services are summarized here.

Identity Change

According to the caregiver identity theory, the caregiving role emerges out of an existing role relationship, usually a familial role such as daughter, wife, or husband. As the needs of the care recipient increase in quantity and intensity over time, a change takes place in the dyadic relationship between the caregiver and the care recipient. The initial familial relationship gives way to a relationship characterized by caregiving. As caregivers move through their caregiving career, they change not only their behaviors but also their role identity in relation to the care recipient. This identity change occurs because the care tasks that are required to maintain the health of the care recipient become inconsistent with the expectations associated with the caregiver's initial role that has established the context for caregiving in the first place. To a large degree, this shift in identity is necessitated by significant changes in the care context, most often an increase in the level of dependency of the care recipient. Other significant changes in the care context, however, might include an increase or decrease in the availability of informal or formal supports or a change in living arrangement.

For most caregivers of persons with chronic conditions or dementia, the change in the role identity that a caregiver experiences in relation to the care recipient is a slow and insidious process. The process occurs in stops and starts and ultimately results in a significant shift from one's initial role relationship (i.e., spouse, daughter, or friend) to that of caregiver. Initially, the care needs of the elder may be relatively small, and the corresponding care tasks may represent only minimal extensions of the initial familial role relationship (i.e., a wife or daughter role).

For example, a daughter may quite easily assist her mother who has some memory impairment with paying bills, shopping, or transportation to appointments without experiencing stress. As the disease progresses, the needs of the mother and resultant demands placed on the daughter increase. As this process unfolds, the daughter's activities gradually increase in intensity and become discrepant with the personal norms that a daughter has internalized with respect to her role as a daughter. Thus, over time, the caregiving activities transform the initial mother–daughter relationship into a caregiving relationship. The daughter may now find herself engaging in activities with respect to her parent that she never engaged in previously, such as assisting with bathing or dressing. Simply put, her activities are now discrepant with her previous role identity. Furthermore, these activities make time demands that limit her other role performances (e.g., time for being a spouse, for being a mother to her own children, for friendship roles, and so on). The end result is incongruence between what the daughter is now doing as a caregiver and the way that she views herself and her obligations (i.e., her identity) as a daughter.

It is the incongruence between caregiving tasks and the meaning attached to these tasks that cause caregivers distress. To the extent that the daughter's behavior is discrepant with her self-view about the types and amount of care she should be providing, the daughter experiences distress (i.e., burden). It is this distress that prompts caregivers to take actions to restore congruence between their care behaviors and their personal expectations, which stem from their role identities. In the caregiver identity model, the personal expectations or rules that individuals use to define appropriate behavior for themselves are referred to as "identity standards" (Burke, 1991). Consequently, it is when a caregiver is experiencing discrepancy between what she is doing and her personal expectations or rules that she is most likely to be open to accepting support services. It is these periods that are "servable moments."

Five Phases of Caregiving

Montgomery and Kosloski (2000) have identified five phases of the caregiving career that are linked to changes in the care recipient's need for assistance. The pie charts shown in Figure 18.1 illustrate the identity change process as it is associated with the five phases.

Phase I of the caregiving career is the period of role onset. This period begins at the point that a caregiver assists the care recipient in a manner that is not a usual part of the initial familial role that connects

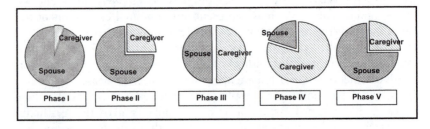

FIGURE 18.1   Caregiver identity mapped to the five phases of the caregiving career.

the caregiver to the care recipient (e.g., daughter or spouse). In this first phase of the care process, caregivers are rarely aware of their caregiver role identity.

Phase II of the caregiving career begins when the caregiver acknowledges that his or her care activities are beyond the normal scope of the initial familial role. This is the point of self-identification as a caregiver (Montgomery & Kosloski, 2000). During this phase of the career, a caregiver is still maintaining his or her primary familial identity in relation to the care recipient but acknowledges the presence of the caregiver role.

Phase III of the caregiving career begins when the care needs of the care recipient increase in quantity and intensity to a level that requires assistance that is beyond the normal boundaries of the initial familial relationship. At this point, the caregiver is often torn between maintaining his or her initial identity as a relative (e.g., daughter, wife, or husband) and assuming the role of caregiver as a primary identity. Caregivers who opt to continue with their caregiving tasks through phase III usually increase the intensity of care they provide over time to such an extent that the caregiver role comes to dominate the dyadic relationship. This shift in identity, which is illustrated by the fourth diagram in Figure 18.1, is usually accompanied by the initial consideration of an alternative living arrangement for the care recipient, which marks the movement into phase IV.

For many spouses, phase IV can continue for an extended time period in which the caregiver continues to revisit the option of nursing home placement.

The final phase of the caregiving career, phase V, begins when the care recipient is moved to a setting that relieves the caregiver of primary responsibility for care. Most often, this phase entails placement in some type of long-term care facility, but it could entail movement to the home of another family member or movement into an assisted living facility. During this final phase, the caregiver is often able to shift his or her primary identity back to the initial familial role and significantly reduce the salience of the caregiver role (Coe & Neufeld, 1999). The salience of the caregiver role, relative to the familial role, would be very similar to that experienced in phase II.

Although Montgomery and Kosloski delineated five phases, they also noted that movement between phases is not a universal experience for caregivers, nor is it a steady, smooth process. Tremendous variation exists in the trajectory of caregiving careers. In fact, many caregivers, especially adult children, exit from the caregiving role during phase II or phase III and move directly into phase V. The type and level of impairment that the care recipient exhibits, the relative stability of functioning level, the physical and social environment in which care is provided, and the initial familial relationship between the caregiver and the care recipient all influence the caregiving trajectory.

What is uniform about caregiving careers is that caregivers experience significant distress at the points of transition between identities. For example, a caregiver who holds an identity consistent with phase II but engages in care tasks that are more consistent with phase III will experience significant distress. This distress will prompt a caregiver to seek support services. Hence, these transition points can be viewed as servable moments.

Using the Caregiver Identity Theory to Guide Practice

When caregiver distress is understood to be linked with incongruence between a caregiver's personal rules for interacting with and helping a care recipient and her actual behavior, the avenues for using support services as mechanisms to relieve stress become more apparent. Social workers can help caregivers avoid or alleviate stress by helping caregivers to (a) change their behaviors to bring them in line with their personal norms or "identity standard, (b) change their negative self-appraisal to affirm the consistency between their identity and their behavior, or (c) change their identity standards. From this perspective, support services such as respite care, education programs, counseling, support groups, or case management are understood to be mechanisms for achieving one or more of these three outcomes.

Respite as a Mechanism to Change Behaviors

Perhaps the easiest means to create congruence between a caregiver's behavior and his or her identity standard is to change the caregiver's behavior to become consistent with an established identity standard. For most caregivers, this means avoiding care tasks that infringe on an initial familial identity (i.e., daughter). The introduction of in-home respite care or day care can serve this purpose. For example, a daughter confronted with her mother's need for constant supervision may maintain her primary identity as a daughter by seeking relief from this obligation through respite services. In this way, the daughter may restrain the time demands placed on her as a result of caregiving responsibility to a level that will allow her sufficient time to meet obligations associated with her role as a spouse, a mother, or an employee. That is, the daughter is able to maintain her initial role identity as daughter by shifting care tasks that are not consistent with this identity to other formal or informal helpers.

The introduction of respite services as a means to change behaviors may not always be an appropriate or viable avenue for relieving stress because using respite may be inconsistent with the personal expectations or rules (i.e., identity standard) that an individual maintains for his or her relationship with the care recipient. Consider, for example, the situation where a care attendant is hired to provide personal care for a dependent husband. While this service may relieve the wife from duty of bathing her husband, it may also create stress if it undermines her ability to comply with a personal identity standard that deems caring for her husband a proper "wifely duty." This example underscores the fact that not all respite services are of equal value. Thus, it is important for social workers to understand the purpose for introducing respite to be certain that the selected service corresponds with the desired goal.

Enhance Self-Appraisal to Facilitate Respite Use

As noted earlier, a major difficulty encountered by social work practitioners is resistance or a reluctance of a caregiver to use respite services in a timely manner. The identity theory offers insights here as well as guidance for practice. This resistance may stem from a caregiver's judgment that use of respite services is inconsistent with her personal norms. One avenue for encouraging respite use, then, is to change that judgment. This can be accomplished by helping the caregiver cognitively reframe his or her situation and thereby counter any negative self-evaluation.

For example, a wife caregiver who is resistant to accepting respite services because she sees all care tasks as her personal duty may be encouraged by a support group or a counselor to reframe her views about the appropriateness of accepting respite care. Sometimes this reframing process may entail countering negative messages caregivers receive from the care recipient or other family members (Levesque et al., 1995). Reframing might also consist of encouraging the caregiver to view the use of an adult day care program as mutually beneficial to the care recipient and the caregiver. To accomplish this, a social worker can emphasize to the caregiver the new opportunities for socialization that day care affords the care recipient and the likelihood that a break or rest from caregiving will improve the caregiver's performance when she is "back on the job." The use of this type of cognitive reframing allows caregivers to transform negative feelings into positive appraisals.

Change in Identity Standard

A third means to reduce distress caused by incongruence between identity standards and behavior is to help the caregiver alter his or her personal rules. When discrepancies are small, providers can help the caregiver "stretch" an identity standard to fit the caregiver's behavior and thereby allow a positive self-appraisal. Essentially, this is the situation described previously where a wife caregiver is encouraged to alter her norms to accept respite services. When, however, distress is high because of significant incongruence between behaviors and identity standards, caregivers may be better helped by encouraging them to *adopt a new identity* that is accompanied by a new set of rules (i.e., a new identity standard). Through education, counseling, or care management, caregivers can be taught about the changing needs of the care recipient and encouraged to embrace an identity in relation to the care recipient that places greater emphasis on the caregiver role than on the initial familial role.

In the case of the wife caring for her husband, the wife may come to define herself primarily as a caregiver. With this shift in identity, the wife may comfortably discontinue activities she previously defined as duties of a wife and accept more help from both formal and informal sources.

Implications for Delivery of Respite Services

The caregiver identity theory has several implications for effectively delivering respite services. First, the caregiver identity model draws attention to the fact that offering respite services as a discrete support mechanism apart from counseling or educational program may be ineffective. While respite is the most widely used and requested service, it may not always be the most appropriate service. As suggested earlier, the goal of respite is to give caregivers time away from the caregiving responsibilities so that they may attend to their own needs. As such, respite may be of little use to a wife who is struggling with the behaviors of her husband with Alzheimer's disease. Granted, respite may provide time away from the difficulties associated with the problem behaviors, but it does not teach the wife how to deal with the behaviors in a constructive manner. Essentially, the wife's presenting problem goes unaddressed. What may be more appropriate for the wife in this situation is attending an education program where she learns about the progression of the disease and what to expect as her husband's abilities decrease.

In addition to helping the social worker determine whether respite is the most appropriate form of support for a caregiver at a given time, the caregiver identity theory also provides some insight for selecting the optimal time in a caregiver's career to provide respite services. During the early phases of the caregiving process, respite is not usually appropriate because caregivers generally are not performing intense care tasks and, in the case of adult children, are often not living with the care receiver. At the same time, spouses may not identify themselves as caregivers until the very late stages of their mate's dependency. Consequently, spouses are likely to perceive information about respite programs that is directed toward caregivers as being largely irrelevant to them.

Only when caregivers reach the point at which they experience a discrepancy between their identity and their care tasks will they be fully receptive to respite programs (Montgomery & Kosloski, in press). This is the servable moment, the time when social workers can best help caregivers maintain their role by offering appropriate services. If services are not made available at the servable moment, caregivers may prematurely consider nursing home placement and move beyond the point at which they would be open to the use of support services. This is the point at which respite programs become "too little too late" and fail to serve a preventive function (Montgomery & Kosloski, 1994). This knowledge about the servable moment can help social workers intervene in a timely manner.

Finally, the caregiver identity theory may help social workers determine the proper type and dose of service. Once a caregiver has reached a servable moment and a determination has been made about the most appropriate type of support service, a social worker must also determine the amount of service that is needed. For example, if it is believed that respite would be the most appropriate service for an adult child caregiver who works full time, the social worker might ask, How much is needed in order to benefit this caregiver? If the caregiver is a full-time employee working 5 days a week, 1 day of respite care may be of little help.

CONCLUSION

After more than two decades of extensive research on caregiving, stress, and respite, practitioners and policymakers are still faced with the challenge of effectively serving a growing population of informal caregivers. This chapter has provided detailed information about the range of respite programs that exist in communities and about our current knowledge of the impact of respite on caregivers. Although a number of questions remain concerning the costs and benefits of respite services, there is general consensus that families can benefit from these services. Knowledge of how to effectively target available respite services to a diverse clientele is a major challenge for social workers. The caregiver identity theory has been introduced as a model useful for guiding social workers as they work with family caregivers.

REFERENCES

Administration on Aging. (2000). Older Americans Act. Retrieved October 1, 2005, from http://www.aoa.gov/about/legbudg/oaa/legbudg_oaa.asp

Alzheimer's Association and the National Alliance for Caregiving. (2000). *Who cares? Families caring for persons with Alzheimer's disease.* Bethesda, MD: Alzheimer's Association and the National Alliance for Caregiving.

Baumgarten, M., Lebel, P., Laprise, H., Leclerc, C., & Quinn, C. (2002). Adult day care for the frail elderly: Outcomes, satisfaction, and cost. *Journal of Aging and Health, 14,* 237.

Burke, P. (1991). Identity processes and social stress. *American Sociological Review, 56,* 836–849.

Clark, M., & Huttlinger, K. (1998). Elder care among Mexican American families. *Clinical Nursing Research, 7,* 64–81.

Coe, M., & Neufeld, A. (1999). Male caregivers' use of formal support. *Western Journal of Nursing Research, 21,* 568–588.

Coon, D. W., Gallagher-Thompson, D., & Thompson, L. W. (2003). *Innovative interventions to reduce dementia caregiver distress: A clinical guide.* New York: Springer.

Cox, C. (1993). Service needs and interests: A comparison of African American and White caregivers seeking Alzheimer's assistance. *Journal of Alzheimer's Care and Related Disorders and Research, 8*(3), 33–40.

Cox, C. (1997). Findings from a statewide program of respite care: A comparison of service users, stoppers, and nonusers. *The Gerontologist, 37,* 511–517.

Delgado, M., & Tennstedt, S. (1997). Puerto Rican sons as primary caregivers of elderly parents. *Social Work, 42,* 125–134.

Dellasega, C., & Zerbe, T. M. (2002). Caregivers of frail rural older adults: Effects of an advanced practice nursing intervention. *Journal of Gerontological Nursing, 28*(10), 40–49.

Dziegielewski, S. F., & Ricks, J. L. (2000). Adult day programs for elderly who are mentally impaired and the measurement of caregiver satisfaction. *Activities, Adaptation and Aging, 24*(4), 51–64.

Family Caregiver Alliance. (2005). *Caregiver statistics.* Retrieved October 5, 2005, from http://www.caregiver.org/caregiver/jsp/content_node.jsp?nodeid=439

Forester, A., Young, J., & Langhorne, P. (1999). Systematic review of day hospital care for elderly people: The day hospital group. *British Medical Journal, 318,* 837–841.

Gaugler, J. E., Edwards, A. B., Femia, E. E., Zarit, S. H., Stephens, M. P., Townsend, A., et al. (2000). Predictors of institutionalization of cognitively impaired elders: Family help and the timing of placement. *Journals of Gerontology. Series B, Psychological Sciences and Social Sciences, 55,* P247–P255.

Gaugler, J. E., Jarrott, S. E., Zarit, S. H., Stephens, M. P., Townsend, A., & Greene, R. (2003). Adult day service use and reductions in caregiving hours: Effects on stress and psychological well-being for dementia caregivers. *International Journal of Geriatric Psychiatry, 18,* 55–62.

Gaugler, J. E., Kane, R. L., Kane, R. A., Clay, T., & Newcomer, R. (2003). Caregiving and institutionalization of cognitively impaired older people: Utilizing dynamic predictors of change. *The Gerontologist, 43,* 219–229.

Gwyther, L. P. (1989). Overcoming barriers: Home care for dementia patients. *Caring: National Association for Home Care Magazine, 8*(8), 12–16.

Henderson, J. N., & Gutierrez-Mayka, M. (1992). Ethnocultural themes in caregiving to Alzheimer's disease patients in Hispanic families. *Clinical Gerontologist, 11,* 59–74.

Hooyman, N. R., & Gonyea, J. (1995a). Introduction. In D. S. Foster (Ed.), *Feminist perspectives on family care: Policies for gender justice* (Vol. 6, pp. 3–4). Thousand Oaks, CA: Sage.

Hooyman, N. R., & Gonyea, J. (1995b). Social services and social support. In D. S. Foster (Ed.), *Feminist perspectives on family care: Policies for gender justice* (Vol. 6, pp. 271–272). Thousand Oaks, CA: Sage.

Ishii-Kuntz, M. (1997). Intergenerational relationships among Chinese, Japanese, and Korean Americans. *Family Relations, 46*, 23–32.

Kagan, J. (2001). *Lifespan and respite*. Retrieved August, 28, 2006, from http://www.archrespite.org/NRC-Lifespan.htm

Knight, B. G., Lutzky, S. M., & Macofsky-Urban, F. (1993). A meta-analytic review of interventions for caregiver distress: Recommendations for future research. *The Gerontologist, 33*, 240.

Kosloski, K., & Montgomery, R. J. V. (1994a). The impact of respite use on nursing home placement. *The Gerontologist, 35*, 67–74.

Kosloski, K., & Montgomery, R. J. V. (1994b). Investigating patterns of service use by families providing care for dependent elders. *Journal of Aging and Health, 6*, 17–37.

Kosloski, K., Montgomery, R. J. V., & Karner, T. X. (1999). Differences in the perceived need for assistive services by culturally diverse caregivers of persons with dementia. *Journal of Applied Gerontology, 18*, 239–256.

Kosloski, K., Montgomery, R. J. V., & Youngbauer, J. (2001). Utilization of respite services: A comparison of users, seekers, and nonseekers. *Journal of Applied Gerontology, 20*, 111–132.

Laditka, J. N., & Laditka, S. B. (2001). Adult children helping older parents: Variations in likelihood and hours by gender, race, and family role. *Research on Aging, 23*, 429.

Levesque, L., Cossette, S., & Laurin, L. (1995). A multidimensional examination of the psychological and social well-being of caregivers of a demented relative. *Research on Aging, 17*, 332–361.

Montgomery, R. J. V. (1996). Examining respite care: Promises and limitations. In R. Kane & J. Dobrof Penrod (Eds.), *Family caregiving in a caring society: Policy perceptions* (pp. 29–45). Thousand Oaks, CA: Sage.

Montgomery, R. J. V. (2005). *Findings from care manager focus groups conducted in Wisconsin, Michigan, Washington, and Florida*. Unpublished manuscript, University of Wisconsin–Milwaukee.

Montgomery, R. J. V., Karner, T. X., Schaefer, J. P., Hupp, K., Klaus, S., Schleyer, M., et al. (2001). *Further analysis and evaluation of the Administration on Aging: Alzheimer's demonstration grant to states*. Lawrence: University of Kansas.

Montgomery, R. J. V., & Kosloski, K. (1994). A longitudinal analysis of nursing home placement for dependent elders cared for by spouses vs adult children. *Journal of Gerontology: Social Studies, 49*(2), S62–S74.

Montgomery, R. J. V., & Kosloski, K. (1995). Respite revisited: Re-assessing the impact. In P. R. Katz, R. Kane, & M. D. Mezey (Eds.), *Quality care in geriatric settings* (pp. 47–67). New York: Springer.

Montgomery, R. J. V., & Kosloski, K. (2000). Family caregiving: Change, continuity, and diversity. In R. Rubinstein & M. Lawton (Eds.), *Alzheimer's disease and related dementias: Strategies in care and research* (pp. 143–171). New York: Springer.

Montgomery, R. J. V., & Kosloski, K. (2001). *Change, continuity, and diversity among caregivers*. Milwaukee: University of Wisconsin, Milwaukee, National Family Caregiver Support Program.

Montgomery, R. J. V., & Kosloski, K. (in press). Pathways to a caregiver identity for older adults. In R. C. Talley & R. J. V. Montgomery (Eds.), *Caregiving across the lifespan*. New York: Oxford University Press.

Montgomery, R. J. V., Marquis, J., Schaefer, J., & Kosloski, K. (2002). Profiles of respite use. *Home Health Care Services Quarterly, 3/4*, 33–64.

Montgomery, R. J. V., & Rowe, J. M. (2003). *Findings from care manager focus groups conducted in Savannah and Atlanta, Georgia.* Unpublished manuscript, University of Wisconsin–Milwaukee.

Montgomery, R. J. V., & Williams, K. N. (2001). Implications of differential impacts of care-giving for future research on Alzheimer care. *Aging and Mental Health, 5*(Suppl. 1), S23–S34.

Montoro-Rodriguez, J., Kosloski, K., & Montgomery, R. J. V. (2003). Evaluating a practice-oriented service model to increase the use of respite services among minorities and rural caregivers. *The Gerontologist, 43,* 916–924.

Pearlin, L. I., Mullan, J. T., Semple, S. J., & Skaff, M. M. (1990). Caregiving and the stress process: An overview of concepts and their measures. *The Gerontologist, 30,* 583–594.

Pearlin, L. I., Turner, H., & Semple, S. (1989). Coping and the mediation of caregiver stress. In E. L. Light & D. Barry (Eds.), *Alzheimer's disease treatment and family stress: Directions for research* (pp. 198–217). Rockville, MD: U.S. Department of Health and Human Services.

Pillemer, K., Suitor, J., & Wethington, E. (2003). Integrating theory, basic research, and intervention: Two case studies from caregiving research. *The Gerontologist, 43*(Special Issue 1), 19–28.

Sorensen, S., Pinquart, M., & Duberstein, P. (2002). How effective are interventions with caregivers? An updated meta-analysis. *The Gerontologist, 42,* 356–372.

Spector, W. D., Fleishman, J. A., Pezzin, L. E., & Spillman, B. C. (2000). *The characteristics of long-term care users.* Rockville, MD: Agency for Healthcare Research and Policy.

Stryker, S. (1994). Identity theory: Its development, research base, and prospects. *Studies in Symbolic Interaction, 16,* 9–20.

Townsend, D., & Kosloski, K. (2002). Factors related to client satisfaction with community-based respite services. *Home Health Care Services Quarterly, 21*(3–4), 89–106.

Warren, S., Kerr, J. R., Smith, D., Godkin, D., & Schalm, C. (2003). The impact of adult day programs on family caregivers of elderly relatives. *Journal of Community Health Nursing, 20,* 209–221.

Zarit, S. H., Stephens, M. A. P., Townsend, A., Greene, R., & Leitsch, S. A. (1999). Patterns of adult day service use by family caregivers: A comparison of brief versus sustained use. *Family Relations, 48,* 355–362.

PART V

Residential Care and Other Models

CHAPTER NINETEEN

Information to Promote Quality Dementia Care in Residential Settings

Sheryl Zimmerman

INTRODUCTION

As dementia progresses, care needs sometimes become too demanding for the informal caregiving network; in such cases, residential care is required. Over the past decade, residential care options for individuals with dementia have expanded from traditional nursing home (NH) care, to that provided in special care units in NHs, to that provided in residential care/assisted living (RC/AL) communities, to that provided in special care units in RC/AL. RC/AL communities are those that provide room, board, 24-hour oversight, and assistance with activities of daily living (Zimmerman, Sloane, & Eckert, 2001). Today, there are more than 1.8 million NH beds and 800,000 RC/AL beds (Institute on Medicine, 2001). Approximately half of these beds are filled by older adults with dementia, suggesting that almost 1 million individuals with dementia are receiving residential long-term care.

Soon after data became available on the merits of special care, it became clear that it was not a panacea to address the needs of long-term care residents with dementia. Instead, "special" care was not always provided in these settings, nor did it necessarily translate to better outcomes. Research on the quality of special care has shown both positive and negative findings related to resident outcomes (such as

363

cognition, function, and hospitalization), staff outcomes (including stress and burnout), and family outcomes (e.g., depression and satisfaction) (Zimmerman & Sloane, 1999).

Whether NHs provide better care than RC/AL communities for persons with dementia has not been clear, either. While NHs offer some clear advantages, such as ongoing supervision and medical oversight, the medical and skilled nursing needs of individuals with dementia tend to be minor until late in the disease process. Alternately, the social model of RC/AL might better fit the needs of these individuals. Information is now coming available that indicates that, overall, RC/AL settings provide care that results in similar outcomes to NHs, except as related to medical care (Sloane, Zimmerman, Gruber-Baldini, et al., 2005).

Thus, the matter of setting is less compelling in the discussion of residential care for persons with dementia than is the matter of quality of life and quality of care within the setting. Consequently, this chapter focuses on three key areas: the quality of life of residents with dementia in NHs and RC/AL settings, evidence-based components of care that relate to quality of life, and the role of staff and families in care and in promoting quality of life. It closes with implications for social work practice. Throughout, the chapter incorporates evidence from a study of quality of life and quality of care in RC/AL communities and NHs and by so doing ties together these important considerations.

QUALITY OF LIFE OF RESIDENTIAL CARE/ ASSISTED LIVING AND NURSING HOME RESIDENTS WITH DEMENTIA

There are good reasons to assess the quality of life of long-term care residents with dementia. The most obvious is that if it can be determined in what ways quality of life is deficient, steps can be taken to improve it. Of course, we already know that quality of life for persons with dementia is less than optimal; who can argue that life is better for those in full control of their cognition and function? Instead, these assessments are helpful because they can provide a benchmark of sorts: the quality of life of one individual with dementia can be compared to that of another, thereby suggesting areas in which it can be improved. Another use of these assessments is that they can indicate change in quality of life over time, which also can guide strategies for care.

Numerous measures are available to assess quality of life, each of which approaches the definition somewhat differently. To a large extent, the choice of measures depends on how one chooses to conceptualize quality of life and whether the assessment will be conducted through the eyes of an outsider or of the person with dementia. It is helpful to consider the range of assessment options because the way in which quality of life is measured will affect the findings and the resulting suggestions for care.

For example, *Quality of Life in Dementia (QOL-D)* (Albert et al., 1996) focuses on restriction in activity and narrowing of affect as the fundamental components of quality of life; it includes 15 items and is completed by a care provider. The *Alzheimer Disease Related Quality of Life (ADRQL)* (Rabins, Kasper, Kleinman, Black, & Patrick, 2000) is also completed by a care provider but is markedly longer (47 items) and addresses five domains: social interaction, awareness of self, feelings and mood, enjoyment of activities, and response to surroundings. At the other extreme, the *Dementia Quality of Life (DQoL)* (Brod, Stewart, Sands, & Walton, 1999) was developed for completion by persons with dementia; it includes 29 items within five domains that evaluate feeling states that are thought to represent the subjective experience of dementia (self-esteem, positive affect/humor, negative affect, feelings of belonging, and sense of aesthetics). The *Quality of Life in Alzheimer's Disease (QOL-AD)* (Logsdon, Gibbons, McCurry, & Teri, 2000) can be completed by either a care provider or a person with dementia; it has 13 or 15 items (the longer version being the one used in long-term care) (Edelman, Fulton, Kuhn, & Chang, 2005) and assesses physical condition, mood, interpersonal relationships, ability to participate in meaningful activities, and financial situation. There are also measures specific to stage of disease, such as the *Quality of Life in Late-Stage Dementia Scale (QUALID)* (Weiner et al., 2000).

All the measures noted above are interview based, but those that assess QOL through observation also exist, such as *Dementia Care Mapping (DCM)* (Bradford Dementia Group, 1997; Brooker, 2005), which observes behavior and well-being; the *Philadelphia Geriatric Center Affect Rating Scale (PGC-ARS)* (Lawton, Van Haitsma, & Klapper, 1996), which assesses quality of life by observing affective states through facial expression and body movement; and the *Resident and Staff Observation Checklist—Quality of Life Measure (RSOC-QoL)* (Sloane, Zimmerman, Williams, et al., 2005), which records appearance, location, activity, behavior, affect, restraint use, and interactions of residents in long-term care settings.

The fact that many measures are available is fortunate because these different measures of quality of life are not highly correlated (Sloane, Zimmerman, Williams, et al., 2005). Instead, they reflect different perspectives and components of quality of life; consequently, the use of multiple measures is recommended to allow for a more comprehensive assessment. In addition, to the extent possible, residents themselves should be asked to provide data on their quality of life. In general, those with Mini-Mental State Exam (MMSE) (Folstein, Folstein, & McHugh, 1975) scores higher than 10 are able to reliably and validly provide this information (Mozley et al., 1999).

Despite the availability of measures, quality of life for residents with dementia in long-term care has not been studied extensively. An exception is the work conducted by the Collaborative Studies of Long-Term (CS-LTC). The CS-LTC visited 45 NHs and RC/AL communities across four states and obtained data from 121 residents and their care providers about quality of life. The 15-item *Quality of Life in Alzheimer's Disease (QOL-AD)* used a 4-point Likert scale ranging from 1 (poor) to 4 (excellent) to rate physical health, energy, mood, living situation, memory, relationship with family, relationships with people who work here, relationships with friends, personality overall, ability to keep busy, ability to do things for fun, life overall, ability to take care of self, ability to live with others, and ability to make choices in life. Scores averaged 2.9 (per item) as rated by residents and 2.7 as rated by staff caregivers (Sloane, Zimmerman, Williams, et al., 2005).

This finding, of poorer scores reported by proxy respondents, is a common finding across many studies (Magaziner, Zimmerman, Gruber-Baldini, Hebel, & Fox, 1997). Regardless of the difference between the two, however, both scales had good reliability (alpha = 0.89–0.92), and both scores were close to a rating of "good" quality of life for residents with dementia in long-term care. However, there was virtually no agreement between the two raters, with a correlation of $r = 0.02$. Analyses indicated that care provider ratings somewhat reflected their assessment of the resident's cognition and function, whereas residents' ratings of their own quality of life were not at all reflective of their cognitive or functional status (Sloane, Zimmerman, Williams, et al., 2005).

In sum, for both the staff and the residents, the quality-of-life ratings were much more than a reflection of the resident's abilities. Thus, the quality of life of residents in long-term care reflects more than their own limitations—paving the way to consider how care may relate to quality of life.

QUALITY OF CARE THAT RELATES TO BETTER QUALITY OF LIFE

The conceptual model of health care quality posits that the structure of care (the capacity to provide care) and the process of care (the manner in which care is provided) relate to outcomes of care (in this case, quality of life) (Donabedian, 1966). In long-term care settings, components of structure include things such as facility demographics (e.g., type, proprietary status), the physical environment (e.g., personalization, safety features), and staffing (e.g., staffing ratios, assignment practices). Components of the process of care include things such as policies and practices (e.g., discharge policies, staff training practices), care provision (e.g., having a dementia care unit, using restraints), and staff behaviors (e.g., hopeful or person-entered approaches to care). Some of these components of care are evidenced at the facility level and therefore affect all residents. For example, a policy of accepting problem behaviors applies to all residents in a facility. Other components express themselves at a resident level; for example, in a facility that uses physical restraints to manage behavior, only some residents would actually be put in restraints.

When examining the relationship of the structure and process of care to outcomes, another matter to take into consideration is timing. Causal relationships require that the action precede the outcome; thus, it is desirable to assess care first and then determine how it relates to change in quality of life over time. However, in cross-sectional studies of long-term care residents, such an examination would be insensitive to the effects that the care environment had been exerting since the time of admission and that were already being reflected in the resident's quality of life. By way of example, a resident living in an abysmal facility would likely have an abysmal quality of life; the effect of care on outcomes would already have occurred. For this reason, cross-sectional studies that adjust for resident differences are also informative.

The previously cited CS-LTC study compared 56 components of the structure and process of care to the quality of life of 421 residents with dementia in 45 long-term care facilities. Table 19.1 summarizes those components of care that relate to resident quality of life, all of which have implications for care practices. One finding that is evident at quick glance is that there are indeed facility-level components of care that relate to resident quality of life, both longitudinally and cross sectionally—although no one component was significant at both time points. Resident-level components of care related to cross-sectional quality of life but not to change in quality of life over time. This point should not be taken to mean that person-centered care is not important for ongoing quality of life, however; instead, it may be that this study did not have a sufficient number of subjects or may have not been assessing all the important components of individualized care.

Table 19.1 indicates that residents have a better quality of life over time in facilities in which staff have specialized roles and more training and encourage activity participation. They have a better quality of life if nurse staffing is stable and if professional and direct care staff are involved in care planning. These types of findings are consistent with

TABLE 19.1   Components of Long-Term Care That Relate to Quality of Life for Residents With Dementia (Zimmerman, Sloane, et al., 2005)[a]

	Quality of Life	
Components of Care	Change Over 6 Months	Cross Sectional
Facility level	Specialized staff	Less nurse turnover
	Staff who have more training	Staff involved in care planning
	Staff who encourage activity participation	More contract aides
		Less stable staff–resident assignment
		Accept problem behavior
Resident level		Staff who are dementia sensitive
		Staff who practice positive person work
		Better-groomed residents
		Family involvement as related to activities

[a] All comparisons are significant at $p < .05$ using linear models that adjust for facility clustering and facility type as well as resident age, race, marital status, tenure, cognition, behavior, depression, function, and comorbidity.

work that speaks to the importance of continuity and involvement in care as related to better outcomes (Zimmerman, Gruber-Baldini, Hebel, Sloane, & Magaziner, 2002). On the other hand, facilities that have more contract aides and less stable staff–resident assignment also have residents with a higher quality of life. Findings such as this suggest that that newer staff–resident relationships are beneficial in some cases—perhaps when the alternative would be that care is provided by workers who are experiencing burnout or stress. This interpretation is supported by the finding that, on a resident level, those whose care providers are more dementia sensitive and who practice positive person work (e.g., verbal and nonverbal interactions such as facilitation, collaboration, negotiation, and recognition) have a better quality of life.

Also related to a better quality of life is being in a facility that is more accepting of problem behavior, being better groomed, and having family involvement. Finally, it is worth noting that while there were few differences in care between special care facilities/units and non–special care facilities/units, the former had a somewhat worse environmental quality but reported more acceptance of problem behaviors and encouragement of activities, and staff in these areas were more often observed practicing positive person work and having physical contact with residents ($p < .05$) (Zimmerman, Williams, et al., 2005).

THE ROLE OF STAFF IN THE PROVISION OF LONG-TERM CARE

Table 19.1 makes it quite clear that staff are important to the quality of life for residents with dementia who reside in long-term care. In this regard, the well-being of the staff is important because it affects the quality of care they provide. Furthermore, staff who feel stressed have less job satisfaction and increased turnover, which relates to resident quality of life. Fortunately, staff stress is modifiable, especially in those cases when it results from lack of training and low self-efficacy in perceived ability to provide care (Evers, Tomic, & Brouwers, 2001; Mackenzie & Peragine, 2003; Schaefer & Moos, 1996). Thus, there is good cause to understand the role and well-being of staff when working to promote resident quality of life.

Unfortunately, while there is a substantial body of research considering the stress on families of caring for people with dementia, little work has investigated the stressors placed on long-term care staff and how to counteract them. The CS-LTC project studied the stress, satisfaction, and attitudes toward dementia of 154 direct care providers in the 45 long-term care facilities. Overall, staff did not report much stress, scoring 1.8 on a scale ranging from 1 to 5; similarly, they reported being rather satisfied (scoring 62.3 on a scale ranging from 0 to 84) and having positive attitudes toward dementia (scoring 70.7 on a scale ranging from 19 to 95) (Zimmerman, Sloane, et al., 2005). Their attitudes were especially positive in reference to person-centered care, exemplified by endorsing statements such as "it is important for people with dementia to be given choice" and "people with dementia need to feel respected, just like anybody else."

The facility and staff characteristics that relate to stress, satisfaction, and attitudes are shown in Table 19.2. Working in a special care unit is related to both more stress and less satisfaction, perhaps due to providing care to a more challenging clientele and experiencing organizational challenges and expectations that are difficult to meet. Facility characteristics that relate to more positive attitudes (hope and person-centered care) are working in a newer facility, a for-profit facility, and one that serves fewer non-White residents. Recognizing that hope and person-centered attitudes are promoted by the new culture of care (Weiner & Ronch, 2003), it is understandable that they are first evident in these facilities; the task will be

TABLE 19.2 Facility and Staff Characteristics That Relate to Staff Stress, Satisfaction, and Attitudes About Dementia (Zimmerman, Williams, et al., 2005)[a]

Characteristic	More Stress	More Satisfaction	More Positive Attitudes
Facility	Work in a special care unit	Not work in a special care unit	Newer facility
			For-profit facility
			Lower non-White case mix
Staff	Younger workers	Feel better trained	Female
	Working 6–24 months[b]		White
			College education
			Working 12–24 months[b]
			Feel better trained

[a] All comparisons are significant at $p < .05$ using linear models that adjust for facility clustering.

[b] Compared to staff who have been working more than 2 years.

to diffuse these attitudes to other facilities. Turning to staff characteristics, these more positive attitudes are more often espoused by female, White, college-educated workers who have some experience but less than 2 years of experience and feel better trained. Again considering that these attitudes are taught as part of the new culture of care, the task is to help males, non-Whites, and those without a college education to embrace these positive attitudes. The training is likely to have a second benefit, as those who feel better trained are more satisfied. Finally, special attempts might be made to provide support to younger workers and those who have been working for less than 2 years, as these staff feel more stress than those who have been working for a longer period of time (Zimmerman, Williams, et al., 2005).

THE ROLE OF FAMILIES IN THE PROVISION OF LONG-TERM CARE

One way to reduce staff stress and increase staff satisfaction is through their relationships with family members; indeed, satisfaction is increased when staff perceive genuine family efforts to help provide care (Looman,

Noelker, Schur, Whitlatch, & Ejaz, 2002). Family members are typically present in long-term care; it is the norm that long-term care residents were cared for by family before their placement and that caregiving does not end after placement (Dempsey & Pruncho, 1993; Hopp, 1999).

Families constitute an important resource to staff because they have knowledge of the resident's history, and they are important to the resident for emotional connectedness and psychosocial health. Indeed, family presence improves resident psychological and psychosocial well-being as well as the accuracy of diagnosis and so the resultant care (Janzen, 2001; McCallion, Toseland, & Freeman, 1999). In addition, family members are called on to make decisions regarding care for cognitively impaired residents and to provide continuity that may otherwise be lacking because of staff turnover.

The family's role in long-term care provision is increasingly recognized, although it differs somewhat depending whether the resident is living in a NH or a RC/AL community. In the CS-LTC study, families of residents with dementia were found to visit for an average of 4.3 hours per week (NHs) to 4.7 hours per week (RC/AL communities). Family members of RC/AL residents rated themselves as being highly and significantly more involved than those of NH residents, and while both groups reported feeling only a little burdened, the RC/AL families were significantly more burdened than the NH families. Overall, however, neither group desired change in their level of involvement (Port, Zimmerman, Williams, Dobbs, Preisser, & Williams, 2005).

Figure 19.1 illustrates some of the differences between these two groups of family care providers. Families of RC/AL residents were significantly more involved in monitoring medical care, monitoring well-being, and monitoring finances than were families of NH residents. It seems that in these less medically intense settings, caregivers fulfill those functions that they presume are not being completed by staff. In this way, the family may be an especially important component of care for residents with dementia, allowing them to remain in RC/AL communities rather than transitioning to NHs.

IMPLICATIONS FOR SOCIAL WORK PRACTICE

Issues related to quality of life, quality of care, and staff and family involvement in the care of long-term care residents with dementia are relevant to social workers to the extent that they provide services in these settings. Federal law requires that NHs with more than 120 beds employ a full-time social worker who has a bachelor's degree (or higher) in social work or similar qualifications. Smaller NHs must provide social

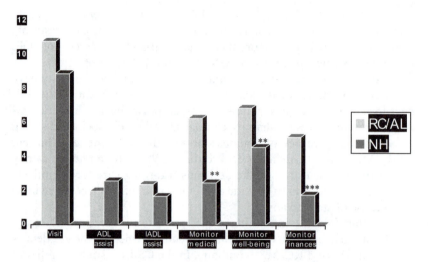

FIGURE 19.1   Family involvement in care tasks (times per month) by
setting (Port et al., 2005)[a].

[a] RC/AL = residential care/assisted living; NH = nursing home; ADL = activities of daily
living; IADL = instrumental activities of daily living.
** $p < .05$.
*** $p < .01$.

services but are not required to have a full-time social worker on staff.
Availability is not at all ensured in RC/AL, where, despite need, social
work presence is not required. However, some of these residents do
receive social work services, including by those not directly employed
by the RC/AL setting (e.g., Medicaid case managers or hospital discharge planners) (Zimmerman, Munn, & Koenig, 2006).

Nursing home social workers are charged with providing quality psychosocial care, including addressing needs related to quality of life (Department of Health and Human Services, 2003). In actuality, they are well
positioned to promote improved quality of life based on their person-in-
environment perspective and knowledge of group processes to foster resident, staff, and family involvement. Further, the National Association of
Social Workers expressly recommends that social workers in long-term care
not only provide direct services to residents and their families but also be
responsible for fostering a climate and policies that enhance quality of life,
including advocating on a case, policy, and program level (National Association of Social Workers, n.d., 2003).

In addition, there is a call to action to monitor and measure psychosocial care and quality of life in long-term care—including engaging social

workers in the use of applied measurement tools—and to examine attributes of social workers in leadership and management roles in NHs (Vourlekis, Zlotnik, & Simons, 2005). All these suggested roles and responsibilities provide support and guidance for implementing the evidence-based care practices presented in this chapter.

Individuals with dementia who reside in long-term care settings do have quality to their lives, but that quality is variable. In the CS-LTC study, ratings of quality of life ranged from 18 to 60, in a scale that had a theoretical range of 15 to 60. Thus, some residents had an extremely poor quality of life, and others had an extremely good quality of life. Social workers in direct care could administer the same measure to all residents and/or their caregivers, with the results providing clues as to areas in which one individual's quality of life is deficient and might be improved. For example, if two residents with similar levels of cognitive and functional impairment score differently on items such as relationships with friends or ability to take care of self, care planning could consider strategies to maximize quality of life in the indicated area.

Administered over time, quality-of-life measures can identify when change is occurring. In some instances, change in quality of life might pre-date other indicators and so could be a marker for decline. In other cases, change in function might not trigger a change in quality of life, which might suggest a particular strength of the individual worth preserving as long as possible. Regardless the use, the choice of which measure of quality of life to use should be consistent with the resident's level of impairment and his or her values and preferences.

Staff rate quality of life more poorly than do the residents themselves. The extent to which such ratings affect care provision is unknown. On the one hand, it is plausible that those who consider quality of life to be worse might work harder to improve it. On the other, it is also plausible that they might choose to direct their efforts to others who still have perceived quality in their lives. Thus, social workers might strive to better understand the implications of these ratings and also the factors that relate to these ratings, as they, too, may have implications for improving care. For example, there is indication that care providers minimize quality of life if they perceive cognitive, affective, functional, and behavioral status to be poor. It may well be that in these instances, care providers need to better understand how quality of life can overcome such deficits. This point is supported by findings indicating that these same staff rate quality of life more highly if they themselves have more training and if they have attitudes that are more person centered (Winzelberg, Williams, Preisser, Zimmerman, & Sloane, 2005). Thus, there is good cause to teach staff how to appreciate the unique nature of each resident. This training would focus on person-centered care, where staff are taught to form relationships that address residents' individual needs despite functional and cognitive deficits (Touhy, 2004).

A number of components of care were related to resident quality of life. Social workers could effect these components of care in their role as leaders and advocates. For example, there is indication that facilities should consider using rotating worker assignments or use a specialized worker perspective. However, both of these findings are not consistent with practice wisdom, and many states promote the use of universal workers (Mollica & Johnson-Lamarche, 2005); thus, social workers might better understand what it is that benefits rotating workers or what specialized workers are doing and the instances in which their care is favorable to that provided by others. They also might serve as advocates in shaping facility policies accordingly and encouraging staff participation in care planning, which is related to better resident quality of life.

Social workers could most definitely provide helpful service at the level of the staff. Frontline work involves complex tasks ranging from providing intimate care to making judgments about the meaning of subtle clinical signs; juxtaposed against this complexity is the fact that standards for staff training and experience are minimal (Zimmerman, Walsh, et al., 2001). The data indicate that staff training is related not only to resident quality of life but also to staff well-being. Social workers might thus approach in-service training empowered with this dual perspective. In addition, in attending to the well-being of staff, social workers might be open to mediating in staff conflicts that relate to stress; this is an area in which social workers have influence (Kruzich & Powell, 1995). Finally, the data also suggest that social workers might want to work with the long-term care administrator to reduce the stress that is concomitant with special care as it is currently provided.

Finally, family involvement is related to resident quality of life. Further, it relates to their own level of well-being and burden as well. For example, there is evidence from other studies that family depression relates to how well both they and the older adult adjust to the long-term care environment (Whitlatch, Schur, Noelker, Ejaz, & Looman, 2001). The findings in this chapter suggest that family members might be helped to understand, in advance, the types of caregiving in which they will be active after the resident's placement; furthermore, social workers might themselves help in some of the monitoring functions that families enact or garner other social supportive services to do so.

CONCLUSION

The social worker who provides care for residents with dementia in long-term care settings may impact quality of life directly or through services provided to staff or families or through system-level intervention within the long-term care facility. Fortunately, evidence exists to provide guidance and options to improve care and quality of life. To a great extent, then, the social worker's success will depend on how much time is available for this work and how amenable the system is to change. It is fortunate indeed that we have some clear direction for the future; all that remains is the support to pursue it.

Acknowledgments

The work on this chapter was supported by a grant from the National Institute on Aging (K02 AG00970), and much of the data that are reported were obtained in a study funded by the Alzheimer's Association.

REFERENCES

Albert, S. M., Del Castillo-Castaneda, C., Sano, M., Jacobs, D. M., Marder, K., Bell, K., et al. (1996). Quality of life in patients with Alzheimer's disease as reported by patient proxies. *Journal of the American Geriatrics Society, 44,* 1342–1347.

Bradford Dementia Group. (1997). *Evaluating dementia care: The DCM method* (7th ed.). Bradford: Bradford Dementia Group.

Brod, M., Stewart, A. L., Sands, L., & Walton, P. (1999). Conceptualization and measurement of quality of life in dementia: The Dementia Quality of Life instrument (DQoL). *Gerontologist, 39,* 25–35.

Brooker, D. (2005). Dementia care mapping: A review of the research literature. *Gerontologist, 45*(Special Issue I), 11–18.

Dempsey, N. P., & Pruncho, R. A. (1993). The family's role in the nursing home: Predictors of technical and non-technical assistance. *Journal of Gerontological Social Work, 27,* 127–145.

Department of Health and Human Services. Office of Inspector General. (2003). *Psychosocial services in skilled nursing facilities* (OEI-020–01–00610). Washington, DC: Author.

Donabedian, A. (1966). Evaluating the quality of medical care. *Milbank Memorial Fund Quarterly, 44*(3, Suppl.), 166–206.

Edelman, P., Fulton, B. R., Kuhn, D., & Chang, C-H. (2005). A comparison of three methods of measuring dementia-specific quality of life: Perspectives of residents, staff, and observers. *Gerontologist, 45*(Special Issue I), 27–36.

Evers, W., Tomic, W., & Brouwers, A. (2001). Effects of aggressive behavior and perceived self-efficacy on burnout among staff of homes for the elderly. *Journal of Mental Health Nursing, 22,* 439–454.

Folstein, M. F., Folstein, S. E., & McHugh, P. R. (1975). "Mini-mental state"—A practical method for grading the cognitive state of patients for the clinician. *Journal of Psychiatric Research, 12,* 189–198.

Hopp, F. (1999). Patterns and predictors of formal and informal care among elderly persons living in board and care homes. *Gerontologist, 39,* 167–176.

Institute on Medicine. (2001). *Improving the quality of long-term care.* Washington, DC: National Academy Press.

Janzen, W. (2001). Long-term care for older adults: The role of the family. *Journal of Gerontological Nursing, 27,* 36–43.

Kruzich, J. M., & Powell, W. E. (1995). Decision-making influence: An empirical study of social workers in nursing homes. *Health and Social Work, 20,* 215–222.

Lawton, M. P., Van Haitsma, K., & Klapper, J. (1996). Observed affect in nursing home residents with Alzheimer's disease. *Journal of Gerontology B: Psychological Sciences and Social Sciences, 51,* P3–P14.

Logsdon, R. G., Gibbons, L. E., McCurry, S. M., & Teri, L. (2000). Quality of life in Alzheimer's disease: Patient and caregiver reports. In S. M. Albert & R. G. Logsdon (Eds.), *Assessing quality of life in Alzheimer's disease* (pp. 17–30). New York: Springer.

Looman, W. J., Noelker, L. S., Schur, D., Whitlatch, C. J., & Ejaz, F. K. (2002). Impact of family members on nurse assistants: What helps, what hurts. *American Journal of Alzheimer's Disease and Other Dementias, 17,* 350–356.

Mackenzie, C. S., & Peragine, G. (2003). Measuring and enhancing self-efficacy among professional caregivers of individuals with dementia. *American Journal of Alzheimer's Disease and Other Dementias, 18,* 291–298.

Magaziner, J., Zimmerman, S. I., Gruber-Baldini, A. L., Hebel, J. R., & Fox, K. M. (1997). Proxy reporting in five areas of functional status: Comparison with self-reports and observations of performance. *American Journal of Epidemiology, 146,* 418–428.

McCallion, P., Toseland, R. W., & Freeman, K. (1999). An evaluation of a family visit education program. *Journal of the American Geriatrics Society, 47,* 203–214.

Mollica, R., & Johnson-Lamarche, H. (2005). *State residential care and assisted living policy: 2004.* Portland, ME: National Academy for State Health Policy.

Mozley, C. G., Huxley, P., Sutcliffe, C., Bagley, H., Burns, A., & Challis, D. (1999). "Not knowing where I am doesn't mean I don't know what I like": Cognitive impairment and quality of life responses in elderly people. *International Journal of Geriatric Psychiatry, 14,* 776–783.

National Association of Social Workers. (n.d.). NASW Clinical indicators for social work and psychosocial services in nursing homes. Retrieved June 6, 2006, from http://www.socialworkers.org/practice/standards/nursing_homes.asp

National Association of Social Workers. (2003). *NASW standards for social work services in long-term care facilities.* Washington, DC: Author.

Port, C. L., Zimmerman, S., Williams, C. S., Dobbs, D., Preisser, J. S., & Williams, S. (2005). Families filling the gap: Comparing family involvement for assisted living and nursing home residents with dementia. *Gerontologist, 45*(Special Issue I), 87–95.

Rabins, P. V., Kasper, J. D., Kleinman, L., Black, B. S., & Patrick, D. L. (2000). Concepts and methods in the development of the ADRQL: An instrument for assessing health-related quality of life in persons with Alzheimer's disease. In S. M. Albert & R. G. Logsdon (Eds.), *Assessing quality of life in Alzheimer's disease* (pp. 51–68). New York: Springer.

Schaefer, J. A., & Moos, R. H. (1996). Effects of work stressors and work climate on long-term care staff's job morale and functioning. *Research in Nursing and Health, 19,* 63–73.

Sloane, P. D., Zimmerman, S., Gruber-Baldini, L., Hebel, J. R., Magaziner, J., & Konrad, T. R. (2005). Health and functional outcomes and health care utilization of persons with dementia in residential care and assisted living facilities: Comparisons with nursing homes. *Gerontologist, 45*(Special Issue I), 124–132.

Sloane, P. D., Zimmerman, S., Williams, C. S., Reed, P. S., Gill, K. S., & Preisser, J. S. (2005). Evaluating the quality of life of long-term residents with dementia. *Gerontologist, 45*(Special Issue I), 37–49.

Touhy, T. A. (2004). Dementia personhood, and nursing: Learning from a nursing situation. *Nursing Science Quarterly, 14,* 43–49.

Vourlekis, B., Zlotnik, J. L., & Simons, K. (2005). *Nursing homes: Toward quality psychosocial care and its measurement: A report to the profession and blueprint for action.* Washington, DC: Institute for the Advancement of Social Work Research.

Weiner, A. W., & Ronch, J. L. (Eds.). (2003). *Culture change in long-term care.* Binghamton, NY: Haworth.

Weiner, M. F., Martin-Cook, K., Svetlik, D. A., Saine, K., Foster, R., & Fontaine, C. S. (2000). The quality of life in late-stage dementia (QUALID) scale. *Journal of the American Medical Directors Association, 1,* 114–116.

Whitlatch, C. J., Schur, D., Noelker, L. S., Ejaz, F. K., & Looman, W. J. (2001). The stress process of family caregiving in institutional settings. *Gerontologist, 41,* 462–473.

Winzelberg., G., Williams, C. S., Preisser, J. S., Zimmerman, S., & Sloane, P. D. (2005). Factors associated with nursing assistant quality of life ratings for residents with dementia in long-term care facilities. *Gerontologist, 45*(Special Issue I), 106–114.

Zimmerman, S., Gruber-Baldini, A. L., Hebel, J. R., Sloane, P. D., & Magaziner, J. (2002). Nursing home facility risk factors for infection and hospitalization: Importance of RN turnover, administration and social factors. *Journal of the American Geriatrics Society, 50,* 1987–1995.

Zimmerman, S., Munn, J., & Koenig, T. (2006). Social work practice in assisted living settings. In B. Berkman & S. Ambruoso (Eds.), *Handbook of social work in health and aging* (pp. 677–684). Oxford: Oxford University Press.

Zimmerman, S. I., & Sloane, P. D. (1999, Fall). Optimum residential care for people with dementia. *Generations,* 62–68.

Zimmerman, S., Sloane, P. D., & Eckert, J. K. (Eds.). (2001). *Assisted living: Needs, practices and policies in residential care for the elderly.* Baltimore: Johns Hopkins University Press.

Zimmerman, S., Sloane, P. D., Williams, C. S., Reed, P. S., Preisser, J. S., Eckert, J. K., et al. (2005). Dementia care and quality of life in assisted living and nursing homes. *Gerontologist, 45*(Special Issue I), 133–146.

Zimmerman, S., Walsh, J. F., Sloane, P. D, Duke, C., & Lea, K. (2001). Screening for a high-quality paraprofessional workforce: The state of the field. *Seniors Housing and Care Journal, 9,* 61–71.

Zimmerman, S., Williams, C. S., Reed, P. S., Boustani, M., Preisser, J. S., Heck, E., et al. (2005). Attitudes, stress and satisfaction of staff caring for residents with dementia. *Gerontologist, 45*(Special Issue I), 96–105.

CHAPTER TWENTY

Quality Care in Residential Settings: Research Into Practice

Jeanne Heid-Grubman

INTRODUCTION

The Alzheimer's Association is the largest voluntary health care organization dedicated to finding a cure for Alzheimer's and providing support for those living with the disease and their care partners. Since its inception in 1980, the Alzheimer's Association has continually demonstrated its commitment to quality care for persons with dementia through various initiatives and programs. *Guidelines for Dignity* (Alzheimer's Association, 1992) and *Key Elements of Dementia Care* (Alzheimer's Association, 1997) were published to provide guiding principles for residential care providers involved in the care of people with dementia.

In 2005, the Alzheimer's Association launched a multi-year initiative, the Campaign for Quality Residential Care, to provide support, guidance, and practical tools for residential care organizations and their staff. The foundation of this campaign was a set of practice recommendations that were based on the latest evidence in dementia care research (Alzheimer's Association, 2005a). These recommendations were developed with input from researchers, dementia care experts, and association staff who collectively developed what may be considered a common definition of quality care for persons with dementia. Twenty-four leading national organizations formally expressed their acceptance or support, including the National Association of Social Workers, the primary membership organization in the field of social work.

As director of education and outreach, my primary role on the team was to help shape the messages and translate them into a national training program for residential care staff. It was my responsibility to coordinate the development of *Foundations of Dementia Care*, a standardized curriculum to be delivered throughout the country through the association's network of 80 chapters (Alzheimer's Association, 2005b). My participation in the campaign was informed by years of experience in residential settings, first as a social worker and then in various management roles over a 20-year period. Several other members of the development team were social workers as well, ensuring that the perspective of the social worker was well represented in the development of the recommendations and development of the curriculum that is being used to teach them.

This chapter focuses on the role of the social worker in providing quality care for residents with dementia. The primary recommendations of the Campaign for Quality Residential Care are considered from the point of view of the social worker's role in the implementation of these recommendations. A number of the obstacles preventing providers from reaching their goals are discussed, and concrete and practical approaches are proposed. Finally, social workers are challenged to rethink their current roles and approaches and to assume clear positions of leadership in the field of dementia care.

SCOPE OF CONCERN

Before discussing specific issues related to social workers and dementia care, it is important to define the scope of the concern. Many residences function as if all residents with dementia reside within special care units. Although the social worker assigned to the special care unit may be recognized as a critical member of the dementia care team and may have a clear impact on the quality of care provided, social workers working in areas outside the special care unit are not required or even expected to have any expertise in dementia care. The problem with this approach is that, in reality, most nursing home residents with dementia do not reside in special care units. In 2003, for example, there were about 700,000 nursing home residents with dementia but only about 92,000 beds in special care units. At most, therefore, 13% of nursing home residents with dementia were in special care units, and 87% were living in other areas of the residence (Alzheimer's Association, 2004).

Likewise, most assisted living residents with dementia do not live in special care units. A study of 193 assisted living residences in four states found that, depending on the size of the facility, only 11% to 32% of assisted living residents with moderate to severe dementia were living in special care units. Thus, 68% to 89% were living in other areas of the residence (Rosenblatt et al., 2004). It is clear that social workers throughout the continuum must develop a level of expertise in dementia care and assume leadership positions accordingly.

CORE THEMES OF THE PRACTICE RECOMMENDATIONS

Regardless of the setting, the social worker is pivotal to the implementation of the Alzheimer's Association's practice recommendations and to ensuring the provision of quality care for residents with dementia. The field of dementia care has led a movement away from the more traditional medical model with its illness orientation to a social model of care in which each person is seen in his or her entirety. The new model of residential care is one that reflects the cardinal values of social work, with a focus on the individual and promotion of self-determination (Hepworth & Larsons, 1993). Social workers have played an important leadership role in this culture change movement as they should in the implementation of the person-centered approach recommended by the Alzheimer's Association.

In order to examine the social worker's leadership role, I have identified three core themes or beliefs that are woven throughout the practice recommendations. These three are not all-inclusive, as the practice recommendations address various aspects of care, but they are areas in which social workers play a particularly important role:

1. Staff must know each resident as a unique person.
2. The focus should be on the resident's remaining abilities and potential for independence.
3. Resident behavior must be seen as a way to understand how a resident is seeing the world.

The experienced dementia care practitioner will note that these are not new issues. They have been discussed for years as fundamental to quality care. Some organizations have created successful dementia care programs closely adhering to these themes. Other organizations have not even begun to apply the principles. The majority, however, fall somewhere in between. Although they insist that these themes are integral to their mission, they have not truly committed to their implementation. The social worker may play an important role in all three of these areas.

A Challenge to Social Workers

The previously mentioned core themes that serve as the foundation of the Alzheimer's Association's dementia care practice recommendations appear at surface to be quite simple. In reality, however, each one of them requires deep-seated culture change. Unless this is realized, successful implementation is unlikely.

The culture of a particular residence may be defined in terms of its organizational culture, including its group norms, values, formal philosophy, and written as well as unwritten rules. Gibson and Barsade (2003) describe culture as consisting of layers, the top and most visible one being the "artifacts" or behaviors and attributes that are easily apparent. The second layer is the organization's behavioral norms or unspoken rules regarding what is considered acceptable behavior. The third layer, the deepest and most important one, holds the values and beliefs of the culture. This is where one finds the vision of how things "ought to be."

For example, consider the layers involved in the first theme mentioned previously: knowing each resident as a unique person. Whenever I have the opportunity to meet with a group of residential care staff, I ask them how they get to know the residents—their backgrounds, interests, and who they are. I have always believed that this information is fundamental to quality care. In skilled care settings, one of the most common answers is that either the social worker or the admissions coordinator prepares a social history that contains much of this information. The social history is at what we refer to as the outer or most visible layer, and, because it is required by regulation in this setting, one can be fairly confident that it exists. So, on the surface, it appears as if the goal of knowing the resident is met, at least in part.

If one were to peel through to the second layer, or the "unspoken rules of behavior," however, some obstacles are likely to surface. When I ask the direct care staff if they have access to the social history, they often indicate that they are "allowed" to look in the chart to read it if and when they have time. The unspoken rule is that the social history must be in the chart but the staff is not required to know it or to have even read it. The problem is that this extremely valuable document is often buried in the chart, inaccessible to those who are in most need of the information it provides. In reality, the resident's obituary is sometimes the first glimpse into many aspects of the resident's past life.

In these situations, if one peels through to yet another layer, the innermost layer, one may find lacking a fundamental belief in the importance of knowing the resident as a unique person. At this deepest and most important layer may instead be the belief that most residents are alike and that if you know one, you know them all. This layer may also reveal a fundamental lack of respect for the direct care worker, for whom critical information may be deemed unimportant.

My fear as an experienced social worker and residential care professional is that, for many reasons, including overwhelming documentation requirements, many social workers in residential settings may be trapped in the outer, or surface, layer of the culture. They may be so intent on meeting the regulation of writing a social history, for example, that they lose sight of its purpose, which is that all staff know this critically important information. We bemoan the task orientation of direct care staff who are said to lose sight of the resident when faced with so many tasks to accomplish. Yet there's a real possibility that professionals, including social workers, are just as guilty of this task orientation. A social worker who completes all social history forms despite the fact that few staff actually read the document is focusing on the task rather than on its purpose.

I am not encouraging social workers to ignore the paperwork but rather to remember its intent. I am challenging them to be strong in their values and beliefs and to champion those values and beliefs. I implore social workers in residential settings to recognize their positions of leadership in order to influence the inner beliefs of the organization.

According to the National Association of Social Workers (2003), two of the social worker's key functions are to "participate in planning and policy development for the facility" and to assist "the facility to achieve and maintain a therapeutic environment essential to the optimal quality of life." Accordingly, social workers must delve beneath the surface to examine the behavioral norms and unwritten rules that are ruling the organization. They must challenge those rules when necessary and help to rewrite them. It is their responsibility to identify those values that are at the core of person-centered care and to share their beliefs with others. Social workers must be champions for quality care for residents with dementia.

The three previously identified core themes of the Alzheimer's Association's practice recommendations are now examined in light of this challenge to social workers to assert leadership. The substance of the recommendations are explored and obstacles to implementation identified. There is a focus on the special role social workers may play in ensuring success.

Know Each Resident as a Unique Person

The Alzheimer's Association is committed to the belief that, in order to provide quality care for a resident with dementia, it is essential to know as much as possible about the person. This value is a common thread throughout the practice recommendations, based on the conviction that "each person with dementia is unique, having a different constellation of abilities and needs for support, which changes over time as the disease progresses." In order to understand a resident's behavior, you need to know the person. In order to understand his or her pain, you need to know the person. In order to bring simple joys into his or her life, you need to know the person. This is a deep-seated belief of what "ought to be."

This is the case regardless of a person's physical, social, or cognitive status, and it is one of the basic premises of person-centered care. It is even more important, however, for people with dementia, whose communication limitations often prevent them from being able to express their own needs. They rely on others to know who they are as people.

The social history, as discussed previously, is just one tool for getting to know the resident. The Alzheimer's Association recommends as critical to quality care a comprehensive holistic assessment that addresses the many aspects of the person. This assessment should include an understanding of the person's cognitive health, physical health, physical functioning, behavioral status, sensory capabilities, decision-making capacity, communication abilities, personal background, cultural preferences, and spiritual needs and preferences.

In skilled care settings, the government-mandated minimum data set (MDS) provides a significant amount of valuable information, and it is routinely completed. If one were to look at this as evidence, it would seem that the goal of making sure that staff really know the resident is well met. Again, it is important to peel through to the next layer to examine the unwritten rules of the organization in order to understand the reality of the situation. In many organizations, the reality is that the direct care staff, those individuals who are providing most of the hands-on care, seldom see the MDS.

If social workers are to be champions for person-centered care, therefore, they must be willing to peel away the surface layer of the culture and examine the reality of the systems with objective and open minds. I would suggest that they start by examining three areas in particular: what is being done at time of admission, how transitions to other levels of care are being handled, and the dissemination of the care plans. These three areas in particular have a formidable impact on the goal of knowing each resident as a unique person.

It is important to recognize that the admission process is critical to person-centered dementia care. My first job in social work was as director of social services in an Episcopalian skilled care facility on the shore of Lake Erie. In those days, the position entailed both social work and admissions responsibilities. It was then that I came to understand what a traumatic event the day of admission could be for resident, family, and staff alike. I pledged to do everything within my power to ensure that residents and their families were walking into a group of friends, not strangers. For this purpose and to ease the stress of the caregivers as well, I made every effort to provide staff with a detailed profile of each resident prior to his or her taking a step into the door. Although the admissions process may now be handled by others, the social worker may still help to set the tone for the organization.

Without someone with conviction overseeing the admission process, the goal of knowing each new resident as a unique person may be easily lost. I worked at another residence that had, prior to my arrival, developed an exemplary preadmission assessment form that was completed with families and distributed to staff before the resident was admitted. It captured the individual's personality, lifestyle, personal history, and current concerns in rich detail. A new admissions director came in and discarded the form because it took too much time to complete. From that time on, staff complained that they knew almost nothing about the new residents when they arrived. If the social worker or someone else within the organization had set the tone and helped establish the standard through formal policy and procedure, this may not have happened.

Even those residences that are good at collecting and sharing information prior to admission may not be as good about moving the information with residents as they move along the continuum. Caregivers of residents with dementia learn fine nuances about the individual that make the care partnership work. One resident may not feel comfortable unless he has his *Wall Street Journal* in his hand even though he hasn't been able to read in years. Another may refuse to eat her meal until all of her tablemates have been served. A third may cross and uncross her legs repeatedly when she needs to use the bathroom. These nuggets of information are absolutely invaluable for quality dementia care. Yet they often do not accompany the resident when he or she moves.

The dilemma regarding passing on valuable information is repeated with the care plans. Most organizations can be considered to have performed exceptionally well in meeting the goal of developing a written care or service plan. The mere existence of this written document, however, should not suffice. The practice recommendations insist that "all staff involved in resident care needs to be familiar with this plan of care." This is where the obstacles again present themselves. In many organizations, direct care staff are not involved in the care plan meetings and, in fact, rarely even lay eyes on the care plan. Even when they do, it is often written in language that is not easy to understand or interesting to read, which again limits access for the caregiver. The care plan, a potentially invaluable document for knowing the resident as a unique person, often falls short of its potential in practice.

The often-solo social worker is not in a position to hand deliver the information from one area of the building to another when the resident moves within the continuum or to ensure that all staff know the care plans. She or he should be in the position, however, to influence the written policies and unspoken rules of behavior, that second layer of the culture that determines the standard of practice. The social worker should be in a position to identify the flaws in the system of communication and assist in the development of new procedures for ensuring that the goal is met.

Social workers may demonstrate their conviction in the importance of knowing each resident as a unique person through their everyday responsibilities. Because their reach is limited in scope and time, however, it is perhaps even more important that they find their voices within their organizations and establish positions of leadership through which they can influence the organization and its core beliefs. There are many ways that organizations may demonstrate their commitment to knowing the resident. These programs, policies, and approaches, sometimes delivered by the social worker and other times with the social worker's support, influence the behavioral norms or unspoken rules about what is considered acceptable behavior by the staff of this organization. Among those to be considered are the following:

- Inviting families to share what they know about the resident; tape recording or videotaping these sessions to be available for all care staff regardless of their shift or assignment
- Making sure that families meet the primary caregiver to open lines of communication
- Conducting an evaluation of communication flow; studying paperwork and its use as well as the need for information and whether it is met; placing forms where staff have ready access
- Informing family members of potential residents about the consumer Web-based tool for families developed by the Alzheimer's Association, which provides an extensive personal profile form for families to provide detailed information about their relative to any care provider in need of information (Alzheimer's Association, 2006)
- Making a commitment to primary assignments in order to ensure familiarity with the residents and developing a system that ensures that relief staff members are well-trained and orientated to the residents

- Creating templates for life storybooks that are given to families to complete prior to admission; organizing scrapbooking parties for residents and families to elaborate on the book's contents
- Revising the hospital transfer form to include more detailed information about the resident as a person
- Creating alternative means of communication to written reports and forms so as to address issues of literacy

The social worker is in a position to demonstrate a true commitment to the importance of knowing each and every resident as a unique person. She or he must champion that belief, helping to ensure that it takes root in the deepest level of the organization's culture.

Focus on the Resident's Remaining Abilities and Potential for Independence

In addition to knowing each resident as a unique person, the dementia care practice recommendations also claim as fundamental for effective care and understanding that "people with dementia are able to experience joy, comfort, meaning and growth in their lives" and that they should be enabled to remain as independent as possible for as long as possible. This requires a dramatic adjustment in perspective and approach, shifting the focus from one of loss and illness to one of remaining strengths, abilities, and potential for enjoyment of life. As leaders, social workers have a responsibility to integrate these beliefs into the daily life of the organization.

Loss and illness have long been the focal point in the field of long-term care. When looking at residents' functional levels, how much assistance they need is discussed much more often than how much they are capable of doing. When written care plans are developed, areas of weakness (vision loss, incontinence, forgetfulness) are identified much more frequently than areas of strength (good interpersonal skills, ability to comb hair and brush teeth). Likewise, when particular behaviors become a concern, they begin to define the person. The person who frequently attempts to leave the premises is seen as a "wanderer" or an "exit seeker," overshadowing all the other positive aspects of the person. Loss and illness take precedence over the rest of the person.

Social workers have many opportunities to help shift the perspective from the negative to the positive. The assessment process is a natural place to begin. One way to ensure a positive shift is to closely examine the source of assessment information. It is not unusual for professionals to ask the direct care staff for information regarding the resident's abilities. When assessing a resident's ability to dress herself, for example, the nurse's aide is considered most likely to know the answer. It is important to realize, however, that this answer may address what is being done for the resident but not the individual's actual potential. After all, it is often considered quicker to do for the residents than to help them help themselves. The source of assessment information may greatly impact the understanding about a resident's strengths, abilities, and overall potential.

When assessing residents' abilities, it is important to include multiple perspectives and not rely solely on the caregiver. When possible, therapists—occupational, speech, and physical—should be included in the team both for purposes of assessment as well as for follow-up treatment. Also essential to this assessment is the family, who may have valuable information regarding the resident's strengths and abilities. Social workers, through their traditional role of family liaison, are in the position to seek input from family members and to communicate what they have learned to the other members of the team.

One disturbing but critical conversation that I had with a family member comes to mind. Staff was challenged by a resident who, for days after admission, was urinating all over the residence—in wastebaskets, flowerpots, drawers, and the like. I met with the resident's wife and asked her how she handled her husband's incontinence when he was still at home. She informed me that he had never been incontinent in his life, not even one time. Unfortunately, this is not at all atypical, but this particular incident was the one that opened my eyes. I wondered how many thousands of times this had happened, with staff just assuming that the new resident was unable to be independent and then making certain that he always wore his incontinence briefs and could not easily remove them, minimizing the possibility of independent toileting forever more. In reality, this particular resident was just having difficulty finding the bathroom, as this was a new environment. With support and time, he was once again able to toilet himself.

Just as a different perspective may be gained from the family, likewise different staff may offer different perspectives. Day staff may describe a complete different functioning level than the evening staff as resident functioning varies throughout the day. Functioning may also vary from day to day, so assessments need to take place over a period of time. It is important to realize that thorough assessment is essential to maintaining independence and that the source of information is critical to this assessment.

Careful assessment provides an excellent opportunity for the social worker to steer the focus toward residents' strengths, abilities, and potential for independence. Proposing actual approaches to care that maximize independence provides another opportunity to shift the focus. The practice recommendations suggest incorporating "strategies such

as task breakdown, fitness programs and physical or occupational therapy to help residents complete their daily routines and maintain their
functional abilities as long as possible." Dependency may be minimized
by giving residents the tools they need to remain independent, such as
offering verbal reminders, allowing additional time, providing adaptive equipment, sequencing, and exercising patience in the caregiving
approach. Social workers play significant roles in care plan meetings,
at which time many approaches are determined. Their commitment to
empowering residents and enhancing the quality of their lives should be
clearly demonstrated at this time and whenever the opportunity arises.

Even more fundamental than a change in perspective during assessment and the special attention to approach, a change in the caregiver–
resident relationship is essential to shifting the focus from one of loss and
dependency to one of ability, growth, and potential. Rather than the staff
being the givers of care and the residents being the recipients, the practice
recommendations suggest that staff consider themselves "care partners"
with residents, helping residents achieve optimal quality of life. Residents
and their care partners need to work together, making use of the resident's
remaining strengths, abilities, and drive to enhance the quality of life. This
is true culture change, and the social worker needs to show leadership in
this shift in attitude.

If there is to be a focus on residents' abilities and potential for
independence, the common programs, policies, and approaches must reflect
that commitment. The social worker may be directly involved in their
implementation, or she or he may influence their development through
leadership and deep-seated belief. Among the ways that various residences have demonstrated their belief in the need to focus on resident's
remaining abilities and potential for independence are the following:

- Identifying meaningful roles for residents, such as hostess in the
  dining room, clerical assistant, and so on
- Revising assessment tools and care planning documents with a
  focus on strengths and abilities
- Adapting activity programming to ensure opportunities for
  success and to minimize passive activities
- Developing effective systems of follow-through after completion
  of therapy treatments
- Minimizing activity programming that does not involve the
  resident, such as making party decorations while all residents
  only watch
- Developing communication logs or other systems of communication between direct care staff to identify resident accomplish-
  ments, abilities, and sources of enjoyment

There is clearly potential for the social worker to influence, support, and help to sustain all of these. After all, one of the primary goals of the long-term care social worker is to "promote an optimal level of psychological, physical and social functioning" (National Association of Social Workers, 2003).

Understand That Resident Behavior May Help Explain How a Resident Sees the World

Just as the other two themes, knowing the resident and focusing on strengths, are woven throughout the practice recommendations, so too is this theme. Distinct patterns of behavior are recognized in residents with dementia, such as periods of agitation, attempts to leave the premises, increased evening restlessness, and repetitive vocalizations or movements, among numerous others. These patterns of behavior are seen so often that staff learn to react in patterned ways. With residents who repeatedly try to leave the premises, for example, staff have learned to respond, sometimes through a behavioral approach such as distracting and redirecting and sometimes through pharmaceutical intervention.

The critical step that is often forgotten, however, is to try to understand the meaning of the behavior. The behavior provides a glimpse into the world as seen through the lens of dementia. The Alzheimer's Association defines resident behavior as a "form of communication" and an "expression of preference." The resident who is repeatedly trying to leave the premises may believe that her young children are waiting for her at home. A resident who is going in and out of another resident's room and rummaging through the drawers may be bored, or she may be searching for something she lost. Someone else who swings at the caregiver during morning care may be uncomfortable with the way the caregiver approached her. When the caregiver understands how a resident is seeing the world, it is much easier to determine if the behavior is a problem in the first place, to prevent the behavior if it is problematic, and to determine a successful approach.

Again, this is certainly not new information, yet the reality is that we often make more effort to contain the behavior than to understand the meaning behind it. In order to minimize the potential negative impact of a resident's behavior, "care partners" must understand the meaning of the behavior. They must make an effort to understand what may be triggering a certain behavior and how to approach the resident while the behavior is being manifested. The social worker may play an important role in both of these areas.

Let's begin by discussing the assessment process. There are at least two important steps in the assessment process: the tracking of behavioral patterns and the analysis of the behavior. If one were to look at the culture's outer or surface layer for most skilled care facilities, one would probably find solid evidence that some degree of assessment was taking place. Most have a behavior log or observation form of some type that tracks frequency and time of certain behaviors, at least for those residents on psychotropic medications. A behavioral analysis form may also exist. So, at first glace, if one were to look at only the outer and most visible layer, one would certainly find indications that most skilled care facilities appreciate the importance of understanding the resident's behavior.

Peeling through to the next layer, however, one gets a glimpse of the unspoken rules for what is acceptable regarding resident behavior. Organizations that truly believe in the importance of understanding resident behavior use these tools in the actual analysis of the behavior. They use them as guides for discussion in special team meetings where key members of the caregiving team gather to attempt to understand the meaning of the behavior and discuss interventions. They refer to these tools in care plan meetings. And they share them with behavioral specialists called in for consultation. Organizations that are not truly convinced at the deepest level that knowing why the behavior is happening actually matters are not likely to commit staff time to an analysis of the behavior.

There may be many reasons for this lack of belief in the importance of understanding what the behavior is telling us about the person. One reason most certainly may be a lack of knowledge or expertise in analyzing and working with the behavior. If the organization does not have the skill or competence internally or the external resources on which to call, it is easy to see how they would develop a lack of faith in the importance of understanding the behavior.

Professional dementia care specialists may be hired to provide the needed expertise, but the reality is that most organizations do not choose to do so. Direct care workers are more likely to turn to professionals who are already on staff, including the social worker as the organization's mental health professional. In order to meet the organization's need, however, the social worker must have a level of competence that many admit they lack (Naito-Chan, Damron-Rodriguez, & Simmons, 2004).

There is no required competency in dementia care, and schools of social work do not consistently include the topic in their required curriculum. In 1987, the federal Omnibus Budget Reconciliation Act legislation mandated training in geriatrics for certified nursing assistants, but social service staff had no such mandate. It is my belief, however, that social workers in any long-term care setting, not just in special care areas, have an obligation to develop a degree of competence in dementia care, particularly in how to assess behavior and intervene appropriately.

Through so doing, the care team may be led to a better understanding of the world that the residents are experiencing.

Social workers should not only commit to developing their own competence but encourage the development of others as well. Training of caregiving staff is essential. I have worked with many experienced caregivers who, when a coworker is absent, would prefer working short staffed than to work with someone who has not been trained. They have seen too many episodes of increased agitation and aggression as well as other caregiving issues to convince them otherwise. Studies indeed suggest that properly trained and supervised staff may have a significant impact on resident behavior (Burgio, Stevens, Burgio, Roth, Paul et al., 2002). These caregivers develop sensitivity to the resident's perception of the world.

Learning is not likely to take place in the vacuum of the classroom without being reinforced when the staff member returns to the floor. The Alzheimer's Association's Campaign for Quality Residential Care promotes the creation of a learning environment where opportunities to gain insight are abundant and team leaders are well prepared to support the process of learning. Social workers play an important role in this learning environment. First, they are in a position to role model the process of examining the behavior in order to understand its meaning. Second, they may praise staff for successful interventions, such as when an aide recognizes that a resident is agitated because she is worried about her "young children" being at home alone and comforts the resident accordingly. Positive reinforcement is an effective tool for ensuring success.

The social worker plays an important leadership role in encouraging the organization to develop a deep-seated commitment to understanding the world in which residents with dementia live. This commitment may be demonstrated through programs, approaches, and initiatives that are incorporated into the routines of the organization, such as the following:

- Establishing clear guidelines for when and how behavioral assessments will take place
- Holding "grand rounds" with a psychiatrist or behavioral specialist on a regular basis
- Developing an intensive mentoring program with staff as mentors who have expertise in understanding resident behavior and developing effective approaches
- Developing policies that minimize the possibility of premature use of medications, such as assigning responsibility for changes in medication to one nurse clinician who reviews staff requests or changing medications

- Developing a restraint reduction program that is coupled with mobility and restorative efforts
- Routinely considering pain as the fifth vital sign and a potential trigger for agitation and other forms of behavior

Through demonstrating commitment to the goal, social workers play an important leadership role in the organization.

CONCLUSION

In this chapter, we have discussed the critical role of the social worker in ensuring quality care for residents with dementia. This discussion recognized the different layers of a culture of care: the surface layer of what appears to be, the second layer of what actually is, and the inner layer of what the organization believes "ought to be." The challenge faced in the field of dementia care is that commitment to many of the core concepts, as described in the Alzheimer's Association's dementia care practice recommendations, is apparent on the surface layer of the organization but has not yet been absorbed into the inner layer of the culture. In this chapter, we have challenged social workers to assume leadership roles in keeping the core concepts of dementia care visible to the organization and in encouraging their absorption into the organization's deep-seated inner beliefs.

We have reviewed three core themes or beliefs that are woven throughout the practice recommendations, identified for their particular relevance to the role of the social worker. Regarding the first theme, knowing each resident as a unique person, social workers were asked to explore beyond the visible artifacts of the social history form, MDS, and care plan to the inner layers of the culture. Three particular periods of time were identified as significant for exploration: at admission, during transition to another level of care, and during the care plan process.

Pertaining to the second theme, focusing on the resident's remaining abilities and potential for independence, social workers were asked to play a leadership role in shifting the focus from one of loss and illness to one of remaining strengths, abilities, and potential for enjoyment in life. They were asked to examine three key aspects of caregiving: the source of assessment information, the approach to caregiving, and the role of the caregiver. Each holds potential for a change in everyday procedures as well as a shift in the organization's inner beliefs.

And in regard to the third theme, considering resident behavior as a means to understand how a resident is seeing the world, social workers were asked to help others understand the importance of attempting to see reality from the perspective of the resident. Social workers were challenged to develop their own expertise in understanding resident behavior as well as to contribute to the creation of a learning environment that reinforces the demonstration of successful dementia care.

Examples of successful programs, approaches, and initiatives were provided to offer avenues for impact, emphasizing that the social workers cannot and need not make all these happen on their own. Rather, they must assume leadership roles, championing their values and beliefs in order to influence their organizations. This support is essential to the success in implementation of the Alzheimer's Association's dementia care practice recommendations and to their absorption into the innermost layer of each organization's culture.

REFERENCES

Alzheimer's Association. (1992). *Guidelines for dignity.* Chicago: Author.

Alzheimer's Association. (1997). *Key elements of dementia care.* Chicago: Author.

Alzheimer's Association. (2004). *People with Alzheimer's disease and dementia in nursing homes.* Washington, DC: Alzheimer's Association Public Policy Division: K. Maslow.

Alzheimer's Association. (2005a). *Dementia care practice recommendations for assisted living residences and nursing homes.* Chicago: Author.

Alzheimer's Association. (2005b). *Foundations of dementia care.* Chicago: Author.

Alzheimer's Association. (2006). *Personal facts and insights.* CareFinder. Available at http://alz.org/carefinder/support/documents/personalfacts.pdf

Burgio, L., Stevens, A., Burgio, K., Roth, D. L., Paul, P., Gerstle, J., et al. (2002). Teaching and maintaining behavior management skills in the nursing home. *The Gerontologist, 42,* 487–496.

Gibson, D., & Barsade, S. (2003). Managing organizational culture change: The case of long-term care. In A. Weiner & J. Ronch (Eds.), *Culture change in long-term care* (pp. 5–16). Binghamton, NY: Haworth Social Work Practice Press.

Hepworth, D., & Larsons, J. (1993). *Direct social work practice: Theory and skills.* Pacific Grove, CA: Brooks/Cole.

Naito-Chan, E., Damron-Rodriguez, J., & Simmons, W. (2004). Identifying competencies for geriatric social work practice. *Journal of Gerontological Social Work, 43,* 59–78.

National Association of Social Workers. (2003). *NASW standards for social workers in long-term care.* Washington, DC: Author.

Rosenblatt, A., Samus, Q. M., Steele, C. D., Baker, A. S., Harper, M. G., Brandt, J., et al. (2004). The Maryland Assisted Living Study: Prevalence, recognition, and treatment of dementia and other psychiatric disorders in the assisted living population of central Maryland. *Journal of the American Geriatrics Society, 52,* 1618–1625.

PART VI

Conclusions

CHAPTER TWENTY-ONE

Concluding Remarks: The Challenge for Social Work

Carole B. Cox

INTRODUCTION

As the chapters in this book underscore, Alzheimer's disease and dementia are major concerns for older persons and their families. Moreover, as with all major public health problems, the impact of dementia reaches beyond those immediately affected; it creates immense costs to society in terms of the care required and the concomitant financial burden, expenditure, and often lost wages of those providing care. As is common with all public health problems, dementia is not a condition that can be treated by only one profession or specialty. The many ramifications of the illness necessitate a plurality of interventions that focus on the person with the illness, the caregiver, and the systems within which they interact.

Consequently, social work—with its concentration on the individual, the environment, and the interactions between them—encompasses the perspectives and skills that are directly applicable to many phases of the illness. Unfortunately, recent data indicate that social workers may not be receiving the education necessary to work with older persons with dementia. A survey of more than 200 licensed clinical social workers in Florida, found that most did not feel adequately prepared to work with this population. The understanding and skills that they used in their work were a result of their own years of professional experience and their work within a service agency serving older persons (Kane, Hamlin, & Hawkins, 2004). This finding suggests that their education prior to practice had not sufficiently prepared them for work with persons with dementia or their families. Thus, an immediate challenge for the profession is to assure that practitioners have the necessary knowledge base that can enable them to work effectively with this population.

The first step must be to encourage the involvement and interest of students in gerontology. Efforts are underway to accomplish this task such as those by the National Association of Social Workers (NASW), the Hartford Foundation, and the Council on Social Work Education (CSWE). The NASW has recently established a specialty certification for clinical social workers in gerontology that requires specialized gerontology courses and experience in working with older adults. The Hartford Foundation, through its geriatric social work initiative and its National Center for Gerontological Social Work Education, is working toward stimulating student interest in gerontology by encouraging the infusion of gerontological content throughout the curriculum and also providing funding for doctoral students and faculty (Hartford Foundation, 2006). Through the CSWE and its Gero-Ed Forum, resources are also available online that include discussions, role plays, resources, and quizzes that can be incorporated into social work courses to increase students' knowledge and understanding of aging.

But such efforts will not be successful until social workers themselves overcome their own biases and negative attitudes toward working with older persons. As stated in the CSWE blueprint (CSWE, 2001), effective gerontological infusion within the curriculum can be accomplished only when efforts are made to combat ageism within society and within the profession itself. As long as the profession itself denies the reality of aging, the needs of those with dementia, as well as those of many other older persons, will remain unmet.

Individuals confronting dementia and their families are extremely diverse and have a myriad of needs that demand interventions on many levels. The person with the diagnosis requires skilled counseling by a practitioner who is familiar with the stages of the illness and their impact. The family requires practitioners who are sensitive and empathic and also knowledgeable about dementia and its manifestations, resources, and support systems. Equally important is that the practitioner works with the family in a culturally competent framework, thus assuring that interventions are appropriate and acceptable to their values and tradition.

ASSESSMENT AND DIAGNOSIS

Social workers can play major roles in ensuring that persons are accurately diagnosed. As discussed in chapters in this book, dementia can be a symptom of many different diseases or conditions, implying that social workers must be aware of the required medical exams and assessment tools to confirm its specific cause. As treatment in the early stage can have significant impact on behavior and symptoms, social workers need to assume assertive roles in reaching out to persons with dementia symptoms and helping them to link with appropriate services. In order to do this, practitioners themselves must be knowledgeable about the resources that exist within their communities, such as diagnostic and treatment centers and programs offered by local hospitals, clinics, and the Alzheimer's Association.

As with all social work practice, it is necessary to begin where the client is. The initial diagnosis is usually accompanied by emotions such as grief and anger; helping clients cope with these feelings is critical for their own adjustment and the establishment of a therapeutic relationship. Moreover, it is important to understand that dementia may be only one of the conditions that the person has. Care is often further complicated by the fact that dementia may be accompanied by other chronic illnesses common in older persons, making assessment and treatment more difficult. Practitioners both in the community and in institutions such as hospitals and residential care can play important roles in helping ensure that the care the person receives is appropriate and that their multiple needs are addressed.

TREATING THE PERSON WITH DEMENTIA

As frequently happens in social work, it may be difficult to decide who the client is. The emotional and psychological concerns of the person with dementia are vulnerable to being overshadowed by those of the caregiver. In this instance, there is an imminent risk of focusing on the pressing needs of the caregiver while ignoring those of the care receiver. But, by doing so, the quality of life of the person with dementia can be seriously jeopardized. For example, the practitioner who concentrates on relieving the burden and stress of the caregiver by recommending institutionalization when the person with the illness is still able to manage in the community may be focusing primarily on the goals and needs of the caregiver. Doing this further undermines the care receiver's sense of autonomy and self-determination, values that are at the core of social work practice.

As stated in many chapters, people with dementia still hope to have pleasurable life experiences, to be treated with dignity and care, and to communicate with others. Understanding the desire for meaningful relationships and activities and helping them realize those desires can prolong their quality of life. Moreover, the decision as to who is the client can have major ramifications on the selection and use of services.

TREATING AND FAMILY CAREGIVERS

Families confront many issues as they encounter the diagnosis and learn to cope with the progression and demands of the illness. As their needs continue to change, they present challenges to social workers who must help them adapt to the process of the illness. As discussed in several of the chapters, caregivers are often at risk of isolation, depression, and even physical problems. Assessing the ongoing status of the caregivers is a prerequisite for offering appropriate and supportive interventions. It is also critical to recognize that the needs of caregivers frequently differ with regard to their roles. For example, studies indicate that women may be more stressed than men and that employed caregivers are particularly stressed as they attempt to juggle multiple roles and responsibilities. Practitioners must respond to caregivers and their unique situations and characteristics in order to ensure that they are providing assistance that can help them adjust and cope.

An ongoing challenge is to empower caregivers so that they have a sense of mastery that can enable them to deal with the demands and decisions associated with caregiving. Using a strengths perspective, the practitioner can help families to focus on their capacities and resources rather than their difficulties and weaknesses. Helping caregivers reframe obstacles that they are facing into challenges to be met can reinforce their sense of accomplishment and competency. At the same time, allowing them to vent their fears and concerns is important in helping them adjust to their ever-changing roles. Chapters in the book provide specific tools and techniques that can be incorporated into interventions in working with families.

Services are available that can assist families in their roles, and a challenge here is to ensure that these services are sensitive to the special needs associated with dementia and that they are properly used. Skilled case managers continually assess and evaluate caregivers and work with them toward enhancing their caregiving abilities. A major challenge for these managers is not to usurp the roles and abilities of the caregivers themselves but to learn from them, trust in them, and offer them continued support.

An underlying challenge is making sure that services are utilized. Many barriers deter persons from using programs, including a lack of knowledge or understanding of existing programs, a denial of the diagnosis, or a refusal to accept that one is indeed a caregiver. As has been discussed in many chapters, programs such as care management, day care, and support groups can provide relief to caregivers while also helping to enable their caregiving capacity. Each can be an important asset in the caregiving relationship as they offer counseling, relieve isolation, and educate families about the ever-changing needs of their relatives.

Many of the chapters in this book suggest strategies that may facilitate service use by caregivers. The challenge for practitioners is to keep current with this literature and research so that they can apply such findings and intervene effectively to help ensure that needed services are appropriately used. Social workers must be willing to take a proactive stance with caregivers, reaching out to them so that they are knowledgeable of the help and resources they can offer. Although it may take some time before their services are accepted, this outreach is important, as it provides the vital link to accessing programs. Indeed, the knowledge that people and services are available may in itself be supportive.

CULTURAL ISSUES

Persons respond to dementia in diverse ways, and ethnicity and culture remain major sources of these responses. Thus, an important challenge is to ensure that services are culturally sensitive. This means recognizing differences and developing interventions and programs that are accessible and acceptable to diverse groups. Concomitantly, social workers must guard against stereotyping on the basis of cultural differences, as persons vary in their adherence to traditional beliefs and values. Moreover, there is great heterogeneity within groups, and factors such as social class and gender can be important forces in determining service use that must be considered when exploring the impact of ethnicity on the dementia experience.

Language can present an immediate barrier to diagnosis and service utilization. Persons must be able to communicate with practitioners and understand the terminology that they are using. Understanding the values and traditions of a specific culture is critical so that practitioners can reframe services when appropriate to ensure that they are congruent with them. As an example, by stressing the way a program such as day care will benefit the person with dementia rather than the caregiver, caregivers with a strong sense of filial responsibility may be more encouraged to use that program than if they felt the benefit was mainly to themselves.

Networking within the ethnic community can also be important in promoting service use. This involves educating and involving many community programs that can distribute information or brochures and make referrals. Reaching out to these agencies and educating their workers about dementia and available resources can further promote program development and effective outreach to ethnic families. Local health fairs, churches, and even schools can provide formats for dementia outreach and education.

As new service models are developed, they must be shared to ensure further replications. Journal articles, continuing education courses, and conferences are primary means of disseminating information about new programs. Practitioners must stay informed regarding new developments in the field that can offer important suggestions for service delivery. Moreover, learning should not be restricted to programs in the United States. Models used in other countries, as discussed in the chapters in this book, can offer important suggestions for comprehensive delivery systems.

CHALLENGES FOR RESEARCH

Research is critical in the area of dementia, and such research must not be restricted to the medical profession. Social work research is essential in order to further understand the variations in the experiences of both the individual with the illness and the caregiver. It is only through good research that effective interventions can be designed. Parallel to the biomedical research being conducted on dementia, social work research is essential to ensure the highest quality of life for those affected. Until both prevention and cures are found, such research is crucial.

In all phases of this research, it is important to recognize the role of cultural diversity, as findings from one group may not be generalized to others. Consequently, there is often a need to replicate studies within specific populations to ensure that services and interventions are indeed appropriate.

One area in which social work research is particularly relevant is identifying the factors that impede persons from seeking assessments when symptoms of cognitive impairment first occur. Studies continue to indicate that people wait as long as 3 or more years after symptoms are noticed before they seek professional advice. By identifying the reasons for such delays, appropriate strategies can be developed that encourage more timely responses, enabling treatments and interventions to be offered in the early stages of the illness.

As persons confront the diagnosis of dementia, they undergo many challenges that threaten their emotional well-being. Further research can assist social work practitioners in developing their skills in discussing the diagnosis with the individual and the family so as to assist them in coping and in their decisions. Such research can help in the formation of relationships that can strengthen the coping abilities of families throughout the course of the illness.

Social work research can also make important contributions with regard to the many factors contributing to caregiver resiliency. Increasing our knowledge of both risk factors and factors that strengthen adjustment and coping is necessary for the further development of interventions. Moreover, replicating these studies with diverse populations is essential to ensure that interventions are congruent with the needs and values of specific groups.

As services for families continue to expand, research on the factors that promote utilization of these programs is required. Many programs remain underutilized, as persons fail to equate them with their own needs or resist using them. Further research on service utilization can help identify the most effective ways of fostering service use and linking families to services. The overall goal must be to maximize service access and use.

Within residential settings, research can help in understanding the factors that are conducive to the adoption of new interventions and practices that can increase the quality of life for residents with dementia. As more is learned about staff training in dementia care and ways to improve the environment for residents, studies should begin to focus on the factors that may act as barriers to their implementation. Such research is required in order to ensure that the settings in which many with dementia reside are environments that support them and enhance their independence and well-being.

Improving the quality of life of the person with dementia, whether in the community or in a residential setting, must become a priority for social work research. Tools that are sensitive to the person's needs and to their abilities to respond are beginning to be developed, and persons with the illness are increasingly being incorporated into care planning and decision making. The continual development of person-centered measures that are responsive to their changing status and the implementation of such instruments are fundamental for ensuring quality care. Social work involvement in the creation of these measures can add to their sensitivity in measuring these important changes.

Developing systems of dementia care require students and practitioners who are committed to this area of practice. An important area for research is that of developing educational models and programs that stimulate this involvement. This must include research on effective strategies for combating ageism in the profession itself. Until social workers' own ageist attitudes are confronted and challenged, their ability to provide competent care and interventions as discussed throughout this book will be severely limited.

CHALLENGES FOR POLICY ADVOCACY

The macroperspective of the profession that translates case into cause forms a basis for social work advocacy. This necessitates not only advocating for the individual client but also advocating for changes in policies and programs so that they can adequately address the needs of all persons coping with dementia and its related issues.

Silverstein and Peters-Beumer give an example of the pressing need for policy advocacy in their chapter on mobility. Having alternative transportation for persons with dementia may assist in helping them be less resistant to ceasing their own driving. Policies that promote such transportation can be important in reducing the burden on both the individual and their families, but such policies struggle to become reality. As policy advocates, social workers should assume active roles in seeking changes that would benefit this population.

At the state and federal levels, advocacy is needed for increased funding for both research and services. Ensuring that grants are available for studies that can impact on care and support is critical for the continuing improvement of programs. Funding for services that can relieve families, including providing them with financial assistance, is essential if they are to effectively continue in their roles as caregivers. As such funds remain limited and inadequate to meet the financial expenses faced by many caregivers, their options for services and relief remain limited and their burdens continue to increase.

Medicare, which could assist many with dementia, is restricted in its ability to help. Mental health care, under which most dementia treatment is classified, continues to be reimbursed at lower rates than other types of care, while Medicare's requirements for home care make most persons with dementia ineligible for the service. Expanding the coverage under this nearly universal program is basic to assisting many with dementia and their families obtain the support that they require. In addition, Medicare should encourage early detection and care through complete geriatric assessments so that changes may be diagnosed and early intervention offered.

Social workers as advocates must work toward influencing legislators so that the interests of these persons and their needs are recognized and met. Using the knowledge from their own work, they must work to underscore the impact that policies have on persons with dementia and their families. Involving clients, those who are impacted by the policies, in these efforts further strengthens these advocacy efforts.

An example of the role that advocacy can play in bringing attention to the illness and to the needs of persons is offered in the example given by Jenny Knauss, a health advocate who at the age of 65 developed Alzheimer's disease. Working with her coauthor, she started an advocacy organization, spoke at the Alzheimer's Association policy forum, and posted a Web site about advocacy efforts. But, at she clearly states, those who have the illness need others to follow up on their efforts and to continue their struggle with policymakers (Knauss & Moyer, 2006). As advocates, social workers can play key roles in stimulating these efforts.

Improving the quality of the staff caring for persons with dementia must also be a policy concern. Such improvement depends on staff receiving appropriate training and education in dementia care. It also requires that these persons be given salaries that are commensurate with the work and services that they provide. As the numbers of persons requiring their assistance continues to increase, policies must be enacted that recognize and reward the critical roles played by these staff and thus further motivate them to remain in their critical caring roles.

As advocates, social workers can continually ensure that attention is given to the concerns of these persons and that programs such as in-service training on dementia care are offered. The Alzheimer's Association, at both the national and state levels, maintains advocacy networks that work for changes in public policies so that they meet the needs of patients and their families. Participation in the organization is an important means for social workers to become involved as advocates working for change.

As underscored throughout this book, dementia impacts individuals, families, and society. To date, there is no known prevention or cure for the most common type, Alzheimer's disease, and thus the number of persons with the illness can be expected to increase along with its demands. Social workers can play major roles as counselors, educators, researchers, and advocates to ensure that these demands are met. Social justice, a core value of the profession, demands that social workers assume these roles so that society, through its policies and institutions, recognize and respond to the rights of this ever-increasing population. This is an overriding challenge that the profession must not fail to meet.

REFERENCES

Council on Social Work Education/SAGE-SW. (2001). *A blueprint for the new millennium.* New York: Author.

Hartford Foundation. (2006). *Geriatric social work initiative.* New York: Author.

Kane, M., Hamlin, E., & Hawkins, W. (2004). How adequate do social workers feel to work with elders with Alzheimer's disease? *Social Work and Mental Health, 2,* 63–84.

Knauss, J., & Moyer, D. (2006). Role of advocacy in our adventure with Alzheimer's. *Dementia, 5,* 67–72.

Resources

Alzheimer's Disease Education and Referral Center (ADEAR)

- http://www.alzheimers.org/adcdir.htm
- Lists current NIA-sponsored AD centers for clinical services and research
- Provides a list of available clinical trials and research updates

NINCDS-ADRDA diagnostic criteria for Alzheimer's disease, vascular dementia, and dementia with Lewy bodies

- McKhann, G., Drachman, D., Folstein, M., Katzman, R., Price, D., & Stadlan, E. (1984). Clinical diagnosis of Alzheimer's disease: Report of the NINCDS-ADRDA Work Group under the auspices of Department of Health and Human Services Task Force on Alzheimer's Disease. *Neurology, 34,* 939–944.
- Roman, G., Tatemichi, T., Erkinjuntti, T., Cummings, J., Masdeu, J., Garcia, J., et al. (1993). Vascular dementia: Diagnostic criteria for research studies. Report of the NINDS-AIREN International Workshop. *Neurology, 43,* 250–260.

- McKeith, I., Galasko, D., Kosaka, K., Perry, E., Dickson, D., Hansen, L., et al. (1996). Consensus guidelines for the clinical and pathologic diagnosis of dementia with Lewy bodies: Report of the consortium on DLB international workshop. *Neurology, 47,* 1113–1124.

American Psychological Association, Presidential Task Force on the Assessment of Age-Consistent Memory Decline and Dementia (APA)

- http://www.apa.org/practice/dementia.html
- Guidelines for the evaluation of dementia and age-related cognitive decline.

Quality Standards Subcommittee of the Academy of Neurology, clinical practice guidelines. (Abstracted from the AAN's Guidelines for early detection, diagnosis, and management of dementia)

- http://www.americangeriatrics.org/products/positionpapers/aan-dementia.shtml

Mini-Mental State Exam

- http://en.wikipedia.org/wiki/mini_mental_state_examination

Informant Questionnaire on Cognitive Decline in the Elderly—short form (IGCODE)

- http://www.anu.edu.au/iqcode/doc/shortEnglish.pdf

Katz Index

- http://www.hartfordign.org/publications/trythis/issue02.pdf

Lawton IADL Scale (Physical Self Maintenance Scale)

- http://www.chcr.brown.edu/pcoc/Functi.htm
- See also Lawton, M. P., & Brody, E. (1969). Assessment of older people: Self-maintaining and instrumental activities of daily living. *Gerontologist, 9,* 180.

Pfeffer Functional Activities Questionnaire (FAQ)

- http://www.hospitalmedicine.org/geriresource/toolbox/pdfs/function_status_questionnai.pdf
- The FAQ is the last instrument located on this page.

Neuropsychiatric Inventory Questionnaire

- Cummings, J. (1997). The neuropsychiatric inventory: Assessing psychopathology in dementia patients. *Neurology, 48,* S10–S16.

Geriatric Depression Scale (GDS) (Sheikh & Yesavage)

- http://www.merck.com/mrkshared/mmg/tables/33t4.jsp

Cornell Scale for Depression in Dementia (Alexopoulos et al.)

- http://www.emoryhealthcare.org/departments/fuqua/CornellScale.pdf

Clinical Dementia Rating Scale (Berg, 1988)

- http://www.adrc.wustl.edu/edrScale.html

Global Deterioration Scale (GDS) (Reisberg)

- Reisberg, B., Ferris, S., de Leon, M., & Crook, T. (1982). The global deterioration scale for assessment of primary degenerative dementia. *American Journal of Psychiatry, 139,* 1136–1139.

Brief Cognitive Rating Scale (BCRS) (Reisberg & Ferris, 1998)

- Reisberg, B., & Ferris, S. (1998). Brief Cognitive Rating Scale. *Psychopharmacology Bulletin, 24,* 629–636.

Behavioral Pathology in AD Rating Scale (BEHAVE-AD) (Reisberg)

- Reisberg, B., Franssen, E., Sclan, S., Kluger, A., & Ferris, S. (1989). Stage specific incidence of potentially remediable behavioral symptoms in aging and Alzheimer's disease: A study of 120 patients using the BEHAVE-AD. *Bulletin of Clinical Neuroscience, 54,* 95–112.

Functional Assessment Staging Scale (FAST)

- Reisberg, B. (1988). Functional assessment staging (FAST). *Psychopharmacology Bulletin, 24, 653–659.*

RESOURCES FOR CAREGIVERS

Mather Lifeways—Powerful Tools for Caregivers

- http://www.matherlifeways.com/re_powerfultools.asp

The Caregiver Guide—National Institute on Aging

- http://www.nia.nih.gov/Alzheimers/Publications/caregiverguide.htm

Caregiver Resources from the Alzheimer's Association

- http://www.alz.org/Resources/TopicIndex/Caregivers.asp

Alzheimer's Caregivers: How to Cope (Mayo Clinic)

- http://www.mayoclinic.com/health/alzheimers-caregiver/AZ00038

Alzheimer's Caregiver Support Online

- http://alzonline.net/

National Alzheimer's Association

- http://www.alz.org
- Information about AD for caregivers and professionals

Alzheimer's Disease Education and Referral Service

- http://www.alzheimers.org

NIA site

- Information about AD and related disorders

Ageless design

- http://www.agelessdesign.com
- Caregiver support and information

Eldercare Online

- http://www.ec-online.net
- Caregiver support and information

Alzheimer's Resource Room

- http://www.aoa.gov/alz/index.asp

U.S. Administration on Aging site

- Information about AD, patient and caregiver support

The Fisher Center for Alzheimer's Research

- http://www.alzinfo.org
- Information about AD and research

Duke Family Support Program

- A series for professionals and family caregivers addressing anger issues in Alzheimer's care:
- *Pressure Points: Alzheimer's and Anger:* A book for families and professionals about the sources of anger in Alzheimer's care and suggested anger management strategies. May be ordered from The Duke Family Support Program, http://www. dukefamilysupport.org, or ordered from the ADEAR Center, National Institute on Aging Alzheimer's Information http:// www.alzheimers.org.
- *Wait A Minute! When Anger Gets Too Much:* A high-impact brochure adapted from the book, *Pressure Points: Alzheimer's and Anger.* Offers tips for managing anger using the voices of Alzheimer's caregivers reporting typical anger-producing scenarios. May be downloaded from http://www.dukefamilysupport. org or ordered from the Duke Family Support Program, Box 3600 Duke Medical Center, Durham, NC, 27710.

- *"Hit Pause" Helping Dementia Families Deal With Anger:* A booklet for professionals or aging staff working with Alzheimer's or dementia family caregivers with anger issues. May be downloaded from http://www.dukefamilysupport.org or ordered from the Duke Family Support Program, Box 3600 Duke Medical Center, Durham, NC, 27710.

DRIVING AND MOBILITY

(Source: modified from http://www.asaging.org/drivewell)

National Highway Traffic Safety Administration

- http://www.nhtsa.gov
- This site has information for consumers and professionals on older driver safety, including educational materials about driving with particular medical conditions or diseases, health professionals working with older adult drivers, and an online library of research studies, references, and policy statements relating to NHTSA's older-driver safety initiative.

AAA Foundation for Traffic Safety

- http://www.seniordrivers.org
- This site has tips and information to keep an older driver's driving skills sharp. The site includes video clips covering some of the trickiest situations drivers might encounter and also gives professionals information on supplemental transportation programs for seniors as well as information about current research on older driver safety.

AAA (Motor Clubs)

- http://www.aaapublicaffairs.com
- This Web site provides an overview of the AAA priority issue, Lifelong Safe Mobility. Included are educational programs and resources for senior drivers as well as state legislation. Also available from this site is information about AAA Roadwise Review. Developed by AAA and notable transportation researchers, this computer-based screening tool allows seniors to measure the eight functional abilities most correlated to safe driving in the privacy of their own home.

Administration on Aging

- http://www.aoa.gov/prof/notes/notes_older_drivers.asp
- This site links to various articles for professionals regarding older driver health and safety, including information on disability, low vision, transportation and mobility, and Alzheimer's disease and related dementia.

American Occupational Therapy Association

- http://www.aota.org/olderdriver
- This site has an array of materials for professionals and consumers about driver evaluation and retraining and the role of occupational therapy driver rehabilitation specialists in keeping individuals connected to their communities. The site also has the nation's most comprehensive and searchable national database of driver rehabilitation specialists.

AARP

- http://www.aarp.org/life/drive
- This site gives consumers information about the nation's largest driver refresher course for older adults as well as some quick, informal tests that individuals can take to begin assessing their fitness to drive safely.

American Medical Association

- http://www.ama-assn.org/ama/pub/category/10791.html
- This site gives viewers electronic access to the *Physician's Guide to Assessing and Counseling Older Drivers,* a publication developed by the American Medical Association in cooperation with the National Highway Traffic Safety Administration.

At the Crossroads: A Guide to Alzheimer's, Dementia, and Driving

- http://www.thehartford.com/alzheimers
- The Hartford Financial Services Group, Inc., the MIT Age Lab, and the Connecticut Community Care, Inc., have developed this guide as a tool to help individuals and caregivers determine when it is time to stop driving.

Beverly Foundation

- http://www.beverlyfoundation.org

- This site highlights the research and technical assistance provided by the foundation older adult mobility and transportation. The Resource STORe found on the site highlights reports, articles, brochures, and pamphlets prepared by the Beverly Foundation to public, private, and nonprofit organizations as well as professionals in health, aging, and transportation and communities across the nation. The foundation covers four areas: mobility and senior mobility, traditional transportation, supplemental transportation, and off-the-road care and services.

Community Transportation Association of America (CTAA)

- http://www.ctaa.org
- CTAA' s site provides an overview of their technical assistance programs in transit design and solutions and Transportation Lending service. The Information Station connects viewers with community transportation news, resources, and ideas, including transportation options. It provides categorical guides, a glossary of terms, online publications, links to related Web sites, and a powerful search engine.

Compendium of Law Enforcement Older Driver Programs

- http://www.aamva.org/drivers/drv_AgingDrivers.asp
- The National Highway and Traffic Administration has compiled a listing by state of each older driver safety program sponsored by law enforcement (2004).

Easter Seals Project ACTION

- http://www.projectaction.org
- This national program addresses transit accessibility issues through technical assistance, resource development, and training. Easter Seals Project Action's popular bus familiarization training consists of 2 days of instruction for travel trainers, teachers, job coaches, and bus operators. Funded by the Federal Transit Administration and administered through Easter Seals, Easter Seals Project ACTION has supported research and demonstration projects to provide solutions to accessibility challenges since 1988. This site also contains information on the new National Center on Senior Transportation. The center's goal is to increase the capacity and use of transportation options for older Americans throughout the U.S.

ITNAmerica™

- http://www.itnamerica.org
- This site describes a model transportation program using automobiles and both paid and volunteer drivers to provide dignified service 24 hours a day, 7 days a week. The site describes how ITN is sustained entirely by fares from the people who use the service and voluntary local community support with no public subsidy for capital or operating expense. Program participants become members of the organization and pay for their rides from personal transportation accounts.

National Association of Area Agencies on Aging

- http://www.n4a.org/older_driver_safety.cfm
- This site for professionals gives information about n4a's Older Driver Safety Project, which is funded by the National Highway Traffic Safety Administration. It includes a brochure about community-based approaches to promoting older driver safety.

South Carolina Geriatric Education Center (SC-GEC)

- http://www.musc.edu/scgec/
- SC-GEC has produced several training modules in geriatrics and gerontology for audiences (faculty, students, and practicing health and social service professionals), including two 1-hour training modules on driving and the older adult and driving and Alzheimer's disease.

United We Ride

- http://www.unitedweride.gov
- United We Ride is an interagency federal national initiative that supports states and their localities in developing coordinated human service delivery systems.

We Need to Talk: Family Conversations With Older Drivers

- http://www.thehartford.com/talkwitholderdrivers
- The Hartford Financial Services Group, Inc., and the MIT AgeLab developed information to help families initiate productive and caring conversations with older adults about driving safety. These suggestions are based on research with drivers over the age of 50. This valuable booklet serves as a great tool in driving discussion sessions or to present to families and loved ones.

Index